MEDICAL MASTERCLASS

Cardiology and Respiratory Medicine

Disclaimer

Although every effort has been made to ensure that drug doses and other information are presented accurately in this publication, the ultimate responsibility rests with the prescribing physician. Neither the publishers nor the authors can be held responsible for any consequences arising from the use of information contained herein. Any product mentioned in this publication should be used in accordance with the prescribing information prepared by the manufacturers.

The information presented in this publication reflects the opinions of its contributors and should not be taken to represent the policy and views of the Royal College of Physicians of London, unless this is specifically stated.

Every effort has been made by the contributors to contact holders of copyright to obtain permission to reproduce copyright material. However, if any have been inadvertently overlooked, the publisher will be pleased to make the necessary arrangements at the first opportunity.

Medical Masterclass

EDITOR-IN-CHIEF

John D. Firth DM FRCP

Consultant Physician and Nephrologist
Addenbrooke's Hospital
Cambridge

Cardiology and Respiratory Medicine

EDITORS

Michael I. Polkey MRCP PhD

Consultant Physician
Royal Brompton Hospital
London

Paul R. Roberts MB ChB MRCP MD

Specialist Registrar, Cardiology
Southampton General Hospital
Southampton

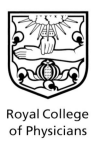

Royal College
of Physicians

© 2004 Royal College of Physicians of London

First published 2001 Blackwell Science Ltd
Reprinted 2004 Royal College of Physicians of London

Published by:
Royal College of Physicians of London
11 St. Andrews Place
Regent's Park
London NW1 4LE
United Kingdom

Set and printed by Graphicraft Limited, Hong Kong

ISBN: 1-86016-221-5 (this book)
ISBN: 1-86016-210-X (set)

Distribution Information:
Jerwood Medical Education Resource Centre
Royal College of Physicians of London
11 St. Andrews Place
Regent's Park
London NW1 4LE
United Kingdom
Tel: 0044 (0)207 935 1174 ext 422/490
Fax: 0044 (0)207 486 6653
Email: merc@rcplondon.ac.uk
Web: http://www.rcplondon.ac.uk/

Contents

List of contributors, vii
Foreword, viii
Preface, ix
Acknowledgements, x
Key features, xi

Cardiology

1 Clinical presentations, 3
  1.1 Paroxysmal palpitations, 3
  1.2 Palpitations with dizziness, 6
  1.3 Syncope, 9
  1.4 Stroke and a murmur, 12
  1.5 Acute central chest pain, 15
  1.6 Breathlessness and ankle swelling, 19
  1.7 Hypotension following myocardial infarction, 23
  1.8 Breathlessness and haemodynamic collapse, 25
  1.9 Pleuritic pain, 28
  1.10 Breathlessness and exertional presyncope, 30
  1.11 Dyspnoea, ankle oedema and cyanosis, 33
  1.12 Chest pain and recurrent syncope, 35
  1.13 Fever, weight loss and new murmur, 38
  1.14 Chest pain following a 'flu-like illness, 42
  1.15 Elevated blood pressure at routine screening, 46
  1.16 Murmur in pregnancy, 48
2 Diseases and treatments, 51
  2.1 Coronary artery disease, 51
    2.1.1 Stable angina, 51
    2.1.2 Unstable angina, 53
    2.1.3 Myocardial infarction, 55
  2.2 Cardiac arrhythmia, 58
    2.2.1 Bradycardia, 58
    2.2.2 Tachycardia, 59
  2.3 Cardiac failure, 63
  2.4 Diseases of heart muscle, 66
    2.4.1 Hypertrophic cardiomyopathy, 66
    2.4.2 Dilated cardiomyopathy, 69
    2.4.3 Restrictive cardiomyopathy, 70
    2.4.4 Acute myocarditis, 71
  2.5 Valvular heart disease, 71
    2.5.1 Aortic stenosis, 71
    2.5.2 Aortic regurgitation, 72
    2.5.3 Mitral stenosis, 74
    2.5.4 Mitral regurgitation, 75
    2.5.5 Tricuspid valve disease, 77
    2.5.6 Pulmonary valve disease, 78

2.6 Pericardial disease, 78
  2.6.1 Acute pericarditis, 78
  2.6.2 Pericardial effusion, 80
  2.6.3 Constrictive pericarditis, 82
2.7 Congenital heart disease, 84
  2.7.1 Tetralogy of Fallot, 85
  2.7.2 Eisenmenger's syndrome, 86
  2.7.3 Transposition of the great arteries, 87
  2.7.4 Ebstein's anomaly, 88
  2.7.5 Atrial septal defect, 89
  2.7.6 Ventricular septal defect, 90
  2.7.7 Patent ductus arteriosus, 90
  2.7.8 Coarctation of the aorta, 91
2.8 Infective diseases of the heart, 92
  2.8.1 Infective endocarditis, 92
  2.8.2 Rheumatic fever, 94
2.9 Cardiac tumours, 95
2.10 Traumatic heart disease, 97
2.11 Diseases of systemic arteries, 99
  2.11.1 Aortic dissection, 99
2.12 Diseases of pulmonary arteries, 101
  2.12.1 Primary pulmonary hypertension, 101
  2.12.2 Secondary pulmonary hypertension, 103
2.13 Cardiac complications of systemic disease, 104
  2.13.1 Thyroid disease, 104
  2.13.2 Diabetes, 105
  2.13.3 Autoimmune rheumatic diseases, 105
  2.13.4 Renal disease, 106
2.14 Systemic complications of cardiac disease, 107
  2.14.1 Stroke, 107
2.15 Pregnancy and the heart, 108
2.16 General anaesthesia in heart disease, 110
2.17 Hypertension, 110
  2.17.1 Accelerated phase hypertension, 113
2.18 Venous thromboembolism, 115
  2.18.1 Pulmonary embolism, 115
2.19 Driving restrictions in cardiology, 118
3 Investigations and practical procedures, 120
  3.1 ECG, 120
    3.1.1 Exercise ECGs, 124
  3.2 Basic electrophysiology studies, 125
  3.3 Ambulatory monitoring, 127
  3.4 Radiofrequency ablation and implantable cardioverter defibrillators, 130
    3.4.1 Radiofrequency ablation, 130
    3.4.2 Implantable cardioverter defibrillator, 131
  3.5 Pacemakers, 132
  3.6 The chest radiograph in cardiac disease, 134

3.7 Cardiac biochemical markers, 135
3.8 Cardiac catheterization, percutaneous transluminal coronary angioplasty and stenting, 136
    3.8.1 Cardiac catheterization, 136
    3.8.2 Percutaneous transluminal coronary angioplasty and stenting, 138
3.9 Computed tomography and magnetic resonance imaging, 140
    3.9.1 Computed tomography, 140
    3.9.2 Magnetic resonance imaging, 140
3.10 Ventilation–perfusion isotope scanning ($\dot{V}/\dot{Q}$), 140
3.11 Echocardiography, 141
3.12 Nuclear cardiology, 143
    3.12.1 Myocardial perfusion imaging, 143
    3.12.2 Positron emission tomography, 144
4 Self-assessment, 145

Respiratory Medicine

1 Clinical presentations, 153
  1.1 New breathlessness, 153
  1.2 Solitary pulmonary nodule, 155
  1.3 Exertional dyspnoea with daily sputum, 158
  1.4 Dyspnoea and fine inspiratory crackles, 160
  1.5 Pleuritic chest pain, 163
  1.6 Unexplained hypoxia, 167
  1.7 Nocturnal cough, 169
  1.8 Daytime sleepiness and morning headache, 172
  1.9 Haemoptysis and weight loss, 174
  1.10 Pleural effusion and fever, 176
  1.11 Lung cancer with asbestos exposure, 178
  1.12 Lobar collapse in non-smoker, 180
  1.13 Breathlessness with a normal radiograph, 182
  1.14 Upper airway obstruction, 184
  1.15 Difficult decisions, 185
2 Diseases and treatments, 188
  2.1 Upper airway, 188
    2.1.1 Obstructive sleep apnoea, 188
  2.2 Atopy and asthma, 190
    2.2.1 Allergic rhinitis, 190
    2.2.2 Asthma, 191
  2.3 Chronic obstructive pulmonary disease, 194
  2.4 Bronchiectasis, 197
  2.5 Cystic fibrosis, 199
  2.6 Occupational lung disease, 202
    2.6.1 Asbestosis and the pneumoconioses, 202
  2.7 Diffuse parenchymal (interstitial) lung disease, 204

    2.7.1 Cryptogenic fibrosing alveolitis, 204
    2.7.2 Bronchiolitis obliterans and organizing pneumonia, 205
  2.8 Miscellaneous conditions, 206
    2.8.1 Extrinsic allergic alveolitis, 206
    2.8.2 Sarcoidosis, 208
    2.8.3 Pulmonary vasculitis, 210
    2.8.4 Pulmonary eosinophilia, 212
    2.8.5 Iatrogenic lung disease, 214
    2.8.6 Smoke inhalation, 215
    2.8.7 Sickle cell disease and the lung, 217
    2.8.8 Human immunodeficiency virus and the lung, 218
  2.9 Malignancy, 220
    2.9.1 Lung cancer, 220
    2.9.2 Mesothelioma, 224
    2.9.3 Mediastinal tumours, 226
  2.10 Disorders of the chest wall and diaphragm, 227
  2.11 Complications of respiratory disease, 230
    2.11.1 Chronic respiratory failure, 230
    2.11.2 Cor pulmonale, 230
  2.12 Treatments in respiratory disease, 231
    2.12.1 Domiciliary oxygen therapy, 231
    2.12.2 Continuous positive airways pressure, 232
    2.12.3 Non-invasive ventilation, 234
  2.13 Lung transplantation, 236
3 Investigations and practical procedures, 237
  3.1 Arterial blood gas sampling, 237
  3.2 Aspiration of pleural effusion or pneumothorax, 237
  3.3 Pleural biopsy, 238
  3.4 Intercostal tube insertion, 239
  3.5 Fibreoptic bronchoscopy and transbronchial biopsy, 240
    3.5.1 Fibreoptic bronchoscopy, 240
    3.5.2 Transbronchial biopsy, 241
  3.6 Interpretation of clinical data, 241
    3.6.1 Arterial blood gases, 241
    3.6.2 Lung function tests, 243
    3.6.3 Overnight oximetry, 244
    3.6.4 Chest radiograph, 244
    3.6.5 Computed tomography scan of the thorax, 245
4 Self-assessment, 250

Answers to Self-assessment, 255
The Medical Masterclass series, 263
Index, 273

List of contributors

Praveen Bhatia MBBS MRCP
Staff Physician
Blackpool Victoria Hospital
Blackpool

Peter E. Glennon MB ChB Hons MD MRCP
BHF Clinical Lecturer
University of Cambridge
Addenbrooke's Hospital
Cambridge

Catherine E.G. Head MA MRCP
MRC Clinical Training Fellow and Specialist Registrar
University of Cambridge
Cambridge

Michael I. Polkey MRCP PhD
Consultant Physician
Royal Brompton Hospital
London

Paul R. Roberts MB ChB MRCP MD
Specialist Registrar, Cardiology
Southampton General Hospital
Southampton

Hamish A. Walker BA Hons MB BS MRCP
Clinical Research Fellow
Specialist Registrar Cardiology
Hammersmith Hospital
London

Veronica L.C. White BSc MSc MBBS MRCP
Research Fellow
Department of Respiratory Medicine
St. Bartholomew's Hospital
London

Foreword

Since its foundation in 1518, the Royal College of Physicians has engaged in a wide range of activities dedicated to its overall aim of upholding and improving standards of medical practice. *Medical Masterclass* is one of the most innovative and ambitious educational resources the College has developed, and while it continues the tradition of pioneering and supporting high quality medicine, it also makes use of modern day technology by offering computer-assisted learning.

The MRCP(UK) examination is crucial to the progress of physicians through their training. Preparation is not only essential for success in the examination, but it is also important for the acquisition of requisite knowledge, skills and attitudes appropriate for further training. With a pass rate of about 40% at each sitting of the written papers, the exam is a challenge. The College wishes to encourage excellence, and with this in mind has produced *Medical Masterclass*, a comprehensive distance-learning package designed to help candidates with the preparation that is key to making the grade.

Medical Masterclass has been produced by the RCP's Education Department. It represents a formidable amount of work by Dr John Firth and his team of authors and editors. I congratulate our colleagues for this superb educational product and wholeheartedly recommend it as an invaluable MRCP(UK) study aid.

Professor Carol M. Black CBE
President of the Royal College of Physicians

Preface

Medical Masterclass comprises twelve paper-based modules, two CD-ROMs and a companion website. Its aim is to help doctors in their first few years of training to improve their medical skills and knowledge.

The twelve paper-based modules are divided as follows: two cover the scientific background to medicine, one is devoted to general clinical issues, one to emergency medicine and practical procedures, and eight cover the range of medical specialities. Medicine is often fairly straightforward when the diagnosis is clear, but patients rarely come to their doctor and say 'I've got Hodgkin's disease': they have lumps. The core material of each of the clinical specialities is defined by case presentations in the first part of each module: how do you approach the man who has lumps? Structured concise notes on specific diseases follow later. All practising doctors know that medicine is much more than knowing lots of facts about diseases: how do you tell someone they've got cancer? How do you decide when to stop treatment? Most medical texts say little about these issues: *Medical Masterclass* does not avoid them, nor does it talk in vague and abstract terms.

The two CD-ROMs each contain 30 interactive cases requiring diagnosis and treatment. The format is remarkably close to real life: you see the patient and are told the story; you have to decide how to investigate and treat; but you can't see all the results before you start to make decisions!

The companion website, which will be regularly updated, includes self-assessment questions and mock MRCP(UK) exam papers. How much do you know, and are you improving? You will see how your score compares with your previous attempts, and also how your performance compares with others who have logged on to the site.

The *Medical Masterclass* is produced by the Education Department of the Royal College of Physicians. It has been specifically designed to support candidates studying for the MRCP(UK) Examination (All Parts). I have no doubt that someone putting effort into learning through the *Medical Masterclass* would be in a strong position to impress the examiners.

John Firth
Editor-in-Chief

Acknowledgements

Medical Masterclass has been produced by a team. The names of those who have written and edited material are clearly indicated elsewhere, but without the efforts of many other people *Medical Masterclass* would not exist at all. These include Professor Lesley Rees and Mrs Winnie Wade from the Education Department of the Royal College of Physicians of London, who initiated the project; Dr Mike Stein and Dr Andy Robinson from Medschool.com and Blackwell Science respectively, who have enthusiastically supported it from the beginning; and Ms Filipa Maia and Ms Katherine Bowker, who have run the office with splendid efficiency and induced authors and editors to perform to a schedule rarely achieved. I and the whole of the team of editors and authors are immensely grateful to all of these people for the energy that they have poured into *Medical Masterclass* in various ways.

John Firth
Editor-in-Chief

Key features

We have created a range of icon boxes to help you identify key information and to make learning easier and more enjoyable. Here is a brief explanation:

Clinical pointer

This icon highlights important information to be noted.

Further information

This icon indicates the source of further information and reference.

Hints

This icon highlights useful hints, tips and mnemonics.

Key points

This icon is used to highlight points of particular importance.

Quote

This icon indicates useful or interesting citations from notable individuals, including well-known physicians.

Think about

This icon indicates what the reader should reflect on after having read a passage from the text.

Warning/Hazard

This icon is used to indicate common or important drug interactions, pitfalls of practical procedures, or when to take symptoms or signs particularly seriously.

Cardiology

AUTHORS:
**P.E. Glennon, C.E.G. Head,
P.R. Roberts and H.A. Walker**

EDITOR:
P.R. Roberts

EDITOR-IN-CHIEF:
J.D. Firth

Clinical presentations

1.1 Paroxysmal palpitations

Case history

A 28-year-old teacher is referred to you in outpatients with a 5-year history of intermittent palpitations. Other than the sensation of palpitations she has no other symptoms. In her family, two relatives have died following a sudden collapse.

Clinical approach

The symptom of palpitations (abnormal awareness of the heart beat) can be caused by a range of clinical conditions from the very benign to the potentially life threatening; approach the patient with this in mind. It is unusual to see someone during a symptomatic episode, so as much information as possible should be gained from the history, with a main aim being to assess the patient's potential risk from life-threatening ventricular arrhythmias. You should always have in the back of your mind a list of the possible causes of palpitations (Table 1). In most situations it will be essential to have investigations during a symptomatic episode. Remember that the severity of symptoms does not always reflect the seriousness of the underlying problem: some patients in sinus rhythm may experience severe palpitations, whereas others may be asymptomatic when in ventricular tachycardia.

Table 1 Potential causes of palpitations.

Type of palpitation	Cause
No arrhythmia	Anxiety
	Panic attacks
	Depression
Extrasystoles	Atrial
	Ventricular
Bradyarrhythmia	Atrioventricular block
	Sinus node disease
Tachyarrhythmia	Ventricular tachycardia
	Atrial fibrillation/flutter
	AVNRT
	AVRT
	Sinus tachycardia

AVNRT, atrioventricular nodal re-entry tachycardia; AVRT, atrioventricular re-entry tachycardia.

In this case the family history should make you particularly keen to exclude significant inherited conditions that may predispose to arrhythmias, e.g. hypertrophic obstructive cardiomyopathy.

History of the presenting problem

 Which came first—the anxiety or the palpitation, the chicken or the egg?
- Palpitations secondary to anxiety-induced sinus tachycardia are common
- Patients with cardiac arrhythmias are frequently anxious about their future.

What are the palpitations like?

The characteristics of the palpitations can provide valuable clues in making the diagnosis. Ask the following:
- 'Tap out' the rhythm—note how fast this is, and whether it is regular or irregular. Irregular means that atrial fibrillation is most likely. A 'missed beat' is typically caused by an extrasystole—after the compensatory pause the next sinus beat is felt with extra force. These missed beats are almost always of no pathological significance. However, they can cause worry that is likely to be reinforced because anxiety is the most common cause of awareness of extrasystoles, which are likely to have been long standing and previously asymptomatic.
- Do you feel the palpitations in your neck? These are suggestive of cannon waves, indicating atrioventricular (AV) block.
- How do they start, what brings them on and how do they stop? Do you get any warning at all? Do they come on gradually or suddenly? Palpitations that come on and go away gradually are most likely to be due to sinus tachycardia.
- Are there accompanying symptoms? Do you feel faint or dizzy with them? Have you ever collapsed? Arrhythmias causing these symptoms are more likely to be of a serious (potentially life-threatening) cause and clearly mandate thorough investigation. Some patients with supraventricular tachycardia (SVT) develop polyuria as a result of atrial stretch causing release of atrial natriuretic peptide.
- How frequent are the palpitations? Palpitations that occur infrequently are likely to be difficult to catch on tape.
- What treatments have been tried already? An SVT may be terminated by a Valsalva manoeuvre.

Other aspects

Ask about the following:
- General health: is there anything to suggest thyrotoxicosis? (See *Endocrinology*, Section 1.13.)
- Smoking, alcohol, tea and coffee consumption—acute excess of these can trigger arrhythmia in those predisposed.
- Drugs, prescribed and non-prescribed: a range of these can cause arrhythmia. Always consult the drug datasheet or *British National Formulary* (BNF).
- Is the patient prone to anxiety? Does he or she ever have anxiety attacks?
- Find out whether he or she has a history of recurrent presentation to doctors with medically unexplained symptoms.
- Family history: this is clearly an important element in this case, but always ask directly about it. A patient is much more likely to be concerned about palpitations, even if of benign cause, if a relative has died at a young age of heart disease.

Examination

Examination of the patient with palpitations:
- A normal examination does not rule out a significant arrhythmia
- Do not focus entirely on the cardiovascular system
- Patients with significant cardiovascular pathology may initially present with palpitations
- Take note of the patient's mental state.

General

As the patient is unlikely to be symptomatic at the time, the purpose of examination is to assess the patient's general well-being, including mental state, and to establish whether there is a cardiovascular or systemic cause for the symptoms. Is there any evidence of thyrotoxicosis, which might predispose to paroxysms of atrial fibrillation? In most patients with an SVT, examination will be entirely normal.

Cardiovascular

Take careful note of the following:
- Pulse rate, rhythm and character
- Blood pressure
- Jugular venous pressure (JVP)
- Heart sounds and murmurs
- Lung bases.

Cardiovascular examination is aimed at evaluating whether there is a structural abnormality that may make the patient susceptible to arrhythmias. Pay particular attention to auscultation of the heart:

- The findings of a diastolic murmur, opening snap and loud first heart sound may indicate mitral stenosis, which predisposes to atrial fibrillation as the size of the atria enlarges.
- The harsh systolic murmur found in patients with hypertrophic obstructive cardiomyopathy may suggest ventricular arrhythmias.
- Signs of congestive heart failure raise the possibility of ventricular arrhythmias and atrial fibrillation.

Approach to investigations and management

This should be guided by facts established from the history and examination. Auscultation may suggest a structural cardiac abnormality, such as valvular disease, and in such patients echocardiography may be warranted.

Investigations

ECG

In most situations only a 12-lead ECG in sinus rhythm is available. However, if an ECG has been recorded during symptoms and documents an arrhythmia, it may not be necessary to investigate further because this alone may enable a precise diagnosis to be made (see Section 3.1, p. 120).

Assessing the 12-lead ECG of a patient with palpitations:
- Look for sinus bradycardia/tachycardia.
- Are there any features suggestive of cardiac structural. abnormality, e.g. P mitrale, left ventricular hypertrophy (LVH) (Fig. 1)?
- Measure the PR interval.
- Look for evidence of AV block.
- Are there δ waves (Fig. 2)?
- Has the patient had a previous myocardial infarction (MI)?
- Measure the QT interval and calculate the QTc (QT adjusted for rate).
- Are there any ventricular/atrial ectopic beats?

Ambulatory monitoring

See Section 3.3 (p. 127). An example of an arrhythmia captured on an ambulatory monitor record is shown in Fig. 3.

Management

In many cases when an arrhythmia has been found to be associated with symptoms, the management will be straightforward.

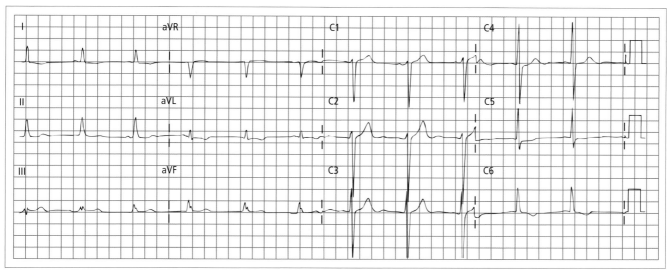

Fig. 1 ECG showing left ventricular hypertrophy with strain (lateral ST/T changes) in a patient with previously undiagnosed aortic stenosis.

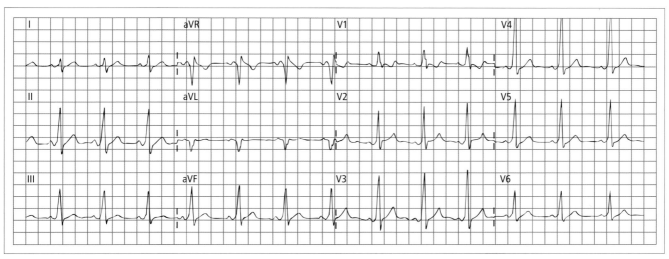

Fig. 2 Twelve-lead ECG of patient with the Wolff–Parkinson–White syndrome. Note the short PR interval and δ waves.

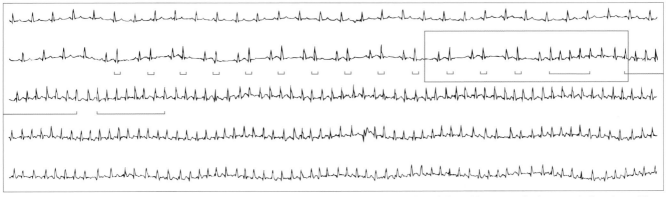

Fig. 3 Ambulatory monitor of a patient with supraventricular tachycardia (SVT). Sinus tachycardia is followed by ventricular bigeminy before the sudden onset of SVT.

Supraventricular arrhythmias

Most SVTs are amenable to pharmacological therapy with class 1, 2, 3 or 4 agents or suitable for radiofrequency ablation. (See Section 2.2.2, p. 59.)

Paroxysmal atrial fibrillation/flutter: initial therapy should be the maintenance of sinus rhythm pharmacologically. Drugs with a class 3 action are most efficacious in this instance, e.g. sotalol, amiodarone. Specific attention should be focused towards the need for anticoagulation. (See Section 2.14.1, p. 108.)

Bradyarrhythmias

See Section 2.2.1, p. 58.

Ventricular arrhythmias

Ventricular arrhythmias may be suitable for ablation or for implantation of an implantable cardioverter defibrillator (ICD). (See Section 3.4, p. 130.)

Others

In many cases a benign arrhythmia is detected, such as ventricular or atrial ectopy, and occasionally symptoms are clearly associated with sinus rhythm. In most cases explanation and positive reassurance to the patient are all that is required. Only in rare instances, where the patient is very debilitated, should a β blocker be prescribed.

Significant symptoms can occasionally be associated with sinus tachycardia; in these circumstances it is important to exclude causes of sinus tachycardia, the most common being anxiety, before attributing the arrhythmia to inappropriate sinus node function.

Brugada P, Gursoy S, Brugada J, Andries E. Investigation of palpitations. *Lancet* 1993; 341: 1254–1258.
Vohra JK. Palpitations: reassurance or more? *Med J Aust* 1999; 170: 442–448.
Zimetbaum P, Josephson ME. Evaluation of patients with palpitations. *N Engl J Med* 1998; 338: 1369–1373.

1.2 Palpitations with dizziness

Case history

A 57-year-old retired policeman presents with a 2-month history of rapid palpitations. Initially he was well during the episodes, but more recently he has noticed that he is dizzy when they go on for a longer time. He made an appointment to see his GP, who referred him directly to the medical admissions unit where you are asked to assess him.

Clinical approach

Your main concern is that this patient gives a history of presyncope, which places him in a higher risk category for life-threatening arrhythmia (see Section 1.1, p. 3). The main objective with this patient is to exclude a significant ventricular arrhythmia. With the little information available, it is apparent that the palpitations are directly related to the presyncope, which would be consistent with the diagnosis of ventricular tachycardia (VT).

It is vital to ensure that the patient is safe while a diagnosis has to be established; he should therefore be admitted for investigation and monitoring. It is essential to document the heart rhythm during an episode. Some patients with VT are asymptomatic, whereas others are extremely symptomatic of only short runs of VT. Both groups are at risk of cardiac arrest as a result of VT or from the VT degenerating into ventricular fibrillation.

 Broad complex tachycardia: do not attribute a broad complex tachyarrhythmia to SVT with aberration unless you are absolutely certain of the diagnosis.

History of the presenting problem

What is the relationship of the presyncope and palpitations?

It is important to determine the order of symptoms; many patients with presyncope or syncope will have a reactive sinus tachycardia after the event that might cause a feeling of palpitation. In this case it is clear that the presyncope is occurring with more prolonged episodes of palpitation.

Aside from ventricular arrhythmia, consider other causes of palpitations and syncope:
- Bradyarrhythmias
- Atrial flutter with 1 : 1 conduction
- Atrial fibrillation and Wolff–Parkinson–White syndrome
- Aortic stenosis.
 And do not forget the following:
- Vasovagal syncope: the most common cause of presyncope and syncope
- Acute blood loss: this will usually be obvious, but it is a mistake to miss the fact that the patient has had melaena!

Relevant past history

Ischaemic heart disease

This is a common cause of VT. Find out the following:

- Is there a previous history of angina/MI?
- Does the patient have symptoms consistent with angina?
- Does the patient have risk factors for ischaemic heart disease (IHD)?

Cardiomyopathy

Most forms of cardiomyopathy can cause VT. Ask the patient the following:
- Is there a history of breathlessness/lethargy?
- Have you had a recent viral illness?
- How much alcohol do you drink? Have you ever drunk heavily in the past?

Drug history

Drug toxicity can provoke VT, e.g. digoxin, quinidine, catecholamines. Check the datasheet or BNF for details of any drug that the patient is taking. Is arrhythmia reported as a side effect?

Family history

Particularly in young patients presenting with arrhythmias, always enquire if anyone in the family has had a similar problem.

Other

Ventricular tachycardia may be part of a primary electrophysiological disturbance or secondary to any pathology that produces structural changes in the ventricles. Any 'cardiac history' could therefore be relevant, e.g. valvular heart disease, congenital heart disease, right ventricular dysplasia, previous cardiac surgery.

Examination

The priorities are to establish the following:
- Is the patient unwell/hypotensive/sweating?
- Is the patient in VT or another arrhythmia at the moment? If the patient is having a symptomatic episode, specific signs may provide clues to the diagnosis.
- Are there any obvious cardiovascular causes for VT?
- Are there any other signs suggesting systemic upset?

General

In most cases the examination will be normal, but it is important to examine all systems thoroughly because many diseases can have an impact on the electrophysiological status of the heart, e.g. renal disease leading to

hyperkalaemia or respiratory disease causing hypoxaemia will both predispose to arrhythmia.

Cardiovascular

The main aim of the cardiovascular examination will be to elicit whether there are any structural abnormalities that may make the patient liable to ventricular arrhythmias. Pay specific attention to:
- pulse rate, rhythm and character
- JVP
- apex beat
- thrills or heaves
- heart sounds and murmurs
- lung bases.

Approach to investigations and management

 A broad complex tachycardia should always be treated as ventricular tachycardia until proven otherwise.

Investigations

12-lead ECG

Obtaining an ECG during an episode is a key objective in establishing a diagnosis (Fig. 4). Beware of confusing VT and SVT with aberrant conduction. (See Section 3.1, p. 120.)

Ambulatory monitoring

If the diagnosis is not apparent, monitoring for longer periods may be necessary. (See Section 3.3, p. 127.)

Electrophysiological study

If symptoms are infrequent or doubt exists as to the diagnosis, then provocation of the rhythm during an electrophysiological study will provide definitive evidence. (See Section 3.2, p. 125.)

Other

If VT is suspected, investigations to identify possible causes should be considered:
- Chest radiograph (cardiomegaly, heart shape, pulmonary oedema) (Fig. 5)
- Check electrolytes: abnormalities of potassium or magnesium can be associated with arrhythmia
- Echocardiogram (cardiac function, valve structure/function, intracardiac masses) (Fig. 6)

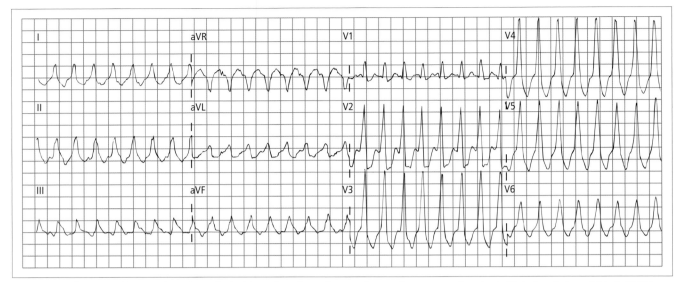

Fig. 4 Twelve-lead ECG of ventricular tachycardia (VT). Note broad complexes and concordance across chest leads. Right bundle-branch block (RBBB) morphology suggests left ventricular origin.

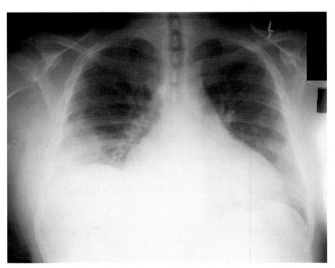

Fig. 5 Chest radiograph of patient with dilated cardiomyopathy. The cardiothoracic ratio is increased. There is a pleural effusion at the right base.

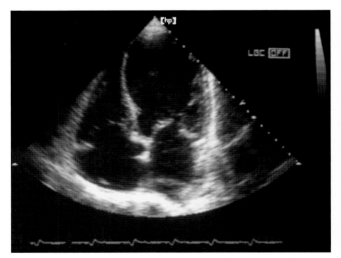

Fig. 6 Echocardiogram demonstrating dilated cardiomyopathy. This is a 'four-chamber' view with both ventricles dilated, particularly the left ventricle (seen in the centre at the top).

- Exercise ECG (ischaemia, exercise-induced arrhythmias)
- Cardiac catheterization (coronary atherosclerosis, valvular function)
- Computed tomography/magnetic resonance imaging (CT/MRI) (mediastinal pathology, pericardial/myocardial disease).

Management

The patient is likely to be having presyncope associated with VT and should be admitted for monitoring and observation. Management will consist of the following:
- Immediate cessation of arrhythmia if in VT (DC shock/pharmacological cardioversion)
- Identification of cause

- Correction of cause
- Antiarrhythmic therapy
- Assessment for ICD.

Immediate management

The priorities are as follows:
- If the patient does not have an output, start emergency resuscitation. (See *Emergency medicine*, Section 1.1.)
- If the patient is haemodynamically compromised, consider DC cardioversion (under general anaesthesia or sedation). (See Section 2.2.2, p. 59.)
- If the patient is not compromised, consider pharmacological intervention (lidocaine, amiodarone).

Correct electrolyte (K^+/Mg^{2+}) imbalances.

Long-term management

IMPLANTABLE CARDIOVERTER DEFIBRILLATOR

All patients with VT should be considered for assessment for an ICD. (See Section 3.4, p. 130.)

ANTIARRHYTHMICS

In those patients who do not have an indication for an ICD, pharmacological therapy should be considered; in many circumstances either sotalol or amiodarone will be the drug of choice. It is essential to monitor the patient to ensure suppression of the arrhythmia; symptomatology is not always adequate because the drugs may slow but not prevent the VT, making it better tolerated or unnoticed. Monitoring will usually be in the form of ambulatory ECG recording, but exercise testing if the arrhythmia is exercise induced or by provocation at electrophysiological study may be appropriate in some cases.

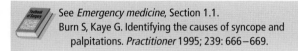

See *Emergency medicine*, Section 1.1.
Burn S, Kaye G. Identifying the causes of syncope and palpitations. *Practitioner* 1995; 239: 666–669.

1.3 Syncope

Case history

A 75-year-old woman presents to you in the accident and emergency (A&E) department with a history of sudden collapse. This occurred unexpectedly while she was shopping and there have been no previous similar episodes. When the paramedic team arrived at the scene she was alert and orientated, and all observations were normal.

Clinical approach

This is a very common clinical problem and accounts for up to 3% of attendances at A&E departments and 1% of hospital admissions. Your aim will be to determine the cause of the syncope, remembering that untreated cardiac related syncope has a 1-year mortality rate of 20–30%. A difficult aspect of managing patients such as this is that there are so many causes of syncope, both cardiac and non-cardiac (Table 2). A carefully taken history may exclude a large proportion of these, and a meticulous examination may elicit the cause. A history from a witness should be obtained if at all possible—it might be invaluable.

Table 2 Causes of syncope.

Type	Cause
Non-cardiac	Seizures
	Postural hypertension
	Cerebrovascular
	Drug induced
	Situational (micturition, defaecation, cough, swallow)
	Psychogenic (anxiety, panic, somatization, depression)
Cardiac	Bradyarrhythmias (including vasovagal)
	Tachyarrhythmias
	Left ventricular outflow obstruction (aortic stenosis, HOCM)
	Myxoma
	Mitral stenosis
	Cardiac ischaemia (MI, angina)
	Pulmonary obstruction (pulmonary stenosis, pulmonary hypertension, pulmonary embolism, Fallot's tetralogy, myxoma)
	Cardiac tamponade
	Aortic dissection

HOCM, hypertrophic obstructive cardiomyopathy; MI, myocardial infarction.

History of the presenting problem

Did the woman really have a syncopal episode, or did she just trip up? If syncope is likely, direct questions should be targeted at excluding all of the causes listed in Table 2. One of the most important of these is seizures.

Seizures or cardiac syncope?

Seizures are associated with the following:
- Blue face (not pale)
- Convulsive movements (usually, but not always)
- Tongue biting
- Incontinence
- Unconsciousness >5min
- Drowsiness and disorientation for a variable length of time on recovery.

A detailed description of the events leading up to the syncopal episode, and a description of the syncopal episode itself and of the recovery phase may provide information to establish the cause. Be very particular: 'Can you remember exactly what you were doing before you collapsed?' Do not accept: 'I was out shopping.' 'Were you sitting down . . . standing up . . . had you just turned your head?' This history should be obtained from the patient, from any witness and preferably from both. You may need to ask specific questions:
- Did you feel sweaty or nauseous before the episodes?
- Did you get palpitations beforehand?
- Did you get chest pain beforehand?
- Did you feel breathless beforehand?

All of these would suggest a cardiac cause, as opposed to seizures. And if someone has had more than one episode:

- How long have you had the symptoms?
- Are the episodes becoming more frequent?
- Have you had fits of any sort before?

Take particular care to consider those conditions that make the patient at high risk of recurrent syncope or death and for which specific treatments are available. These include the following:

- Aortic dissection: was syncope associated with chest pain? Is there a history of hypertension? Has the patient had any previous vascular conditions? (See Section 1.5, p. 15.)
- Pulmonary embolism: has the patient had a period of immobility? Any recent operations? Has there been a previous history of thromboembolism? (See Section 1.9, p. 28.)
- Aortic stenosis: has a murmur been noticed in previous examinations? Is there a history of dyspnoea? Is there a history of exertional presyncope?

Relevant past history

Identification of any underlying cardiac disease places the patient in a high-risk group. Establish whether there are other symptoms suggestive of cardiac abnormality:

- Is there a history of angina/MI?
- Is there any cardiac family history?
- Is there a history of rheumatic fever?
- Are there any risk factors for IHD?
- What medications is she taking? Are there any that might predispose to syncope, e.g. diuretics that could cause postural hypotension, or agents that might predispose to arrhythmia. (See Section 1.2, p. 6.)

Examination

Look for evidence of injury caused by the syncope, and concentrate specifically on cardiovascular and neurological assessment.

Cardiovascular

Take careful note of the following:

- Peripheral perfusion
- Pulse rate and rhythm
- Peripheral pulses, including left radial and femorals
- Pulse character: is it slow rising?
- Blood pressure: is there a postural drop? Is it the same in both arms?
- JVP
- Cardiac apex
- Are there carotid bruits (or bruits elsewhere)?
- Heart sounds and murmurs
- Lung bases
- Liver edge
- Peripheral oedema.

Any abnormal cardiac signs increase the chances of a cardiac cause of syncope.

Ask the patient to move her neck through its full range of movement: does this provoke feelings of presyncope or dizziness, which would suggest vertebrobasilar ischaemia as a likely cause for her syncope?

Consider carotid sinus massage to investigate carotid sinus sensitivity, but be extremely cautious in those patients at risk of atheromatous carotid disease.

Neurological

The presence of any focal neurological signs would raise the possibility that syncope was caused by a cerebro-vascular event, but does not prove that this is the case. A cardiac cause of syncope could have led to cerebrovascular ischaemia.

Approach to investigations and management

Remember that patients with syncope are likely to be in a high state of anxiety and that it is essential that all other explanations are carefully considered before attributing the problem to psychogenic causes.

This woman will need to be admitted to hospital for monitoring and assessment. The history and examination provide the basis for direct investigation and management. If it is felt that syncope is most likely to be neurological in origin then investigation should be pursued as described in *Neurology*, Section 1.20. However, a cardiac cause can never be totally excluded without thorough investigation.

Investigations

Immediate investigations

The immediate investigations of a patient with probable cardiac syncope are discussed below.

ECG

Of patients with a cardiac syncope, 10% will have an identifiable abnormality on the ECG to suggest a cause. Therefore, look for the following:

- Sinus rate
- PR interval
- QRS axis
- QRS width
- Left ventricular hypertrophy
- Right ventricular hypertrophy
- P-wave morphology

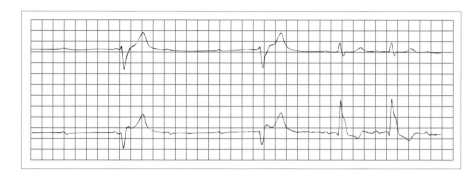

Fig. 7 Complete heart block demonstrated on a Holter monitor.

- Evidence of pre-excitation (Wolff–Parkinson–White syndrome)
- Evidence of acute MI/infarction.

CHEST RADIOGRAPH

Look for the following:
- Cardiac size and shape
- Prominent pulmonary vasculature
- Pulmonary oedema
- Aortic outline: is the mediastinum of normal width?

BLOOD TESTS

These are rarely helpful in establishing a diagnosis, but cardiac enzymes, full blood count (FBC), electrolytes, renal and liver function tests and inflammatory markers will usually be requested as a 'screen'. Electrolyte disturbance (particularly hypokalaemia) might predispose to arrhythmia and syncope (see Section 1.2, p. 6). Raised inflammatory markers may indicate a systemic problem.

Further investigations

DURING HOSPITAL ADMISSION

It is more than likely that the ECG, chest radiograph and screening blood tests will not demonstrate any clear cause of syncope, in which case consider the following:
- Ambulatory monitoring: 24-h Holter monitoring and patient-activated devices may be useful to exclude tachy-/bradyarrhythmias (Fig. 7). (See Section 3.3, p. 127.)
- Echocardiography: this may indicate structural or functional cardiac abnormality—transthoracic echocardiography (Fig. 8) is usually adequate, but in some instances, e.g. when aortic dissection is being considered, trans-oesophageal echocardiography (TOE) may be required.
- If pulmonary embolism is plausible, check blood gases and organize lung ventilation–perfusion scanning or CT angiography. (See Section 1.9, p. 28 and *Respiratory medicine*, Section 1.5.)

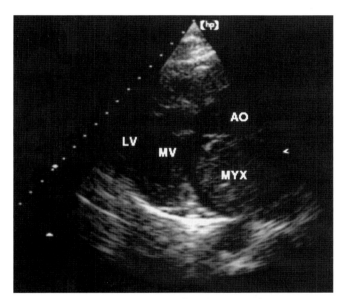

Fig. 8 Transthoracic echocardiogram of atrial myxoma. The myxoma (MYX) is seen to occupy most of the left atrium and is almost prolapsing through the mitral valve (MV) into the left ventricle (LV). The aorta (AO) is seen above the left atrium.

- If aortic dissection is plausible, organize a CT scan of the chest.

FOR THOSE WITH RECURRENT UNEXPLAINED SYNCOPE

Consider the following for patients with recurrent unexplained syncope.

Tilt-table test
A tilt-table test can be helpful in identifying vasovagal syncope, with continuous blood pressure and heart rate monitoring showing abnormal bradycardia and/or hypotension in response to upright tilt. However, the findings on tilt-table testing can be difficult to interpret, particularly in elderly patients, and it is important to adopt a strict protocol and use clear endpoints to define a positive result.

Electrophysiological studies
Abnormalities of sinus and AV node function may be

identified, suggesting a bradycardic cause of syncope. Similarly, provocation of atrial/ventricular arrhythmias may establish the diagnosis. (See Section 3.2, p. 125.)

Management

If a cardiac cause of syncope is established, then management is as indicated:
• Bradyarrhythmias: consider permanent pacemaker. (See Section 3.5, p. 132.)
• Tachyarrhythmias: pharmacological therapy, ablation or an ICD. (See Sections 2.2.2, p. 59 and 3.4, p. 130.)
• Valvular disease: consider surgical intervention. (See Section 2.5, p. 71.)
• Pulmonary embolism: will need anticoagulation. (See Sections 1.9, p. 28, 2.18, p. 115, and *Haematology*, Section 3.6.)
• Hypertrophic obstructive cardiomyopathy: advice on lifestyle changes and pharmacological therapy. (See Section 2.4.1, p. 66.)

If no cause for syncope is established and the patient is agitating to go home ('there's nothing wrong with me, doctor—I just had a faint'), then what should you do? If, after 24–48 h, there has been no recurrence of presyncope or syncope, the patient has 'mobilized' satisfactorily on the ward and serial 12-lead ECGs show no change, most physicians would be willing for the patient to be discharged home with the following:
• Reassurance that nothing terrible has been found, but also a clear statement that no firm diagnosis has been made—meaning that patient and doctors must remain alert.
• A letter for the patient's general practitioner.
• Instructions to report recurrence of presyncope or syncope immediately.
• Arrangements for a 24-h ambulatory monitoring (and perhaps echocardiography) if it has not been possible to obtain this during the patient's inpatient stay (which is preferable, but not always possible).

Most patients will be aware of the serious nature of most cardiac causes of syncope. It is essential to be aware of the psychological needs of such patients. Reassurance and appropriate information at an early stage may prevent problems at a later stage in their management.

See *Medicine for the elderly*, Section 1.1.
See *Emergency medicine*, Sections 1.1, 1.4 and 1.6.
See *Neurology*, Section 1.20.
Kapoor WN. Syncope and hypotension. In: Braunwald E (ed.) *Heart Disease: A textbook of cardiovascular medicine*, 5th edn. Philadelphia, PA: WB Saunders Co., 1997: 863–876.

1.4 Stroke and a murmur

Case history

A 58-year-old woman presents with a left-sided hemiparesis of sudden onset. She had previously been fit and well. However, a murmur had been noted, but not investigated, when she was 45 and undergoing a minor gynaecological procedure.

Clinical approach

A stroke can be a devastating condition with high morbidity and mortality. It is not possible to predict accurately the degree of recovery that this woman will make. It is important to identify whether or not she is at high risk of further events, and in particular whether she is at risk of cardiac embolic stroke. The majority of strokes are related to cerebrovascular atheromatous disease and not to cardiac disease, but most cardiac causes of embolic stroke are treatable, so further events are potentially preventable in this group. In most cases where there is a cardiac cause this will be elicited from the history or examination.

Consider the causes of cardiac embolic strokes when taking a history and examining a patient who has had a stroke:
• 'Non-valvular' atrial fibrillation
• Acute MI with mural thrombus
• Mechanical prosthetic valves
• Rheumatic heart disease
• Dilated cardiomyopathy
• Infective endocarditis
• Paradoxical embolism
• Left atrial myxoma
• Calcific aortic stenosis.

History of the presenting problem

The first priority will be to establish the diagnosis of stroke and then to focus on possible causes.

Identification of cardiac cause of stroke:
• Establish whether there have been any previous thromboembolic events
• Is the patient known to have any cardiac conditions?
• Does the patient have any cardiac symptoms? Specifically, is there a history of palpitations suggestive of atrial fibrillation?

Relevant past history

In most cases, it will be obvious if there is any pre-existing cardiac condition, but ask the patient the following:
• Are you known to have an irregular pulse?
• Have you had angina or a heart attack?
• Have you had rheumatic fever?
• Have you had any heart operations?
• Has a murmur ever been heard?
• Did you have a 'hole in the heart' as a child?

Examination

In the absence of previous cardiac conditions and with an entirely normal clinical examination, the likelihood of the stroke being cardiac in origin is small. It is therefore vital that the examination of the cardiovascular system is thorough. A patient with a recent stroke may have difficulty in co-operating with you during the examination, e.g. rolling the patient on to the side to listen for mitral stenosis may be difficult if he or she has a hemiparesis. However, it is important not to compromise the quality of your examination—seek help in moving the patient if necessary.

General

It is unlikely that there will be many signs from general examination that will help in establishing whether or not the cause was cardiac:
• The patient with a previous MI or dilated cardiomyopathy might be dyspnoeic as a result of cardiac failure, but there are many other causes of breathlessness, including aspiration pneumonia in someone who has just suffered a stroke.
• The patient with infective endocarditis may have fever and peripheral stigmata. (See Section 1.13, p. 38.)
• Look carefully for any signs of previous cardiac surgery, particularly if the patient is unable to give a history.

Do not forget to examine the back and the breast crease where there may be scars from previous mitral surgery (valvuloplasty).

Cardiovascular

Take careful note of the following:
• Peripheral perfusion.
• Peripheral pulses: is it possible that this woman has had an aortic dissection?
• Pulse rhythm and character: in particular, is there atrial fibrillation? Is there aortic stenosis or incompetence?
• Blood pressure: often elevated in someone who has just had a stroke.
• Cardiac apex.
• Heart sounds and murmurs: this woman is said to have a murmur—listen carefully for both mitral stenosis and

aortic incompetence, which are the easy murmurs to miss. You are most unlikely ever to hear the 'tumour plop' of an atrial myxoma, but it is absolutely certain that you will not if you never listen!
• Lung bases.
• Liver edge.
• Peripheral oedema.

Consider non-thromboembolic cardiovascular causes for stroke:
• Aortic dissection involving the carotid arteries
• Vasculitis of the cerebral vessels (very rare).

Approach to investigations and management

In most cases, simple non-invasive investigations will provide the information needed to establish a cardiac cause of stroke.

Investigations

ECG and chest radiograph

Every patient who has a stroke should have a 12-lead ECG and chest radiograph. The ECG may provide valuable clues to the aetiology of thrombus (Fig. 9).

Echocardiogram

Echocardiography should be performed only if there is a clinical, ECG or chest radiographic indication of cardiac abnormality (Fig. 10). (See Section 3.11, p. 141.) CT or MRI of the chest may rarely be required to define a structural abnormality.

Blood tests

Check the FBC (?polycythaemia, ?thrombocytosis), electrolytes, renal and liver function tests, inflammatory markers (if raised, consider endocarditis, myxoma and vasculitis, and perform appropriate specialist blood tests), and blood cultures (if any suspicion of endocarditis).

CT scan of the brain

In any case where anticoagulation is to be considered, a CT brain scan is required to exclude haemorrhage.

Management

The patient will require care appropriate to the disability produced by their stroke. (See *Medicine for the elderly*, Section 1.4, *Emergency medicine*, Section 1.25 and *Neurology*, Sections 1.21 and 2.8.1.)

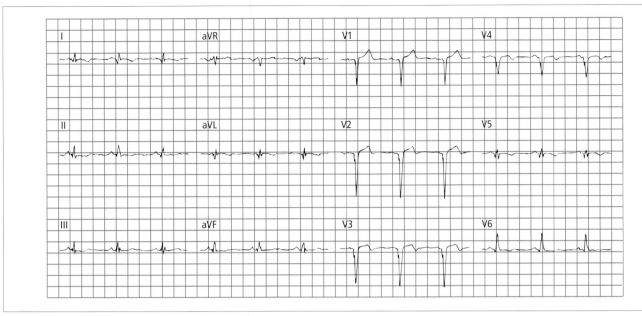

Fig. 9 ECG demonstrating anterior Q waves and poor R-wave progression across the chest leads. This is most probably secondary to a previous large anterior myocardial infarction. Left ventricular mural thrombus is possible in this scenario.

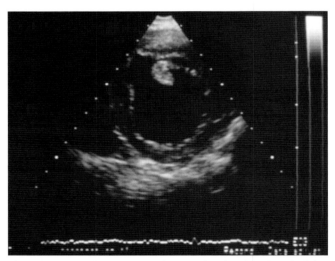

Fig. 10 Transoesophageal echocardiogram of cardiac thrombus. The left ventricle is seen in cross-section with a large mural thrombus.

Particular attention to anticoagulation, restoration of sinus rhythm (in some cases) and surgical correction of cardiac lesions (in rare cases) will be required in patients with a cardiac cause for stroke.

Anticoagulation

If a cardiac cause of stroke has been identified—meaning almost certainly that there is further substantial thromboembolic risk—then, if the stroke is confirmed as ischaemic on CT brain scan, consideration of anticoagulation is required. However, leaving the patient without anticoagulation keeps him or her at risk of further thrombo-

embolism; anticoagulation puts him or her at increased risk of haemorrhagic transformation of a cerebral infarct. There are no good data to determine when anticoagulation should be started. Assuming that the patient is recovering from the stroke, most physicians would begin with heparin (intravenous or low molecular weight) at some time between 7 and 14 days, with a view to longer-term warfarin therapy if the thromboembolic risk persists, and with very careful monitoring of the level of anticoagulation. (See *Haematology*, Section 3.6.)

Strokes may be haemorrhagic, even in those at risk of thromboembolism.
Some features are more likely with cerebral haemorrhages:
- Nausea/vomiting
- Cerebral irritation
- Depressed conscious level.

But ischaemic and haemorrhagic strokes cannot be distinguished with certainty on clinical grounds and a CT brain scan should always be performed before commencing anticoagulation.

Antiarrhythmics

After anticoagulation, restoration of sinus rhythm should be the primary target in those with atrial fibrillation. Pharmacological cardioversion is preferable to DC cardioversion in the short term, because of the risks of a general anaesthetic in the context of a recent stroke. Sotalol or amiodarone are the drugs of choice. (See Section 2.2.2, p. 59.)

Surgical correction of cause

Repair of an aortic dissection, replacement of an infected valve or removal of an atrial myxoma may be necessary immediately. There is increased risk of further cerebral insult when the patient goes on cardiac bypass, but this has to be balanced against the potential risk of not treating the underlying condition. In those with valvular pathology, it is usual to allow time for the patient to make as complete a recovery as possible from the stroke before considering surgery.

See *Medicine for the elderly*, Section 1.4.
See *Emergency medicine*, Section 1.25.
See *Neurology*, Sections 1.21 and 2.8.1.
See *Haematology*, Section 3.6.
Barnett HJM, Eliasziw M, Meldrum HE. Prevention of ischaemic stroke. *Br Med J* 1999; 318: 1539–1543.
Zipes DP. Specific arrhythmias: diagnosis and treatment. In: Braunwald E (ed.) *Heart Disease: A textbook of cardiovascular medicine*, 5th edn. Philadelphia, PA: WB Saunders Co., 1997: 654–656.

1.5 Acute central chest pain

Case history

A 52-year-old lorry driver presents with a tight, aching, central chest pain. This came on while loading his lorry with heavy boxes.

Clinical approach

If the patient is still in pain then your first concern is to decide whether or not he is having an MI. Your initial history must be brief and should be combined with an ECG because timely treatment with aspirin and thrombolytic therapy may be life saving (see Section 2.1.3, p. 55). Dissection of the thoracic aorta is much less common, but should be considered at an early stage because it can be fatal and is potentially remediable, and also because thrombolysis is contraindicated!

The differential diagnosis of central chest pain is set out in Table 3. The brief history given suggests that the pain is not pleuritic, but it is important to confirm this because the differential diagnosis of pleuritic pain is different. (See Section 1.9, p. 28.)

If a firm diagnosis cannot be established on the basis of history, examination and immediately available tests, you should assume that the patient has cardiac ischaemia. The emphasis then switches to assessing the patient's risk of death or MI in the ensuing hours or days.

Table 3 Differential diagnosis of central chest pain.

Common cardiac	Myocardial infarction
	Unstable angina
Common non-cardiac	Oesophagitis
	Musculoskeletal
Must consider	Thoracic aortic dissection
Less common	Pericarditis
	Coronary vasospasm

History of the presenting problem

If the patient is still in pain, you must record an ECG as soon as practicable, not after you have finished the history and examination.

Is the pain the result of cardiac ischaemia?

When, where and how?

This man's pain came on when he was loading heavy boxes on to his lorry, but enquire about the following details if they do not emerge spontaneously in the account of any patient presenting with central chest pain:
- When did it come on?
- What were you doing at the time?
- Where did the pain start? (Ask the patient to indicate where in the chest)
- How did it start? Suddenly (in an instant) or gradually?
- Did it go anywhere else?
  Ischaemic cardiac pain:
- is typically brought on by exercise or emotion, but unstable angina and MI may start at rest or even during sleep
- tends to be felt in the middle of the chest
- does not come on suddenly, but usually builds up over a few minutes
- characteristically radiates to the neck, jaw or left arm.

What?

Ask for a specific description of the character of the pain. Patients sometimes have difficulty finding appropriate adjectives; you may have to make a few suggestions, e.g. aching, burning, stabbing, crushing, sharp, squeezing, tearing, throbbing, tight—but be careful to give enough options so as not to make your suggestions obviously leading. How bad was the pain? Ask the patient to rank it on a scale of 1–10, 10 being the worst pain that they could imagine. In patients with a clear previous history of stable angina, always ask whether the current pain at rest resembles their usual exertional pain.

Ischaemic cardiac pain is typically crushing, squeezing or tight.

Did you notice anything else with the pain?

Are there features that are commonly associated with MI?:
- Did you sweat?
- Were you nauseous? And did you vomit ?
- Did you think you were going to die?

How long did the pain last?

Ischaemic cardiac pain is not fleeting in nature (i.e. a few seconds only), nor does it persist constantly for several days.

Can you make an alternative diagnosis?

Make sure that you consider the options discussed below.

Could the pain be the result of aortic dissection?

If it came on suddenly, is described as 'tearing' or radiates to the back, you must look particularly carefully for evidence of aortic dissection.

Could the pain be caused by oesophagitis, which can be precipitated by bending and lifting?

Ask about belching and reflux, history of indigestion, use of remedies for indigestion or a history of previous investigation for indigestion ('You've never had a barium meal or an endoscopy, have you?'). (See *Gastroenterology*, Section 1.2.)

Could the pain be musculoskeletal?

Unaccustomed physical activity can provoke both ischaemic cardiac pain and musculoskeletal pain. Musculoskeletal pain tends to be less severe and of different character, and can usually be made better or worse by change in position; this is not a feature of ischaemic cardiac pain.

Could the pain result from pericarditis?

Most unlikely in this case—usually a concern in younger patients at low risk of coronary disease, when the most common cause is viral: 'Have you had 'flu or anything like that recently?' The pain often has a superficial quality and may be affected by position, typically improving when the patient leans forward. (See Section 1.14, p. 42.)

Could the chest pain result from anxiety?

Tingling fingers in association with chest pain suggests hyperventilation, but never jump immediately to the diagnosis of 'anxiety'—severe pain (e.g. cardiac ischaemia) may have produced the hyperventilation.

Relevant past history

This provides essential information to judge whether the patient's chest pain is likely to be caused by IHD or, in the jargon, 'to risk stratify the patient'. To put it simply, a young woman with no cardiac risk factors is exceedingly unlikely to have IHD, even if she gives a 'classic' history of angina, whereas it is almost inconceivable that a middle-aged or elderly man who smokes and gives the same history does not have IHD. Focus on the points discussed below.

Previous cardiac events

Ask the patient specifically about the following:
- Angina (stable or unstable)
- MI
- Cardiac catheterization
- Revascularization procedures (percutaneous transluminal coronary angioplasty [PTCA] or coronary arterial bypass grafting [CABG]).

Previous vascular events (non-cardiac)

Ask the patient about a history of the following:
- Stroke/transient ischaemic attack (TIA)
- Peripheral vascular disease.

Risk factors

It is essential to elicit a history of the following:
- Family history
- Smoking
- Hypertension
- Hypercholesterolaemia
- Diabetes.

 Oesophageal pain is often indistinguishable from ischaemic cardiac pain. Both may occur at rest, both may be severe and both are common. Cardiac pain may be associated with, and even relieved by, belching. Beware of discharging a high-risk patient with a clinical diagnosis of oesophageal pain.

Examination

Is the patient well, ill, very ill or nearly dead? Patients having an MI rarely look well; if they look nearly dead, call for intensive care unit (ICU) help immediately! All patients complaining of chest pain need prompt, rapid assessment.

Cardiovascular

Cardiovascular examination in patients presenting with acute central chest pain is frequently normal, which is probably why it is often performed in a cursory manner. Check: peripheral perfusion; pulse rate, rhythm and character; blood pressure; JVP; apex beat; for palpable heaves or thrills; heart sounds and murmurs; lung bases; peripheral pulses; and for ankle swelling. Do not forget key signs that are often missed, including the following:
• Unequal radial pulses and unequal blood pressures in the two arms (?aortic dissection)
• Early diastolic murmur of aortic regurgitation (?aortic dissection)
• Harsh ejection systolic murmur of aortic stenosis
• Pericardial rub.

Abdominal

Do not forget to palpate the epigastrium: is this tender? Is there guarding? Patients with an intra-abdominal catastrophe, e.g. perforated peptic ulcer or pancreatitis, can present with pain in the lower chest and signs of circulatory collapse, making it look very much as though they are having an MI.

Musculoskeletal

If the pain is worse on moving and reproduced by chest wall compression, a musculoskeletal cause is likely.

Approach to investigations and management

 A patient with previously stable angina who presents with increasing frequency and severity of chest pains over a few days ('crescendo angina') is very likely to have an unstable coronary plaque and should be admitted for treatment and further assessment, even if pain free at the time of consultation.

If the patient is hypotensive with poor peripheral perfusion, then proceed as described in *Emergency medicine*, Section 1.2; if not, then proceed to establish a diagnosis as follows.

Investigations

The key investigations are those that will indicate whether or not the patient is suffering from an acute coronary syndrome, i.e. the ECG and biochemical markers of heart muscle damage.

ECG

Look for specific abnormalities:
• ST-segment elevation/left bundle-branch block (LBBB) (MI) (Fig. 11)
• ST-segment depression (unstable angina) (Fig. 12)
• T-wave inversion (may be MI/unstable angina)
• ST-segment elevation concave upwards (pericarditis).

 An entirely normal ECG is associated with relatively low risk but does not rule out serious coronary disease or the presence of unstable angina.

 A patient presenting with a normal ECG, who has had normal coronary angiography within the preceding 5 years, is unlikely to be suffering from an acute coronary syndrome, but this cannot be completely excluded.

Biochemical markers of heart muscle damage

Creatine kinase (CK) and its more specific cardiac isoform, CK-MB, have been used to diagnose MI retrospectively in those with a 'non-diagnostic' ECG. Troponins are more specific and sensitive markers of heart muscle damage and are superseding CK. (See Section 3.7, p. 135.)

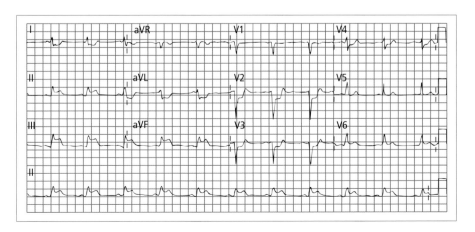

Fig. 11 Acute inferior myocardial infarction. The ECG shows ST segment deviation in the inferior leads (II, III and AVF). ST segment depression in leads V2 and V3 may indicate posterior extension.

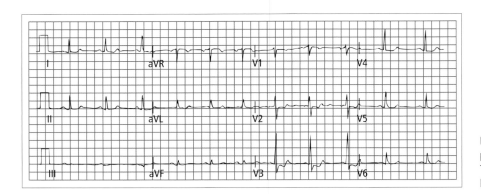

Fig. 12 ECG showing ST depression in a patient presenting with acute chest pain. Thrombolysis is not beneficial, and may be harmful in these circumstances.

Other blood tests

Check FBC, cholesterol, electrolytes, renal and liver function tests. In some cases where there is diagnostic doubt, it will be appropriate to measure the serum amylase.

Chest radiograph

Look for cardiomegaly, pulmonary oedema and mediastinal widening (aortic dissection).

 Consider thoracic aortic dissection (see Section 2.11.1, p. 99) if there is the following:
- History of sudden onset, 'tearing' central chest pain, radiating to the back
- History of hypertension
- Patient looks 'marfanoid'
- Inferior infarction on ECG (dissection extended to right coronary artery)
- Mediastinal widening on chest radiograph.

Management

Give oxygen, analgesia (opiate if necessary) and aspirin 300 mg while the diagnosis is being established. Further treatment depends on the underlying cause:
- MI: see Section 2.1.3, p. 55
- Unstable angina: see Section 2.1.2, p. 53
- Oesophagitis: see *Gastroenterology*, Section 2.2
- Suspected aortic dissection: see Section 2.11.1, p. 99
- Pericarditis: see Section 2.6.1, p. 78
- Coronary vasospasm: treat with high doses of calcium antagonist; avoid β blockers which may exacerbate vasospasm.

Persisting pain of uncertain cause

Reassure the patient that there is no evidence for heart attack at present, but admit for overnight observation and repeat ECG/cardiac markers at 12–24 h.

Pain gone, diagnosis uncertain

Most patients require overnight admission. However, a negative troponin test in conjunction with favourable clinical and ECG criteria is increasingly being used to identify low-risk patients who may be discharged early without the need for overnight stay. However, it is important to realize that a negative troponin test does not rule out coronary disease. Patients discharged early in these circumstances must have more detailed risk assessment within the next few weeks, which should include an exercise test (see Section 3.1.1, p. 124). Patients should be invited to seek medical help again if their symptoms return.

 In difficult cases, consider coronary vasospasm:
- Multiple admissions
- Negative coronary angiogram ('minor irregularities')
- Paroxysms of crushing central chest pain at rest
- Relieved by glyceryl trinitrate (GTN)
- No limitation of exercise
- Pain often associated with profuse sweating, occasionally with syncope
- Usually benign, but patients with significant ECG changes or ventricular arrhythmia during pain must be admitted for urgent treatment and investigation (Fig. 13).

 See *Emergency medicine*, Sections 1.1, 1.2 and 1.3.
See *Gastroenterology*, Section 1.2.
Braunwald E. The history. In: Braunwald E (ed.) *Heart Disease*. Philadelphia, PA: WB Saunders Co., 1996: 3–7.
Crea F, Kaski JC, Maseri A. Key references on coronary artery spasm. *Circulation* 1994; 89: 2442–2446.
Goldman L, Cook EF, Johnson PA *et al*. Prediction of the need for intensive care in patients coming to the emergency department with acute chest pain. *N Engl J Med* 1996; 334: 1498–1504.
Hamm CW, Goldman BU, Heeschen C *et al*. Emergency room triage of patients with acute chest pain by means of rapid testing for cardiac troponin T or troponin I. *N Engl J Med* 1997; 337: 1648–1653.
Hillis SG, Fox KAA. Cardiac troponins in chest pain. *BMJ* 1999; 319: 1451–1452.

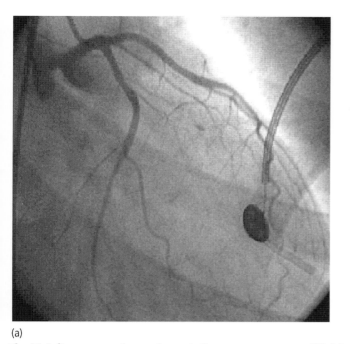

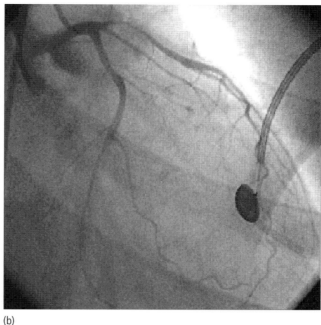

(a)

(b)

Fig. 13 Left coronary angiogram demonstrating coronary vasospasm. This 34-year-old woman presented with chest pain and anterior ST segment elevation on the ECG. Shortly afterwards, she had a VF arrest. After resuscitation, the ECG returned to normal. (a) Initial angiography showed a normal left coronary artery. (b) Intracoronary ergometrine induced localized spasm of the proximal left anterior descending coronary artery, and reproduced the chest pain with ECG changes.

1.6 Breathlessness and ankle swelling

Case history

A 48-year-old professor of mathematics presents with a 6-week history of progressive breathlessness and bilateral ankle swelling.

Clinical approach

These symptoms are most commonly caused by cardiac or pulmonary disease. The cause usually becomes apparent early in the history, and subsequent questions, examination and investigation should be directed to providing confirmatory details. The common differential diagnoses are given in Table 4.

History of the presenting problem

If the following do not emerge spontaneously, make specific enquiry about them:
- Chest pain: if present, does this sound like ischaemic cardiac pain or like pleurisy?
- Cough/sputum, and has there been haemoptysis?
- Wheeze, but note that this is not synonymous with

Table 4 Differential diagnosis of ankle swelling and breathlessness.

Cardiac	Left ventricular dysfunction*
	Valvular heart disease*
	Pericardial effusion/constriction
	Cyanotic congenital heart disease
	High-output cardiac failure secondary to anaemia
Pulmonary	Chronic airway or parenchymal lung disease*
	Chronic, repeated pulmonary embolism
	Primary pulmonary hypertension
Gastrointestinal	Liver failure
	Protein-losing enteropathy
Renal	Nephrotic syndrome
	Chronic renal failure
Endocrine	Hypothyroidism

*Most common causes.

airway disease—it may occur in pulmonary oedema when it is known as 'cardiac asthma'.

Cardiac

Progressive breathlessness associated with orthopnoea, paroxysmal nocturnal dyspnoea and cough productive of clear, frothy sputum would suggest a cardiac cause. The ankle swelling in cardiac failure is usually bilateral and symmetrical, but it is not uncommon for one ankle to swell initially. A preceding episode of severe central chest pain at rest, particularly if occurring against a background of stable angina, would suggest a precipitating MI—the 'really bad episode of indigestion' may have been something different.

Pulmonary

The development of increasing breathlessness and ankle swelling may indicate the development of cor pulmonale in a man with long-standing respiratory disorder. His symptoms are said to have started only 6 weeks ago, but what was he like before then? What is the most vigorous exercise he ever took? Three months ago was his breathing more laboured than that of his wife, family or friends?

Pulmonary embolism

Stepwise progression (sudden deterioration followed by periods of stability) should raise the suspicion of multiple recurrent pulmonary emboli, even in the absence of pleuritic chest pain or haemoptysis.

Relevant past history

Ask about the following:
- Is there anything at all to suggest IHD: heart attack, angina, chest tightness on exercise that may not have been recognized as significant?
- Rheumatic fever or cardiac murmur
- Recurrent asthma/bronchitis or any other respiratory problem
- Smoking, which is obviously a substantial risk factor for both chronic airway disease and IHD
- Alcohol intake
- Thromboembolism.

Examination

A full examination is required, but pay particular attention to the cardiac and respiratory systems. Do not finish your examination until you are absolutely sure where the JVP is.

General

Look for cyanosis, anaemia or stigmata of chronic liver disease.

Cardiac

Look for signs of cardiac dysfunction, check:
- Pulse rate, rhythm, volume and character: a sinus tachycardia may be caused by anxiety or cardiac failure;

consider specifically 'is this man in atrial fibrillation?'. A low-volume pulse might indicate cardiac failure, but is there anything about the character to suggest either aortic stenosis or incompetence?
- Blood pressure, including pulsus paradoxus, which suggests pericardial effusion/tamponade (see Section 2.6.2, p. 80).
- JVP—is this raised?
- Apex beat—is this displaced?
- Is there an S3 gallop?
- Are there murmurs (especially diastolic)?
- Are there basal crepitations? But remember that these are not specific for pulmonary oedema and cardiac failure.

Look for signs of pulmonary hypertension, which is indicated by the following:
- Raised JVP
- Left parasternal heave (palpable right ventricle)
- Loud pulmonary component of the second heart sound.

Also note whether one leg is much more swollen than the other, which might indicate deep venous thrombosis.

Respiratory

Check the shape and expansion of the chest: does this suggest chronic airways disease? Are there any abnormal chest signs (other than basal crepitations)? If there are, a respiratory cause of breathlessness and oedema is likely. Check the peak flow. (See *Respiratory medicine*, Section 1.1.)

 Oedema of the hands and face is a feature of hypoalbuminaemia, and is very rarely the result of congestive cardiac failure (Fig. 14).

Approach to investigations and management

Investigations

These will focus on the heart and lungs. Initial investigations should include an ECG, chest radiograph, urine stick tests for protein and 'screening' blood tests.

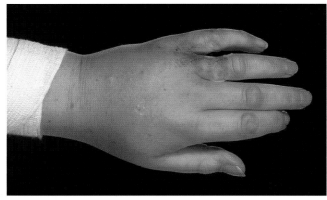

Fig. 14 Hand oedema in a patient with hypoalbuminaemia.

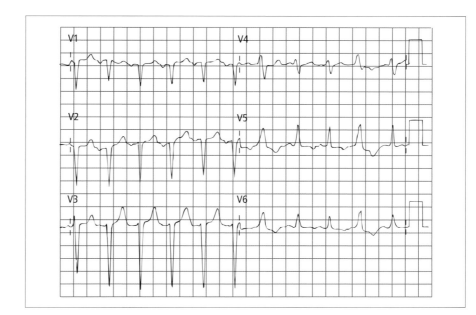

Fig. 15 ECG showing left atrial strain (inverted P wave in V1) and partial left bundle-branch block in a patient with severe congestive cardiac failure secondary to alcoholic cardiomyopathy.

ECG

Look for the following:
• Previous MI, LBBB or poor R-wave progression indicating left ventricular disease.
• A dominantly negative P wave in lead V1, reflecting left atrial hypertrophy—an indirect sign of left heart dysfunction (Fig. 15).
• Right ventricular hypertrophy (right bundle-branch block [RBBB] with dominant R waves in V1) secondary to any cause of pulmonary hypertension.
• Low voltages and electrical alternans, which occur with a large pericardial effusion.
• Atrial arrhythmias: common in both cardiac and pulmonary disease.

Chest radiograph

In the context of an elevated JVP:
• A large heart should prompt echocardiography (Fig. 16).
• Are there signs of pulmonary oedema?
• If the heart size is normal, inspect the lung fields closely for evidence of chronic obstructive airway disease or parenchymal lung disease.
• If the heart size and lung fields are both normal, consider pulmonary embolism or pericardial constriction.

Blood tests

Check the FBC, electrolytes, and renal, liver and thyroid function tests.

Urinalysis

Do not forget this simple test. If there is significant

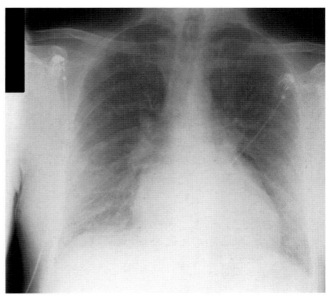

Fig. 16 Chest radiograph showing cardiomegaly and pulmonary oedema in a patient with congestive cardiac failure caused by severe mitral regurgitation. Note cardiomegaly and enlarged left atrium.

proteinuria on dipstick testing (≥2+), the nephrotic syndrome is possible. Check serum albumin and 24-h urinary protein excretion. Remember that proteinuria of up to 1 g/day can be caused by severe cardiac failure.

If the history, examination and tests described above suggest a cardiac cause for breathlessness and oedema, the following cardiac investigations may be needed to make a precise diagnosis.

Echocardiogram

Echocardiography is most useful for ruling out significant valvular or left ventricular disease. Pericardial effusion is commonly found, but careful clinical and echocardiographic assessment is required to judge whether this is contributing to symptoms (see Section 2.6.2, p. 80). Assessment of right heart function is largely subjective, but reasonably accurate indirect measurements of pulmonary artery systolic pressure can be obtained. Echocardiography may suggest pericardial constriction or restrictive cardiomyopathy, which requires cardiac catheterization for confirmation. (See Sections 2.4.3, p. 70 and 2.6.3, p. 82.)

Cardiac catheterization

Right heart catheterization is the most accurate way to measure pulmonary artery pressures. It is useful for detection and quantification of an intracardiac shunt, e.g. atrial septal defect (ASD). It can confirm pericardial constriction and help distinguish it from restrictive cardiomyopathy (see Section 2.4.3, p. 70). It also allows pulmonary angiography if pulmonary embolism is suspected.

Left heart catheterization allows coronary angiography and assessment of valvular dysfunction.

CT of the chest

Spiral CT has a high sensitivity for the detection of pulmonary embolism. It is preferred to ventilation–perfusion scanning if the lung fields are abnormal on a chest radiograph (see Section 2.18, p. 115). It may be helpful in suspected pericardial constriction. (See Section 2.6.3, p. 82.)

- The presence of bilateral basal crackles on auscultation of the chest has a very poor positive predictive value for the presence of pulmonary oedema—a chest radiograph is much more accurate.
- Beware that marked abnormality of renal and liver function tests commonly occurs in congestive cardiac failure, and does not necessarily indicate primary disease in these organs.
- The severity of left ventricular dysfunction on echocardiography correlates poorly with severity of the clinical syndrome of heart failure. However, normal systolic left ventricular function on echocardiography should prompt review of a diagnosis of heart failure.

When the cause of breathlessness is not obvious, consider chronic repeated pulmonary thromboembolism.

This is a commonly missed diagnosis. Multiple small pulmonary emboli lead to progressive occlusion of the pulmonary arteriolar bed, classically presenting with breathlessness that becomes more severe in a stepwise manner. Pulmonary hypertension eventually leads to right ventricular failure and ankle swelling. Prominent pulmonary arteries may be the only finding on a chest radiograph. Diagnosis is made by ventilation–perfusion scan or spiral CT.

Consider primary pulmonary hypertension, particularly in young women with unexplained breathlessness.

This is a rare condition that predominantly affects young women. Although usually idiopathic, there is a link with appetite-suppressant drugs. It presents with progressive breathlessness and fatigue, and is commonly misdiagnosed as asthma. Exertional chest pain ('right ventricular angina') is sometimes a feature. In the later stages, the condition is complicated by peripheral oedema resulting from right heart failure. Diagnosis is by exclusion of recognized causes of pulmonary hypertension, and requires cardiac catheterization. (See Sections 1.10, p. 30, and 2.12.1, p. 101.)

Management

Where breathlessness and oedema are caused by cardiac dysfunction, loop diuretics are central to the relief of symptoms in most cases. Give intravenously if symptoms are severe, but be aware that aggressive diuresis may precipitate circulatory collapse in those who require a high filling pressure, e.g. chronic pulmonary thromboembolism, cor pulmonale, pericardial disease, cyanotic congenital heart disease.

Further management depends on the underlying cause:
- Left ventricular dysfunction: see Section 2.3, p. 63
- Valvular heart disease: see Section 2.5, p. 71
- Pericardial effusion/constriction: see Section 2.6, p. 78
- Cyanotic congenital heart disease: see Section 2.7, p. 84
- Chronic lung disease: see *Respiratory medicine*, Sections 2.3 and 2.11
- Chronic, repeated pulmonary embolism: see Section 2.18, p. 115
- Primary pulmonary hypertension: see Section 2.12.1, p. 101
- Chronic liver disease: see *Gastroenterology*, Section 2.10
- Nephrotic syndrome: see *Nephrology*, Section 2.1.4
- Chronic renal failure: see *Nephrology*, Section 2.1.2.

It is always worth checking that patients with oedema are aware of the need to avoid adding salt to their food. If salt is essential then modest amounts of 'Lo-Salt' (KCl) are better than NaCl. Also check what food they are eating—you would be surprised how many people with oedema insist that they 'do not add any salt to their food', but eat crisps, salted peanuts or tinned soup containing large amounts of it.

See *Emergency medicine*, Section 1.5.

Cohn JN. Drug therapy: the management of chronic heart failure. *N Engl J Med* 1996; 335: 490–498. Review article.

Gaine SP, Rubin LJ. Primary pulmonary hypertension. *Lancet* 1998; 352: 719–725. Review article.

Goldhaber SZ. Pulmonary embolism. *N Engl J Med* 1998; 339: 93–104. Review article.

Watson RDS, Gibbs CR, Lip GYH. ABC of heart failure: clinical features and complications. *BMJ* 2000; 320: 236–239. Review article.

1.7 Hypotension following myocardial infarction

Case history

A 59-year-old man was admitted with an inferior MI for which he was treated with aspirin and thrombolysis. Three hours after admission his condition was judged stable enough to give atenolol. The following morning he was reviewed by a consultant cardiologist on the post-take round, and was felt to have had an uncomplicated course. A CK of 3651 IU/mL was noted, and an ACE inhibitor was recommended. Before this drug could be given, the senior house officer (SHO) was asked to see the patient urgently because he had become drowsy with a systolic blood pressure of 60 mmHg.

Clinical approach

The cause of profound hypotension after MI can usually be established by examining the patient, obtaining an ECG and chest radiograph, and scrutinizing the drug chart. Consider the diagnoses listed in Table 5.

History of presenting problem

Pay particular attention to the following:
- Chest pain: recurrent pain may indicate reinfarction or cardiac rupture.
- Onset: a period of stability followed by an abrupt drop in blood pressure indicates a catastrophic event, but

Table 5 Differential diagnosis of hypotension after myocardial infarction.

Drug induced	Streptokinase infusion
	Intravenous nitrate
	β Blocker
	Angiotensin-converting enzyme inhibitor
Cardiac	Bradyarrhythmia
	Tachyarrhythmia
	Acute left ventricular dysfunction (including reinfarction)
	Acute right ventricular dysfunction (right ventricular infarct)
	Acute mitral regurgitation
	Ventricular septal defect (VSD secondary to septal rupture)
	Cardiac rupture with tamponade
	Aortic dissection
Other (less likely)	Dehydration
	Haemorrhage
	Pulmonary embolus
	Sepsis

hypotension resulting from left ventricular pump failure tends to be more insidious.
- Drugs: look for a temporal relationship of hypotension to administration of drugs—hypotension during infusion of streptokinase is common and usually occurs during the first 20 min.
- Breathlessness: acute breathlessness associated with hypotension may indicate pulmonary oedema.
- Volume depletion: may rarely be caused after MI by vomiting without adequate fluid replacement. This is unlikely to be the explanation, but examine the fluid balance charts.

Examination

General

Assess the general clinical condition of the patient:
- If the patient looks as though he or she is about to arrest, call for resuscitation team help immediately. Do not wait until you are sure that the heart has stopped.
- Conscious level: check the Glasgow Coma Score.
- Pain level.

Cardiovascular

Pay specific attention to the following:
- Peripheral circulation: it is a poor prognostic sign if the patient is shut down—how far up the arms and legs are they cold?
- Heart rate and rhythm
- Blood pressure: measure this yourself. Can you feel the pulse and measure the blood pressure in the left arm? Could the patient have had a dissection, presenting with inferior MI and now progressing?
- JVP: if markedly elevated consider right ventricular infarction, ventricular septal defect (VSD), tamponade or pulmonary embolism.
- S3 gallop.
- New pansystolic murmur: which would suggest VSD or mitral regurgitation, perhaps as a result of chordal or papillary muscle rupture.

Approach to investigations and management

Investigations

The diagnosis should become apparent with the following basic investigations:
- ECG: arrhythmia or reinfarction?
- Chest radiograph: do not assume there is no pulmonary oedema unless you have seen a recent chest radiograph.

• Arterial blood gases: will document hypoxia, which is likely to be the result of pulmonary oedema, but in the presence of a normal chest radiograph would suggest pulmonary embolus.
• Echocardiogram: provides rapid information about left (and to a lesser extent right) ventricular function. Also useful in detection of tamponade, acute mitral regurgitation and VSD.
• Urea and electrolytes to establish renal function.
• Cardiac enzymes: has there been reinfarction?

Differential diagnosis

Consider the diagnoses listed in Table 5—look particularly for evidence of the following:

Acute mitral regurgitation

• Inferior infarction
• Severe pulmonary oedema
• Murmur may not be present as a result of rapid equalization of left ventricular and left atrial pressures
• Echocardiography is diagnostic (Fig. 17).

Acquired ventricular septal defect

• Very high JVP
• Less severe pulmonary oedema than acute mitral regurgitation
• New systolic murmur
• Usually picked up by echocardiography
• Consider a Swan–Ganz pulmonary artery catheter— this will demonstrate a 'step up' in oxygen saturation at the level of the right ventricle, indicating left-to-right shunting.

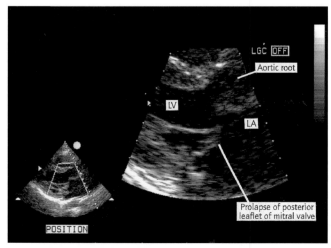

Fig. 17 Transoesophageal echocardiogram showing prolapse of the posterior mitral valve leaflet (indicated) into the left atrium (LA) after papillary muscle rupture. LV, left ventricle.

Ischaemic left ventricular dysfunction

• Severe coronary disease (especially critical left main-stem stenosis)
• Recurrent chest pain accompanied by transient hypotension, pulmonary oedema and widespread ischaemia/ acute infarction on the ECG
• Patients are at high risk of death: refer for cardiac catheterization and appropriate revascularization.

Right ventricular infarction

• Inferior infarction
• Hypotensive patient with high JVP
• Clear lung fields on chest radiograph.

Management

Hypotension after an MI should always be taken seriously and treated quickly, even if the patient appears not to be *in extremis*. Monitor heart rhythm, blood pressure, pulse oximetry, hourly urine output, fluid balance, daily electrolytes and renal function. Then:
• Stop drugs that may contribute to hypotension
• Give high-flow oxygen
• If possible, identify and treat the underlying cause: acute mitral regurgitation and VSD are indications for urgent referral to a cardiothoracic surgeon.

Does the patient require fluid or inotropes? It is often difficult to know. The obvious risk is that fluid could precipitate pulmonary oedema, and monitoring of the pulmonary capillary wedge pressure (PCWP) with a Swan–Ganz catheter is very helpful in this context. As a general rule:
• If the lungs are reasonably clear, the patient is not profoundly hypoxic, and hypotension is the main problem, then give intravenously 250 mL 0.9% saline and reassess, repeating if necessary. This will help those with right ventricular infarction because increasing the preload will increase right ventricular output (See *Physiology*, Section 1.2). Consider inotropes, e.g. dobutamine, epinephrine (adrenaline).
• If there are lots of crackles in the lungs and the patient is hypoxic as well as hypotensive, a bolus of saline will not help and could be fatal. Start inotropes, e.g. dobutamine, epinephrine (adrenaline). Call for ICU help—the patient is likely to die soon if not ventilated electively.

 In a patient who has become breathless and hypotensive with pulmonary oedema on the chest radiograph, inotropic agents may be started without the insertion of a Swan–Ganz catheter because the left atrial filling pressure is almost certainly high. PCWP measurement becomes useful if the clinical situation has not become satisfactory over the next 12–24 h.

Communication

The prognosis of profound hypotension after MI is very poor. You, or one of your colleagues, may have talked to the patient's next of kin when he or she was first admitted and warned of the gravity of the diagnosis. They certainly need to be spoken to now. If they are not present, phone them as soon as management is under way to see if they wish to come up to the hospital. Take your time, speak slowly and do not be afraid of silence or tears:

- 'This is Dr Brown from the hospital . . .'
- 'We promised that we would call if there was any change in the situation . . .' (warning that you are about to give bad news)
- 'I'm calling to say that I'm afraid that your husband has taken a turn for the worse . . .'
- 'His blood pressure has fallen . . .'
- 'We're doing some tests to find out why, and have started to give him some treatment to help the heart, but the situation is serious . . .' (The wife may say 'is he going to die?')
- 'His heart is under a lot of strain; we're doing everything we can; but I don't know whether he is going to pull through . . .' (The wife may say 'how long?')
- 'We have to take things as they come, an hour at a time.'

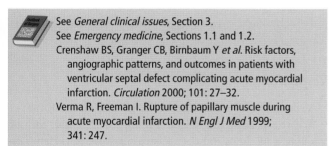

See *General clinical issues*, Section 3.
See *Emergency medicine*, Sections 1.1 and 1.2.
Crenshaw BS, Granger CB, Birnbaum Y *et al*. Risk factors, angiographic patterns, and outcomes in patients with ventricular septal defect complicating acute myocardial infarction. *Circulation* 2000; 101: 27–32.
Verma R, Freeman I. Rupture of papillary muscle during acute myocardial infarction. *N Engl J Med* 1999; 341: 247.

1.8 Breathlessness and haemodynamic collapse

Case history

You are bleeped urgently by A&E to see a 55-year-old woman brought in by ambulance. Her husband called 999 this morning when he found her acutely breathless at home. She had a brief syncopal episode on being moved into the ambulance, but is now conscious, although extremely dyspnoeic, and her blood pressure is only 80 mmHg systolic.

Clinical approach

The following are the priorities:
- Resuscitate (**a**irway, **b**reathing, **c**irculation) and secure venous access while taking the history
- Give high-flow oxygen
- Examine with a clear idea of possible causes of breathlessness and haemodynamic collapse in mind (Table 6)
- Exclude tension pneumothorax—insert a large bore cannula into the silent side of the chest (second intercostal space, midclavicular line) if this is the clinical diagnosis
- Exclude other diagnoses that can be established quickly: arrhythmia, acute MI with definitive ECG changes.

History of presenting problem

If you can obtain a history from the patient and/or her husband, ask particularly about the following:
- Sudden or gradual onset: sudden onset suggests pneumothorax, massive pulmonary embolus (PE), acute valve dysfunction, dissection or arrhythmia
- Central chest or interscapular pain: suggesting MI or aortic dissection
- Pleuritic chest pain or haemoptysis: suggesting smaller PEs preceding a larger one

Table 6 Differential diagnosis of acute dyspnoea and haemodynamic collapse. Note that, although tension pneumothorax is uncommon, this diagnosis should be considered before all others.

General cause	Comment	Specific cause
Cardiac	Common	Myocardial infarction/complications (acute mitral regurgitation, VSD, acute left ventricular failure)
		Arrhythmia (VT)
	Less common	Aortic dissection
		Cardiac tamponade
		Acute aortic regurgitation
Cardiorespiratory	Common	Massive PE (occluding >50% pulmonary vasculature)
Respiratory	Common	Acute life-threatening asthma
	Less common	Tension pneumothorax
Other	Common	Sepsis
	Less common	Intra-abdominal catastrophe
		Severe haemorrhage ('air hunger')
		Anaphylaxis

PE, pulmonary embolism; VSD, ventricular septal defect; VT, ventricular tachycardia.

- Symptoms suggestive of pulmonary oedema: orthopnoea, paroxysmal nocturnal dyspnoea (PND), pink frothy sputum
- Worsening asthma
- Abdominal pain, vomiting, haematemesis, melaena: could there have been an intra-abdominal catastrophe?
- Symptoms suggestive of sepsis: the most common infective cause of hypotension and breathlessness would be septicaemia and acute respiratory distress syndrome (ARDS), but with 'flu-like illness also consider pericardial effusion with sudden decompensation
- Exposure to a known allergen.

Relevant past history

There is not time for a lengthy history, but ask about the following:
- Pulmonary embolism or deep venous thrombosis and relevant risk factors (see Section 2.18, p. 115)
- Cardiac: MI, angina, previously undiagnosed anginal pain, valve disease, rheumatic fever, 'heart murmur' (and if so any recent dental work or surgery—could she have acute valve dysfunction caused by infective endocarditis); hypertension (risk factor for IHD and aortic dissection)
- Respiratory: asthma, chronic airflow obstruction, pneumothorax
- Abdominal: peptic ulcers, pancreatitis, gallstones
- Anaphylaxis: allergy to anything?
- Drugs: a useful rapid marker for past medical history in this context!

 If no history is available, check bags and pockets for inhalers, GTN, etc.

Examination

 This woman will look very ill or nearly dead; if nearly dead, call for ICU help or the cardiac resuscitation team immediately. Do not wait until she has a cardiac arrest if she looks as though she is deteriorating.

Immediate assessment

- Vital signs: pulse (rate and rhythm), blood pressure, respiratory rate, temperature.
- Is there cyanosis? Check pulse oximetry (but do not remove the high-flow oxygen to 'check value on air' in someone who is desperately ill!).
- Conscious level: the Glasgow Coma Score.
- Is there swelling of the lips and tongue (anaphylaxis)?

Is this a tension pneumothorax?

- Chest looks asymmetrical, with side under tension 'blown up'.

- Tracheal deviation away from the side under tension.
- Mediastinal shift: apex beat not in the normal place; cardiac dullness moved to left or right away from the side under tension.
- Side of chest under tension is silent.

Cardiovascular

- Is there paradox? If the pulse becomes impalpable on inspiration, this could be severe asthma or cardiac tamponade.
- Can you feel the left radial pulse? Is the blood pressure the same in the left arm as the right? Could this be an aortic dissection?
- Where is the JVP? This is a critical piece of information: if high, this suggests that the cause of hypotension and breathlessness is cardiac or respiratory; if low, then go for bleeding, intra-abdominal catastrophe or sepsis.
- Are there features to suggest massive pulmonary embolism? High JVP, right ventricular heave, tricuspid regurgitation.
- Could there be acute mitral regurgitation or an acute VSD? Listen for a pansystolic murmur (see Section 1.7, p. 23 for further information). Note that acute aortic regurgitation might not produce an audible early diastolic murmur.
- Can you hear the heart sounds and is there a pericardial rub? Quiet sounds might indicate pericardial fluid and a rub would suggest pericarditis—both making tamponade a likely diagnosis in this context.

Respiratory

- A silent chest would suggest life-threatening asthma.
- Are there any other dramatic signs? A chest full of crackles is likely to indicate severe pulmonary oedema or aspiration. An area of bronchial breathing may indicate that pneumonia is the primary diagnosis.

Abdominal

- Is there tenderness, guarding or an abdominal aortic aneurysm?
- Is there melaena on rectal examination?

Legs

- Signs of a deep venous thrombosis are not necessary for a diagnosis of PE, but would strongly support the diagnosis.

Skin and nails

- Could those spots be meningococcal?
- Are those splinters endocarditic?

Approach to investigations and management

 Always remember that the history, examination, investigation and management should be in parallel, not in series, when dealing with patients who are severely ill.

Investigations

The following investigations are required immediately in all patients who present with severe hypotension and breathlessness.

Blood tests

Check BM stix immediately in anyone who is severely ill. Check arterial gases. Take samples for FBC, electrolytes, renal and liver function tests, cardiac enzymes and blood cultures.

ECG

Perform a 12-lead ECG immediately, and repeat after 1 h (sooner if clinically indicated), looking for the following:
• Arrhythmia (see Section 2.2, p. 58).
• Localized ST segment elevation of acute MI (see Section 2.1.3, p. 55).
• ECG changes compatible with acute PE, the most common being sinus tachycardia and T-wave inversion in leads V1–V4. The 'typical' right axis deviation and 'S1Q3T3' are actually quite unusual (see Section 2.18, p. 115).
• Generalized ST-segment elevation of pericarditis (much less common in this context) or low voltages/voltages of pericardial effusion (see Section 2.6, p. 78).

Chest radiograph

Look for pneumothorax, pulmonary oligaemia (PE), pulmonary oedema, consolidation, effusions, heart size, mediastinal shift and the widened mediastinum of aortic dissection.

 A normal mediastinal width on the chest radiograph does not exclude aortic dissection.

Further investigations may be indicated depending on clinical findings and the results of immediate tests.

Echocardiogram

An echocardiogram is the examination of choice to look for effusion, valve regurgitation and VSD, and to assess ventricular function. Remember that right ventricular dysfunction in the context of acute severe dyspnoea and hypoxia is highly suspicious of a massive PE.

Other investigations

Discuss with a senior colleague whether further imaging is required to establish the diagnosis: tests that may be indicated for suspected PE include ventilation–perfusion ($\dot{V}/\dot{Q}$) scanning, contrast CT of the chest, pulmonary angiography and ultrasound of the leg veins. Check CT abdomen if your assessment suggests an abdominal cause.

Management

'General supportive measures' will be required by all patients:
• First priority is always **a**irway, **b**reathing, **c**irculation
• High-flow oxygen, with monitoring of arterial blood gases
• Rapid restoration of intravascular volume in those who are volume deplete (low JVP, postural hypotension— lying and sitting, as standing will clearly not be possible).

Specific management will depend on the diagnosis:
• Tension pneumothorax: immediate insertion of a wide-bore cannula into the pneumothorax will decompress it and relieve the life-threatening mediastinal shift. (See *Emergency medicine*, Section 1.1; *Respiratory medicine*, Sections 3.2 and 3.4.)
• PE: the two major treatment options for massive PE with haemodynamic collapse are thrombolysis and surgical embolectomy. (See Section 2.18, p. 115.)
• Arrhythmia: see Sections 1.1, p. 3, 1.2, p. 6, 1.3, p. 9 and 2.2, p. 58.
• Complications of MI: see Section 1.7, p. 23.
• Tamponade: urgent pericardiocentesis. (See Section 2.6.2, p. 80.)
• Asthma: see *Emergency medicine*, Section 1.7; *Respiratory medicine*, Section 2.2.2.
• Intra-abdominal catastrophe: call for surgical help immediately; resuscitate while considering surgery and in the anaesthetic room; do not say you will resuscitate and then call the surgeons.
• Anaphylaxis: see *Emergency medicine*, Section 1.29; *Rheumatology and clinical immunology*, Section 1.7.

And, if you do not know the diagnosis, give broad-spectrum antibiotics to cover sepsis. (See *Emergency medicine*, Section 1.28 and *Infectious diseases*, Section 1.2.)

Communication

After making your clinical assessment, performing immediate investigations and initiating management, you will need to speak to her husband to explain the situation. (See Section 1.7, p. 25, for guidance on how to do this.)

British Thoracic Society. Suspected acute pulmonary embolism: a practical approach. *Thorax* 1997; 52: S4.

1.9 Pleuritic pain

Case history

A 36-year-old male computer programmer presents with a 4-h history of moderately severe left-sided pleuritic chest pain. He was well until yesterday but became unusually breathless while cycling to work today.

Clinical approach

Pleuritic pain is the result of pleural irritation (e.g. by air) or inflammation, which may be caused by infarction (peripheral PE), infection (pneumonia) or as part of a systemic inflammatory disorder, e.g. autoimmune rheumatic disease.

The differential diagnosis of the patient presenting with pleuritic pain is shown in Table 7. The two most important acute diagnoses to consider in this case are pneumothorax and PE. Pneumothorax is easily confirmed or excluded on chest radiograph, but the diagnosis of PE may not be so straightforward.

- A low-grade fever (<38°C) does not necessarily indicate infection, it can be associated with inflammation of any cause, including pulmonary infarction
- Pneumonia may present in a variety of ways and sputum production is not generally an early feature
- Rib fracture tends to be associated with a clearly memorable episode of trauma and is therefore not usually a diagnostic difficulty, but remember the possibility of pathological fracture.

Table 7 Differential diagnosis of patient presenting with pleuritic chest pain.

Common causes	Pulmonary embolism
	Pneumothorax
	Pneumonia
	Musculoskeletal: rib fracture, costochondritis, Bornholm's myalgia (Coxsackie B virus, self-limiting), non-specific
Less common causes	Autoimmune rheumatic disease
	Pericarditis
	Neoplasia: primary or secondary
	Herpes zoster ('Shingles' difficult to diagnose before the rash)

History of presenting problem

Bear in mind the diagnoses listed in Table 7 when taking the history—which is most likely?

Description of the pain

Check the following:
- The pain is definitely pleuritic—sharp, localized and exacerbated by deep inspiration and coughing. If not you need to consider other causes of chest pain. (See Section 1.5, p. 15.) If it is exacerbated by movement and associated with tenderness, a musculoskeletal cause becomes more likely.
- Whether the onset of pain was sudden, associated with coughing or straining (pneumothorax, PE) or gradual. Did it follow a 'flu-like illness (pneumonia, Bornholm myalgia) or an incident of chest trauma (pneumothorax, rib fracture)?

Associated symptoms

Ask about the following:
- Dyspnoea: when did this occur in relation to the pain? How severe—'at rest'/'can't walk'/'can't hurry'?
- Cough: non-specific, but production of purulent sputum indicates likely infection and haemoptysis is a feature of PE, pneumonia and (exceedingly unlikely in this case) malignancy.
- Fever: sweats, rigors and temperature >38.5°C would suggest pneumonia.
- Unilateral leg pain, swelling or tenderness, all suggestive of venous thrombosis and strongly supporting the diagnosis of PE in this case.

Relevant risk factors

Pulmonary embolism

Ask about recent immobility/surgery/travel/dehydration, smoking and family history of PE, deep venous thrombosis or hypercoagulable states. In a woman, ask about pregnancy or use of the oral contraceptive/hormone replacement therapy (HRT).

Pneumothorax

Ask about respiratory disease, recent flights or diving.

Relevant past history

Ask specifically about the following:
- Have there been similar previous episodes? (Always a good question to ask—the patient may tell you the diagnosis!)

- Pneumothorax.
- PE or deep venous thrombosis.
- Autoimmune rheumatic disease.

Examination

The first priority is always to establish how unwell the patient is:
- Is he breathless at rest?
- Does he look cyanosed? Check pulse oximetry.
- Can he speak easily?
- Check peripheral perfusion, pulse, blood pressure, respiratory rate and temperature.

This man is not very ill; he noticed his breathlessness when cycling, immediate assessment does not cause concern, and so the examination can be completed before investigation and treatment are considered.

General

Note the following:
- Habitus: tall thin 'marfanoid' young men have an increased risk of spontaneous pneumothorax
- Labial herpes: often seen in pneumonia
- Signs of autoimmune rheumatic disease.

Cardiovascular

Note particularly the following:
- Cardiac rhythm: atrial fibrillation can occur secondary to PE or pneumonia.
- Signs of right ventricular dysfunction: elevated JVP, parasternal heave, loud P2 and pansystolic murmur of tricuspid regurgitation—any or all of these would support the diagnosis of a large PE, but a patient presenting with a small peripheral PE causing lung infarction and pleurisy (as perhaps in this case) would not be expected to have any of these findings.
- Pericardial rub, indicating pericarditis.
- Calf swelling and tenderness: measure both sides—a difference of >2 cm may indicate venous thrombosis and would strongly support the diagnosis of PE in this clinical context.

Respiratory

Note particularly the following:
- Thoracic tenderness or rib crepitus: exquisite local tenderness clearly suggests a musculoskeletal cause, but there can be local tenderness with pleurisy. Rib crepitus proves that a rib has been broken.
- Expansion, percussion and auscultation: is there a pleural rub? These can be very localized; ask the patient to put a finger on the place that hurts most and listen at this point and just around it—you may miss a rub if you do not take care to do this. In pneumothorax, expansion may be reduced, percussion note may be hyperresonant, and breath sounds may be diminished on the affected side, but with a small pneumothorax examination may be normal.

Other

Examine the abdomen for masses and the breasts in a woman.

Approach to investigations and management

Investigations

 In the patient presenting with pleuritic pain, the key initial investigation is the chest radiograph.

Chest radiograph

Look specifically for the following:
- Pneumothorax: look very carefully at the lung apex—is there an area within the chest that does not have any lung markings? Can you see a line indicating the edge of the lung? Are you absolutely sure?
- Lobar oligaemia: a rare sign, but suggesting large PE.
- Pleural effusion: this may be visible only as blunting of the costophrenic angle and would be consistent with the diagnosis of PE or pneumonia.
- Wedge-shaped peripheral infarcts: typical of PE.
- Consolidation: typical of pneumonia.

ECG

Look for arrhythmia, RV strain and pericarditis (see Section 3.1, p. 120). Remember that the ECG is most likely to be normal in someone with PE, and also that pain and fear are the most common causes of sinus tachycardia in a patient presenting to hospital.

Arterial blood gases

If the patient is unwell or pulse oximetry indicates oxygen saturation <95%, check arterial blood gases. Some would recommend that this be performed for all patients presenting with pleuritic chest pain. Typical findings in PE presenting with pleurisy are normal PO_2 (but there may be hypoxia) and reduced PCO_2 as a result of hyperventilation.

 If the probable diagnosis is pulmonary embolism, give anticoagulation (low-molecular-weight heparin) immediately, while waiting for confirmatory investigations.

Further investigations may be indicated depending on clinical findings and the results of immediate tests.

Definitive investigation for pulmonary embolism

Ventilation–perfusion scanning (see Section 3.10, p. 140) is the most common readily available imaging test, but CT angiography is increasingly used.

Blood tests

Full blood count, electrolytes, renal and liver function tests, clotting screen, blood cultures, atypical respiratory serology screen, inflammatory markers and tests for autoimmune rheumatic disease may all be indicated in some patients. In a patient who has recovered from a PE, consider checking thrombophilia screen after the therapeutic course of anticoagulation has been stopped. (See *Haematology*, Section 1.20.)

Sputum

If present, sputum should be sent for microscopy, culture and sensitivity, and also for cytology and acid-fast bacilli (TB) if the clinical picture is appropriate.

Management

This depends on the specific diagnosis:
- PE: see Section 2.18, p. 115; see also *Emergency medicine*, Section 1.8 and *Haematology*, Sections 1.13, 1.20 and 3.6.
- Pneumothorax: see *Emergency medicine*, Section 3.3 and *Respiratory medicine*, Sections 3.2 and 3.4.
- Pneumonia: see *Emergency medicine*, Section 1.9; *Infectious diseases*, Section 1.4; *Respiratory medicine*, Section 1.10.
- Musculoskeletal pain: analgesia and reassurance. Particularly in the case of rib fracture adequate analgesia is essential to allow the patient to inspire fully and avoid hypostatic pneumonia. Local intercostal nerve blocks can be very effective.
- Pericarditis: see Sections 1.14, p. 42 and 2.6.1, p. 78.

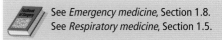 If you diagnose a PE for which there is no obvious cause (e.g. postoperative), perform rectal (and in a woman pelvic) examination and consider pelvic ultrasonography to exclude masses causing deep venous thrombosis by compression.

 See *Emergency medicine*, Section 1.8.
See *Respiratory medicine*, Section 1.5.

1.10 Breathlessness and exertional presyncope

Case history

A 30-year-old woman is referred to outpatients because of gradually worsening fatigue and exertional dyspnoea. A year ago she was fit and active but is now unable to jog or attend her usual exercise classes. There has been no improvement with bronchodilator therapy. She is extremely anxious about an episode last week when she nearly fainted while hurrying for a train to a job interview.

Clinical approach

There are suggestions in this history that stress or anxiety may be contributing to this patient's symptoms, but your primary concern should be to exclude the significant organic conditions that can present insidiously like this, shown in Table 8.

 Exertional syncope or presyncope is a symptom to be taken seriously. It usually indicates an inability to increase the cardiac output appropriately as a result of a fixed obstruction or ventricular dysfunction.

History of the presenting problem

Presenting symptoms

Ask the patient the following:
- Are you limited by fatigue (may indicate low cardiac output), breathlessness or by something else (what)?
- 'How far can you walk/run?' 'How many flights of stairs?' Be specific about this, and try to get a feeling for the pace of progression by asking: 'How does this compare with last Christmas/during your summer holidays?'
- Have there been any other instances of syncope/presyncope, and exactly what were the circumstances?

Associated symptoms

Ask specifically about the following:
- Chest pain: if present, is this pleuritic or anginal? This woman is young for IHD, but anginal pain can be associated with pulmonary hypertension. This is thought to originate from the hypertrophied (and therefore relatively hypoxic) right ventricle.
- Haemoptysis: a feature of pulmonary hypertension, but could also indicate pulmonary embolism.
- Cough/wheeze/sputum: features that would suggest chronic lung disease.

Table 8 Differential diagnosis of exertional dyspnoea and presyncope.

Pathophysiology	Specific conditions
Left ventricular outflow tract obstruction	Hypertrophic cardiomyopathy Aortic subvalvular/valvular/supravalvular stenosis
Pulmonary hypertension	Primary pulmonary hypertension Secondary, e.g. to respiratory disease, pulmonary thromboembolism or mitral valve disease (see Section 2.12.2, p. 103)
Right ventricular outflow tract obstruction	Infundibular/pulmonary stenosis
Left ventricular dysfunction	See Section 2.3, p. 63
Pericardial compromise of cardiac filling	Effusion Constriction
Anaemia	–
Sustained arrhythmia	Atrial fibrillation Complete heart block

- Orthopnoea/PND: suggests pulmonary oedema.
- Palpitations: see Section 1.2, p. 6.
- Ankle oedema/calf swelling or tenderness: unilateral problems raise the possibility of venous thromboembolism; bilateral swelling suggests RV failure.
- Raynaud's phenomenon: this may be present in autoimmune rheumatic disease and also in 10% of women with primary pulmonary hypertension.
- Any features that would suggest autoimmune rheumatic disease, e.g. joint pains, rashes.

Relevant past history

Enquire specifically about a history of the following:
- Venous thromboembolism
- Rheumatic fever or 'heart murmur'
- Chest trauma or TB—may lead to pericardial problems
- Respiratory disease.
  Also ask about the following:
- Smoking
- Alcohol
- Other risk factors for IHD (see Sections 1.5, p. 15 and 2.1, p. 51)
- Other risk factors for PE (see Sections 1.9, p. 28 and 2.18, p. 115)
- If a cause is not obvious, it may also be appropriate to enquire regarding risk factors for HIV infection (see *General clinical issues*, Section 2).

Drug history

Ask directly about the use of the following:
- Oral contraceptive: risk factor for thromboembolism
- Appetite suppressants: implicated in valve disease and pulmonary hypertension
- Cardiotoxic chemotherapy

- Cocaine: can cause LV dysfunction and pulmonary hypertension.

Family history

Ask about any family history of the following:
- IHD
- PE
- Hypertrophic cardiomyopathy
- Pulmonary hypertension.

 Ask broad questions such as 'has anyone in the family died suddenly?'

 Think about pregnancy

Many previously silent cardiorespiratory conditions manifest themselves in pregnancy because of the physiological changes (see Section 1.16, p. 48).

Examination

General

Is she well or ill? Is she breathless at rest or climbing on to the couch? Look for clinical anaemia, clubbing, cyanosis, malar flush, and signs of autoimmune rheumatic disease or endocarditis.

Cardiovascular and respiratory

Full assessment, noting particularly the following:
- Pulse volume, character, rate and rhythm: is the pulse slow rising (left ventricular outflow tract obstruction) or jerky (hypertrophic cardiomyopathy)? If arrhythmia, see Section 1.2, p. 6.

- Blood pressure: is there a narrow pulse pressure suggesting left ventricular outflow tract obstruction?
- JVP: look very carefully for this—you must decide where it is. It could be very high if the right ventricle is hypertrophied or failing or there is pericardial disease (effusion or constriction).
- Heart sounds and murmurs: added sounds suggest ventricular dysfunction; quiet sounds might be the result of chronic lung disease or pericardial effusion. Is that rather loud third sound a pericardial knock?
- Are the lung fields clear?
- Is there any oedema or hepatomegaly: if there is hepatomegaly, is this pulsatile? If it is, there is tricuspid regurgitation and the JVP must be elevated, even if you did not see it the first time around—look again!

Look for the following patterns:
- Pulmonary hypertension: loud P2 and associated RV hypertrophy (parasternal heave), dilatation (pansystolic murmur of tricuspid regurgitation) and dysfunction (raised JVP, oedema and hepatomegaly)
- LV dysfunction: tachycardia, gallop rhythm and fine basal crackles of pulmonary oedema
- PE: pleural rub, calf swelling and tenderness.

Approach to investigations and management

Investigations

The echocardiogram is the key investigation in the patient with dyspnoea and syncope on exertion.

Blood tests

Check pulse oximetry. Perform arterial blood gases if the oxygen saturation is <95% or the patient looks cyanosed. Check FBC, electrolytes, renal and liver function, glucose, cholesterol and inflammatory markers (CRP and ESR). Other tests for autoimmune rheumatic disease may be indicated. (See *Rheumatology and clinical immunology*, Section 3.2.)

Urinalysis

Look specifically for protein, blood and glucose. Could there be a multisystem inflammatory condition?

ECG

Note the rhythm, axis, and any atrial or ventricular hypertrophy (see Section 3.1, p. 120). LBBB is commonly associated with a dilated LV.

Chest radiograph

Note the heart size and shape, pulmonary arteries, lung fields and any valve calcification or pleural effusions.

Echocardiography

Echocardiography allows visualization of ventricular dimensions, hypertrophy and function, together with outflow tracts and valves (with gradients) and any intracardiac shunt or pericardial effusion. If there is significant pulmonary hypertension a dilated, hypertrophied RV, compressing the LV into a D shape (Fig. 18), can usually be seen and the presence of tricuspid regurgitation allows the measurement of pulmonary artery pressure.

Other

- If the echocardiogram suggests pulmonary hypertension but no cause is apparent, further investigations are needed (see Section 2.12.1, p. 101). These are initially directed towards excluding secondary causes of pulmonary hypertension. If a cause is not discovered and the diagnosis of primary pulmonary hypertension is made, other investigations, e.g. right heart catheterization, are used to determine prognosis and optimize treatment.
- Pulmonary function tests.

Management

Further management will depend on the specific diagnosis:

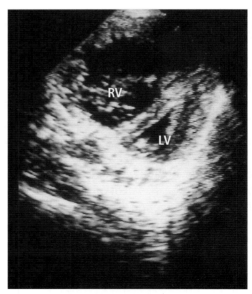

Fig. 18 Short axis echo view of a patient with primary pulmonary hypertension showing the high pressure, dilated right ventricle (RV) compressing the left ventricle (LV) into a characteristic D shape. (Courtesy of Dr LM Shapiro.)

- Pulmonary hypertension: see Section 2.12, p. 101
- Hypertrophic cardiomyopathy: see Section 2.4.1, p. 66
- Valve disease: see Section 2.5, p. 71
- LV dysfunction: see Section 2.3, p. 63
- Pericardial effusion/constriction: see Sections 2.6.2, p. 80 and 2.6.3, p. 82
- Sustained arrhythmia: see Sections 2.2, p. 58
- Anaemia: see *Haematology*, Section 2.1 for discussion.

Examination and investigations normal

Provide reassurance and encourage the patient to maintain activity, but retain an open mind and keep her under review.

 Peacock AJ. Primary pulmonary hypertension. *Thorax* 1999; 54: 1107–1118.

1.11 Dyspnoea, ankle oedema and cyanosis

Case history

A reclusive 45-year-old man is referred by his GP, having sought medical attention for the first time in his life because of ankle swelling that prevented him from putting on his shoes on. The GP was surprised to find that he was centrally cyanosed and moderately dyspnoeic.

Clinical approach

Cyanosis can be of cardiac (right-to-left shunting) or respiratory origin or, rarely, associated with abnormal haemoglobin. Chronically, cyanosis can be reasonably well tolerated, but complications develop (see Section 2.7, p. 84). The differential diagnosis in this man, previously unknown to the medical profession, is wide:
- Respiratory failure and cor pulmonale secondary to chronic obstructive pulmonary disease, but also bronchiectasis, pulmonary fibrosis or hypoventilation syndromes.
- Eisenmenger's syndrome: see Section 2.7.2, p. 86.
- Secondary pulmonary hypertension of another cause.
- Other congenital heart disease: patients with Ebstein's anomaly or mild cases of tetralogy of Fallot may survive to middle age.

You need to determine the cause of the patient's cyanosis by looking for evidence of respiratory disease, pulmonary hypertension and intracardiac shunts.

History of the presenting problem

Ask about the duration and severity of the patient's presenting symptoms:
- How long has his ankle been swelling up for?
- Has he noticed that he has become blue and, if so, when? Has he been a 'funny colour' for as long as he can remember? If this has been very long standing, it suggests a cardiac rather than a respiratory explanation.
- Is he limited by breathlessness? Quantify his functional status—how far can he go on the flat? Can he go up stairs? How many times does he have to stop?

Enquire specifically regarding the following:
- Has he had any symptoms of hyperviscosity? These would include dizziness, headache, visual disturbance or paraesthesiae, probably indicating secondary polycythaemia in this case.
- Has he had any episodes of syncope or presyncope? These are a poor prognostic sign in patients with pulmonary hypertension.
- Does he find it difficult to stay awake sometimes? Has he ever fallen asleep during the day when he was not trying to, e.g. when driving a car? Has anyone ever complained that he snores a lot when he goes to sleep? Does he wake up with headaches in the mornings? Any of these features would make you think that he might have obstructive sleep apnoea.
- Does he smoke, which would put him at risk of chronic lung disease? Does he have chronic cough, sputum or wheeze—all features suggesting that he has chronic lung disease? Is there any history of asbestos exposure?

Ask about features that suggest thromboembolic disease:
- Asymmetrical calf swelling or tenderness
- Pleuritic chest pain
- Haemoptysis.

Also ask about the following:
- Symptoms of liver disease or autoimmune rheumatic disease.
- Use of prescribed medications (unlikely in this man), other drugs and risk factors for HIV (see *General clinical issues*, Section 2).
- History of stroke or transient ischaemic attack: these would be uncommon in a patient aged 45 years, but may be attributable to paradoxical embolism from right-to-left shunting in this case.

Relevant past history

Ask specifically about the following:
- Was he a blue baby? Did he have a heart murmur? Did he have rheumatic fever (try St Vitus' dance)?
- TB and whooping cough: these would put him at risk of bronchiectasis.
- Did any siblings die young? If so, consider cystic fibrosis.

Examination

Concentrate on a full cardiovascular and respiratory examination, noting particularly the following:
• Cyanosis—and check pulse oximetry.
• Neck and oropharynx: is obstructive sleep apnoea likely?
• Clubbing: a feature of congenital cyanotic heart disease, bronchiectasis and fibrosing alveolitis, but not of other causes of secondary pulmonary hypertension or primary pulmonary hypertension.
• Pulse rate and rhythm.
• Blood pressure.
• JVP: this will almost certainly be grossly elevated.
• Is there a left parasternal heave? This would suggest RV hypertrophy (RVH).
• Heart sounds: listen specifically for the fixed split S2 of an ASD, the right ventricular S4 of pressure overload, the loud P2 of pulmonary hypertension or inaudible P2 of right ventricular outflow tract obstruction, e.g. in Fallot's tetralogy.
• Murmurs: listen for the pansystolic murmurs of tricuspid regurgitation and VSD and the ejection systolic murmur of right ventricular outflow tract obstruction, but remember that these may not be dramatic.
• Hepatomegaly: is the liver pulsatile, which would indicate tricuspid regurgitation?
• Oedema.
• Any signs of chronic lung disease, in particular airflow obstruction, fibrosis or bronchiectasis.

Approach to investigations and management

 Cardiac cyanosis will not improve with maximal inspired oxygen whereas respiratory cyanosis generally will.

Investigations

Blood tests

Check arterial blood gases for PO_2 and PCO_2 when the patient is breathing air and (monitoring patient continuously in case he or she is a CO_2 retainer dependent on hypoxic drive) after 10 min on high-flow oxygen (see *Respiratory medicine*, Section 3.6.1.).

Check FBC: is the patient polycythaemic? Check electrolytes, renal and liver function. Other tests, e.g. for autoimmune rheumatic disorders, may be indicated in some cases.

ECG

Look for evidence of RVH. (See Section 3.1, p. 120.)

Chest radiograph

Look for signs of pulmonary hypertension and chronic lung disease, in particular the hyperexpansion of chronic obstructive pulmonary disease and the interstitial shadowing of parenchymal lung disease.

Echocardiography

Echocardiography is a key investigation to assess RV function, RVH and pulmonary pressures, to examine the heart valves, and to look for septal defects and shunts.

Pulmonary function tests

Does the patient have severe obstructive or restrictive lung disease? Check spirometry, lung volumes and gas transfer.

Further investigations

Depending on the initial results consider the following:
• High-resolution CT scan of the chest.
• Transoesophageal echocardiography for ASD if there is pulmonary hypertension and a shunt is suspected but not seen on transthoracic echo.
• Ventilation–perfusion scan or spiral CT if pulmonary thromboembolism is considered possible.
• MRI of the heart to define anatomy more clearly.

Management

Depends on the underlying condition. Note that, in all patients with pulmonary hypertension, great care must be taken with the use of diuretics for oedema—the risk is that overzealous fluid removal can lead to reduction in right ventricular filling pressure and thereby cause circulatory collapse.

 Do not fluid deplete in right-to-left shunting because this increases the shunt.

• Secondary pulmonary hypertension: see Section 2.12.2, p. 103
• Eisenmenger's syndrome and other congenital heart disease: see Section 2.7, p. 84
• Chronic respiratory failure and cor pulmonale: see *Respiratory medicine*, Section 2.11
• Pulmonary thromboembolism: see Sections 1.9, p. 28, and 2.18, p. 115.

 See *Respiratory medicine*, Sections 1.6 and 1.8.

1.12 Chest pain and recurrent syncope

Case history

A 63-year-old retired accountant presents with a 4-month history of syncopal episodes and chest pain on exertion.

Clinical approach

The combination of chest pain and syncope is very suggestive of a cardiac problem. The causes of recurrent syncope are given in Table 9 (see also Table 2, p. 9)—the main differential in this case is between left ventricular outflow tract obstruction from aortic stenosis or hypertrophic obstructive cardiomyopathy, and arrhythmias, which may be supraventricular or ventricular. Complete heart block only rarely causes chest pain, although coexistent IHD may cause angina. Orthostatic hypotension is common in patients treated with antianginal medication, and can lead to syncope. Also remember that pain from any cause, including angina, can cause vasovagal syncope.

History of the presenting problem

Get a good description of the syncopal episodes

Although a patient's recall of the events surrounding a collapse may be limited, try to ascertain as much information as possible from the patient or any witnesses. (See Section 1.3, p. 9 and *Neurology*, Section 1.20.)

When does it happen?

Classically, syncope caused by outflow tract obstruction occurs only on exertion as a result of reflex bradycardia

and vasodilatation. Arrhythmias can occur at any time, but they may happen only on exercise or stress if they are sensitive to increased sympathetic outflow or ischaemia. Syncope from orthostatic hypotension occurs on standing, but may be more prominent after exertion.

Chest pain

The obvious assumption is that this man's pain is the result of angina. This needs to be confirmed—ask specifically: 'Show me where you feel the pain. When do you get the pain? What is it like? Does it go anywhere else? How long does the pain last and what makes it go away?, etc.' (See Sections 1.5, p. 15 and 2.1, p. 51.) Angina with associated dyspnoea on exertion is found in outflow tract obstruction, although not in association with syncope.

Relevant past history

It is obviously important to establish a past history of heart disease. Ask specifically about a history of IHD, valvular disease and arrhythmias:
- Any heart trouble in the past?
- Ever had a heart attack or been told that you have angina?
- Any palpitations or fluttering sensations before?

Try also to ascertain whether there is a history of rheumatic fever. Patients may remember a period of illness as a child with joint pains, or a long period off school or away from sport. Patients with a bicuspid aortic valve may have been told that they have a murmur.

Risk factors

Ask about risk factors for IHD such as hypertension, smoking and family history. A family history of sudden death may reflect hereditary hypertrophic obstructive cardiomyopathy or long QT syndrome with underlying ventricular arrhythmias.

Examination

Examination of a patient with exertional chest pain and syncope:
- General impression: is the patient well or unwell?
- Full cardiovascular examination
- Is the carotid pulse slow rising, suggesting aortic stenosis?
- Is there any arrhythmia?

General

As always, assess whether the patient looks unwell. A patient with critical aortic stenosis or hypertrophic

Table 9 Causes of syncope.

Symptom—syncope with:	Diagnosis to consider
Angina and dyspnoea occurring on exertion	Aortic stenosis or hypertrophic obstructive cardiomyopathy
Associated palpitations	Arrhythmia
Preceded by a definite prodrome with progressive nausea and sweating	Vasovagal syncope
A history of severe dizziness, blurring of vision, weakness or syncope on standing or after exertion in a patient treated with antianginal medication	Orthostatic hypotension
Prolonged episode with involuntary limb movements or tongue biting	Epilepsy

obstructive cardiomyopathy may be dyspnoeic simply on getting undressed.

As you examine the patient with syncopal episodes, consider the following diagnoses:
• Aortic stenosis: slow rising carotid upstroke, undisplaced thrusting apex, ejection systolic murmur radiating to carotids, perhaps with a palpable thrill
• Hypertrophic obstructive cardiomyopathy: jerky carotid pulse, diffuse 'rolling' or double apical pulsation, ejection systolic murmur
• Arrhythmia: look for abnormal rhythm, and for evidence of sinus node disease or ischaemia on the ECG
• Orthostatic hypotension: look for a postural drop in blood pressure.

Cardiovascular

Take careful note of the following:
• Pulse rate and rhythm
• Pulse character
• Blood pressure supine and on standing
• JVP
• Apex
• Heart sounds and murmurs
• Lung bases
• Peripheral oedema.

Approach to investigations and management

Investigations

Investigation of a patient with exertional syncope and chest pain:
• ECG: is there arrhythmia or left ventricular hypertrophy?
• Echocardiography: investigation of choice to exclude severe outflow tract obstruction.

ECG

Look for evidence of left ventricular hypertrophy and ischaemia, also arrhythmias or evidence in support of a rhythm disturbance, e.g. δ waves, long QT interval, bi- or trifascicular block (Fig. 19).

Chest radiograph

Cardiomegaly may suggest severe left ventricular hypertrophy with or without dilatation. Is the aortic valve calcified?

Echocardiography

Assess for evidence of aortic stenosis or hypertrophic obstructive cardiomyopathy and degree of severity. Remember that symptoms are unlikely unless obstruction

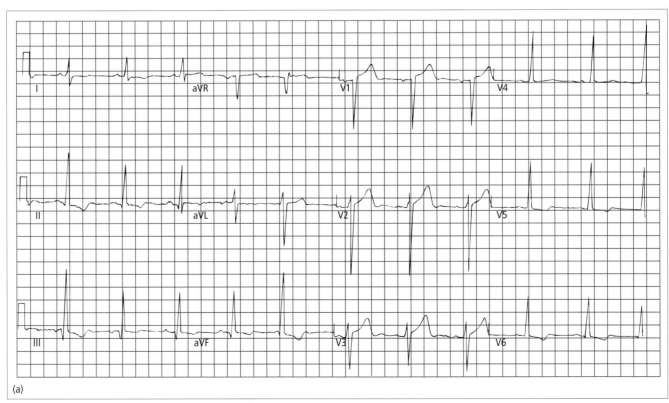

(a)

Fig. 19 Twelve-lead ECGs: (a) left ventricular hypertrophy, (b) old anterior myocardial infarction, (c) long QT.

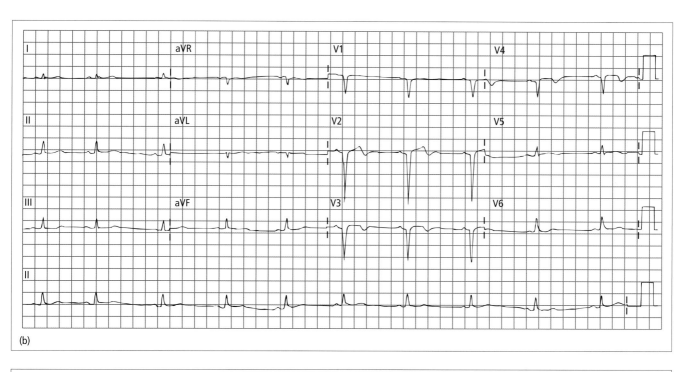

(b)

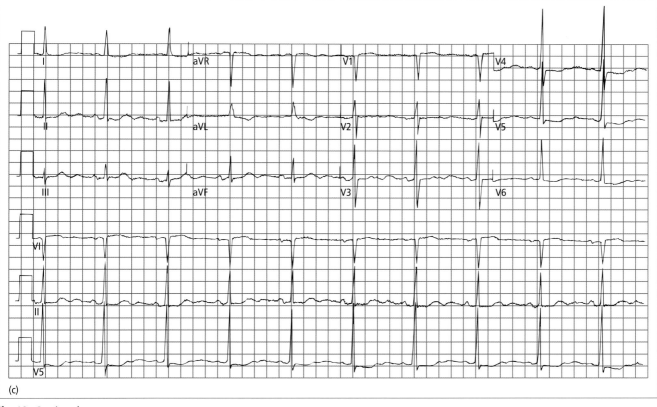

(c)

Fig. 19 *Continued*

is severe. The presence of an old infarct may predispose to ventricular arrhythmia. (See Section 2.1.1, p. 51.)

Twenty-four-hour ambulatory monitor

This may uncover evidence of arrhythmias such as ventricular tachycardia (Fig. 20).

Tilt-table testing

Hypotension with or without bradycardia may be precipitated in a vasovagal syndrome.

For further discussion of the investigation of syncope, see Section 1.3, p. 9.

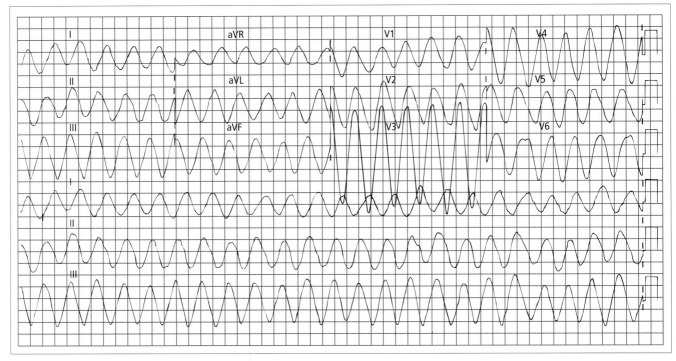

Fig. 20 Twelve-lead ECG showing ventricular tachycardia.

Management

There should be a low threshold for admitting patients with syncope caused by arrhythmia or left ventricular outflow tract obstruction. Remember that it may happen while crossing a road.

- Aortic stenosis: see Section 2.5.1, p. 71
- Arrhythmias: see Sections 1.1, p. 3, 1.2, p. 6, 1.3, p. 9 and 2.2, p. 58
- Hypertrophic obstructive cardiomyopathy: see Section 2.4.1, p. 66
- Orthostatic hypotension: changing antianginal medications to those with less antihypertensive action may reduce the incidence of problems
- Epilepsy and other neurogenic syncope: see *Neurology*, Sections 1.20 and 2.7.

See *Medicine for the elderly*, Section 1.1.
See *Neurology*, Section 1.20.
Abboud FM. Neurocardiogenic syncope. *N Engl J Med* 1993; 328: 1117.
Bradenburg RO. Syncope and sudden death in hypertrophic cardiomyopathy. *J Am Coll Cardiol* 1990; 15: 962.
Grech ED, Ramsdale DR. Exertional syncope in aortic stenosis. *Am Heart J* 1991; 127: 603.
Leitch JW, klein GJ, Yee R *et al*. Syncope associated with supraventricular tachycardia: An expression of tachycardia rate or vasomotor response? *Circulation* 1992; 85: 1064.
Lipsitz L. Orthostatic hypotension in the elderly. *N Engl J Med* 1989; 321: 952.

1.13 Fever, weight loss and new murmur

Case history

A 68-year-old, previously well man with a 6-week history of fever and weight loss is referred to the A&E department by his GP, who has also noticed a heart murmur.

Clinical approach

The list of diagnoses associated with the constitutional symptoms of fever and weight loss that have persisted for more than a few weeks is large—the most common causes are shown in Table 10. However, in the presence of a murmur, whether new or not, the diagnosis of infective endocarditis must go to the top of the list and should initially dominate your approach, even in the absence of any other stigmata. A careful history and examination are essential; other chronic infection, occult malignancy or autoimmune rheumatic disease may be uncovered.

History of the presenting problem

Given the non-specific nature of the symptoms, a careful and thorough history is essential—only scant information is available thus far. The history and examination are

Table 10 Differential diagnosis of 6 weeks' fever and weight loss.

Category	Common example	In presence of a murmur
Infective	Infective endocarditis TB Liver abscess	Infective endocarditis is the number one consideration
Autoimmune rheumatic disorder/vasculitis	SLE Rheumatoid arthritis Polymyalgia rheumatica	SLE (also some other rheumatic disorders) can affect the heart valves and cause substantial diagnostic difficulty
Malignancy	Lymphoma Hypernephroma	Consider atrial myxoma—is this the only case that you will ever diagnose? 'Marantic' endocarditis is possible

SLE, systemic lupus erythematosus; TB, tuberculosis.

dominated by consideration of the most likely diagnosis, infective endocarditis, but clues may emerge that take you off on another tack. Bear the diagnoses listed in Table 10 in mind as you take the history and go on to examine the patient.

General

Gauge the severity of the debilitation. In acute infective endocarditis, the fever is high with rigors and prostration: 'Have you had attacks of really bad shivering and shaking?' 'Have you sweated so much that you had to change your clothes or the sheets on the bed?' The current history is more suggestive of a subacute presentation, which is associated with a low-grade fever, malaise and weight loss.

Cardiac and respiratory symptoms

Ask about symptoms of heart failure:
• Have you been getting breathless going about your business or in bed at night?
• Have your ankles become swollen?

These may be insidious; if present they raise the possibility of haemodynamic compromise from aortic or mitral regurgitation. Sudden episodes of pulmonary oedema can be found in atrial myxoma.

Ask about chest pain, and—if present—get a good description:
• MI is rare in endocarditis, but can arise from coronary artery embolus.
• Pleuritic chest pain and/or haemoptysis may suggest pulmonary abscess or infarction from tricuspid valve endocarditis, as well as TB or other lung pathology. Haemoptysis is also a feature of left atrial myxoma.

Extracardiac manifestations

These may dominate the clinical picture in endocarditis if the patient presents, for example, with an arterial embolus leading to a stroke, or limb or splanchnic infarc-

tion, or more rarely as a result of some other systemic manifestation of endocarditis. This is not so in this case, but enquire about the following:
• Any skin rashes?
• Any changes in your nails recently?
• Have you noticed any blood in your urine?
• Have you had any back or abdominal pain?
• Any changes in your vision?
• Have you had any sudden periods of arm or leg weakness, or episodes of difficulty speaking?

Vasculitic rashes can occur with infective endocarditis, although uncommon, but are not specific and may occur with several of the differential diagnoses. Also rare, but much more suggestive, are transient changes in the hands and feet, which may be painful in the finger or toe pulps (Osler's nodes), or painless in the palms or soles (Janeway's spots or lesions).

Usually causing microscopic haematuria and unnoticed, the glomerulonephritis that may accompany infective endocarditis can cause gross haematuria, as may renal infarction; however, macroscopic haematuria would clearly lead you towards hypernephroma as the diagnosis. Back pain may simply result from myalgia, but severe loin pain suggests renal infarction and could be caused by a renal abscess or tumour. Pain in the left hypochondrium radiating to the left shoulder may result from splenic infarction or an abscess.

Relevant past history

Ask the following:
• Has anyone ever told you that you have a heart murmur, or that they've heard a 'sound' or 'hole' in your heart?
• Have you had rheumatic fever?
• Any recent trips to the dentist for surgery or invasive investigations?
• It may also be appropriate to ask regarding any history of intravenous drug abuse. (See *General clinical issues*, Section 2.)

• Have you had any antibiotics recently? Are you absolutely sure about that? A common reason for it being difficult to make the diagnosis of endocarditis is partial treatment with antibiotics—these can render the blood cultures sterile without effecting a cure.

And, thinking of other diagnoses that present as fever and weight loss:
• Have you ever had TB? Have you been in contact with anyone who has TB?
• Have you had any swollen glands? Have you had any problems with the blood or the lymph glands in the past?
• Have you had arthritis?
• Have you had any odd illnesses in the past?

Examination

> Examination of the patient with chronic fever, malaise and weight loss:
> • How does the patient look?
> • Thorough examination of all systems is essential
> • Look carefully for skin rashes and nail changes
> • Look carefully for signs of embolic phenomena
> • Is there evidence of significant valvular regurgitation?

General

Just as the history may be relatively non-specific, so also may be the examination findings. As always, get an overall impression. Patients with infective endocarditis are likely to look unwell, although elderly patients presenting atypically may simply be confused.

Check the temperature: a low-grade pyrexia (<39°C) is typical, although higher fever spikes are occasionally seen. Pallor and anaemia suggest chronic disease. Look at the hands, feet, skin, conjunctiva and mucous membranes for splinters/vasculitic manifestations of endocarditis.

Cardiovascular

Take particular note of the following:
• Peripheral perfusion.
• Pulse: rate and rhythm.
• Character: is there aortic regurgitation?
• JVP: may be elevated if there is heart failure.
• Apex: is this displaced, suggesting long-standing heart disease?
• Heart sounds and murmurs: give yourself the best chance of hearing the murmurs—switch the ward TV off and stop the vacuuming. For aortic regurgitation, listen with the diaphragm of the stethoscope in the fourth left intercostal space, with the patient leaning forward and having breathed out. For mitral regurgitation and stenosis, listen at the apex with the bell with the patient rolled on

to his or her left side. Could that funny sound really be a 'tumour plop'?
• Basal crackles, suggesting pulmonary oedema in this context.
• Peripheral oedema.

Other systems

Check specifically for the following:
• Lymphadenopathy: check all areas—lymphadenopathy is not a feature of endocarditis and would point towards another infective cause or a lymphoproliferative condition.
• Chest: are there any signs at all? Could this be TB?
• Abdomen: can you feel the spleen? This is often palpable in endocarditis, but a moderately or grossly enlarged spleen would favour lymphoma as the diagnosis. Is the liver palpable or tender? Could this be a presentation of liver abscess? Can you feel a renal mass? It is unlikely that you will, but the diagnosis could be hypernephroma.
• Neurological examination: are there any focal signs, likely to be caused by emboli from an infected valve in this clinical situation.
• Fundi: any evidence of endocarditic lesions?

Approach to investigations and management

Investigations

> Investigation of the patient with chronic fever, malaise and weight loss:
> • Blood cultures: at least three taken 1 h apart from separate well-cleaned sites
> • ESR, CRP, white cell count: is there evidence of systemic inflammation?
> • Urine: look for haematuria and proteinuria, suggesting glomerulonephritis (probably endocarditic)
> • Chest radiograph: look for TB and abscess formation
> • Urgent echocardiography to look for evidence of endocarditis.

Blood cultures

This is the single most important investigation and should be carried out as soon as possible. Three or more blood samples should be taken, from separate sites at different times, ideally over 24 h. Seriously ill patients thought to have endocarditis should have samples taken over 1–2 h and then be given antibiotics.

Blood and urine tests

Check FBC, inflammatory markers (ESR and CRP), electrolytes, renal and liver function, serum complement. Examine the urine with dipstix for haematuria and proteinuria—if positive for blood, examine a specimen microscopically to look for red cell casts. Send urine for laboratory microscopy, culture and sensitivity (but do not rely on this to tell you if there are casts!). A range of other blood tests, in particular serological tests for other infective conditions or autoimmune rheumatic disease, may be indicated if there are appropriate clues from the history or examination.

ECG

Look particularly for evidence of conduction disturbance (if there is, think of aortic root abscess) and atrial fibrillation.

Chest radiograph

Look for pulmonary oedema, heart contour, pulmonary abscess, pneumonia, mediastinal lympadenopathy or lung tumour (Fig. 21).

Echocardiogram

The echocardiogram is crucial for the detection of vegetations or cardiac tumours and the assessment of valvular regurgitation and paravalvular abscesses. If good views cannot be obtained on transthoracic echocardiography, or when there is substantial clinical suspicion despite a normal or non-diagnostic transthoracic study, TOE may be needed (Fig. 22).

Management

This depends on the specific diagnosis:
• Infective endocarditis: see Section 2.8.1, p. 92
• Left atrial myxoma: see Section 2.9, p. 95.
See *Infectious diseases*, *Haematology and oncology*, and *Rheumatology and clinical immunology* modules for further information on the many diseases that can present with fever and are differential diagnoses of infective endocarditis.

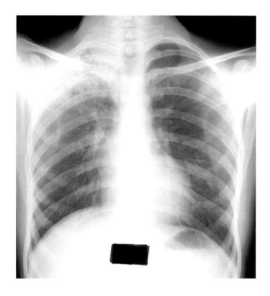

(a)

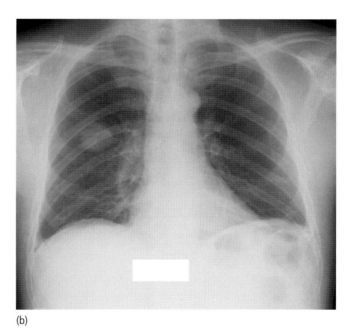

(b)

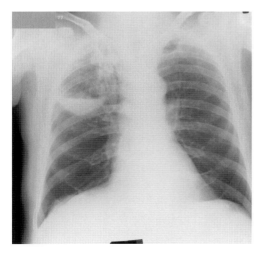

(c)

Fig. 21 Chest radiographs demonstrating (a) TB, (b) lung tumour and (c) abscess.

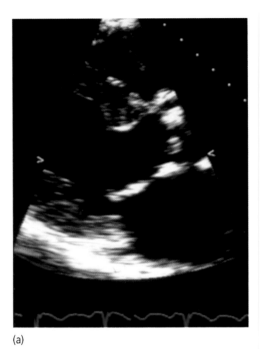

(a)

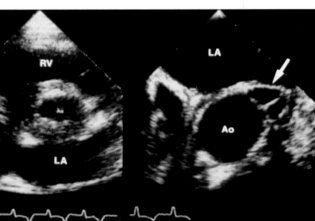

(b)

Fig. 22 (a) Aortic vegetation and (b) para-aortic abscess (arrow). (Courtesy of Dr J Chambers.)

See *Infectious diseases*, Sections 1.8 and 1.10.
See Section 2.8.1, p. 92.
Arnow PM. Flaherty JP. Fever of unknown origin. *Lancet* 1997; 350: 575–580.
Chien JW. Making the most of blood cultures. Tips for optimal use of this time-honored test. *Postgrad Med* 1998; 104: 119–124; 127.
Krivokapich J, Child JS. Role of transthoracic and transesophageal echocardiography in diagnosis and management of infective endocarditis. *Cardiol Clin* 1996; 14: 363–382.
Saccente M, Cobbs CG. Clinical approach to infective endocarditis. *Cardiol Clin* 1996; 14: 351–362.

1.14 Chest pain following a 'flu-like illness

Case history

A 25-year-old woman presents to A&E complaining of a 4-day history of chest pain. She has been unwell with 'flu for the last week. You are referred the patient by the A&E officer who thinks the pain may be pericarditic.

Clinical approach

The history immediately suggests an acute pericarditis of viral aetiology. The risk arises not from this diagnosis, which is usually mild and self-limiting, but from the failure to recognize more serious pathology that presents in a similar manner (Table 11). You must initially decide whether or not the pain is caused by pericarditis, excluding the other causes of chest pain along the way and, if so, whether there is a more serious underlying aetiology. Only then should you assume the diagnosis of viral pericarditis.

As there is some overlap between the symptoms of pericardial and pleural inflammation, you will need to consider pulmonary pathologies, in particular pneumonia and PE. Remember that serositis is also a feature of some autoimmune rheumatic diseases, such as systemic lupus erythematosus (SLE) and rheumatoid arthritis.

In this patient, both MI and aortic dissection would be extremely unlikely, but because of their potentially fatal consequences they should always be borne in mind in any patient presenting with chest pain.

History of the presenting problem

What and where?

Get as much information as possible:
- Show me where you feel the pain?
- What is the pain like?
- Does it go anywhere else?

If a clear description of the pain is not forthcoming, offer suggestions—'like a knife', 'raw'—both of which

Table 11 Differential diagnosis of pericarditic chest pain.

Comment	Diagnosis
Common	Acute pericarditis
	Musculoskeletal
	Oesophagitis
Must consider	Pneumonia
	Pulmonary embolism
	Autoimmune rheumatic disease
Do not completely forget	Myocardial ischaemia
	Aortic dissection

may suggest pericarditic pain, or 'like a heavy weight' or 'squeezing', which do not. The pain of pericarditis is usually located retrosternally, and like angina it may radiate to the neck or shoulders.

How and when?

Ask specifically about the pattern:
- Did the pain start suddenly?
- Do you have pain all the time? If not, when do you get it?
- Does it hurt when you breathe in?
- When you sit forward, does the pain get less?
- Is the pain worse lying in bed?

Pericarditic pain is usually continuous, but does not typically have a sudden onset, unlike PE. It is exacerbated by inspiration, movement and lying supine, and is typically eased by sitting forward. Aside from movement itself, there is no relationship with exertion, unlike angina.

Any other symptoms?

This woman has had 'flu-like symptoms recently, but ask any patient presenting with chest pain the following:
- Have you been feeling 'under the weather' or feverish recently?
- Do you feel breathless?
- Have you coughed up any phlegm? What colour was it? Any blood?
- Any joint pains?
- Do you ever get an acid taste at the back of your mouth?

Acute pericarditis often presents with a story of a recent 'flu-like infection. Although painful breathing may cause dyspnoea in pericarditis, prominent respiratory symptoms are clearly more in keeping with pulmonary pathology. Haemoptysis would suggest pulmonary embolism. The presence of arthralgia may simply reflect the associated viraemia, but could also suggest connective tissue disease. Acid reflux may suggest oesophagitis, as would a history of indigestion.

When taking a history in a young patient, at low risk of IHD, presenting with chest pain—look for the following patterns:
- Pericarditis: sharp or raw retrosternal continuous discomfort, worse on lying down, and relieved by sitting forwards, often with a history of a 'flu-like illness
- Musculoskeletal pain: history of unaccustomed activity with chest wall tenderness
- Oesophagitis: suggested by dyspeptic symptoms, particularly belching and reflux, worse at night
- Pneumonia: fever (sometimes rigors), breathlessness, malaise and (sometimes) pleuritic pain; dry painful cough initially, later productive of sputum
- PE: sudden onset of pleuritic pain with breathlessness and haemoptysis
- MI or aortic dissection: however unlikely you consider these may be in a young patient, think of them if the symptoms are 'ischaemic' or 'tearing' in nature.

Relevant past history

You will obviously ask whether there have been any similar episodes in the past and, if so, what diagnosis (if any) was made.

Although the most likely cause of pericarditis in this case is viral infection and, assuming that the woman is unlikely to have sustained an MI or undergone cardiac surgery, ask about other conditions that are associated with pericarditis:
- Rheumatoid arthritis and other autoimmune rheumatic disease
- Renal failure
- Hypothyroidism
- Rheumatic fever
- Contact with TB
- Malignancy, e.g. breast
- Chest radiotherapy.

Examination

As always, get an overall impression first. A patient with uncomplicated pericarditis is unlikely to look very unwell—he or she will be in pain, which may be severe, and is likely to be sitting forward rather than lying supine. If the patient is unwell, this should prompt a rapid assessment for evidence of tamponade, pulmonary embolism or pneumonia, which may be life threatening.

General

- Check the temperature: pyrexia indicates an inflammatory cause of pain
- Examine the sputum pot: haemoptysis suggests PE
- Does it hurt when I press you on the chest where the pain is? This would clearly suggest a local musculoskeletal cause, but remember that there can be tenderness in pleurisy.

Cardiovascular

Perform a full cardiovascular assessment, taking particular note of the following:
- Peripheral perfusion: is this impaired? It should not be in uncomplicated pericarditis.
- Pulse rate, rhythm and character.
- Blood pressure: does it fall on inspiration?
- JVP: is this elevated?
- Auscultation: is there a pericardial rub?

Respiratory and other systems

- Look for chest signs suggestive of pneumonia or PE.
- Is the patient euthyroid?
- Are there any signs of malignancy, e.g. breast?
- Is there evidence of autoimmune rheumatic disorder, e.g. joint inflammation or deformity, rash?

When examining a young patient, at low risk of IHD, presenting with chest pain, look specifically for the following:

• Pericarditis: is there a pericardial rub? Look for an underlying aetiology.

• Is there evidence of cardiac tamponade? Look for poor peripheral perfusion, elevated venous pressure and tachycardia with a small volume pulse exhibiting pulsus paradoxus (blood pressure falls significantly on inspiration). This is an emergency and requires pericardiocentesis.

• Musculoskeletal pain: pain that is well localized and reproduced by local pressure on the chest wall.

• Pneumonia: fever with signs of focal lung consolidation. Listen for a pleural rub.

• Pulmonary embolism: is there haemoptysis in the sputum pot? Listen for a pleural rub. Are there signs of pulmonary hypertension? (See Sections 1.9, p. 28 and 1.10, p. 30.)

• Aortic dissection: a rank outsider—but does the woman look as though she may have Marfan's syndrome? Can you feel the left radial pulse? Is the blood pressure the same in both arms? (See Section 1.5, p. 15.)

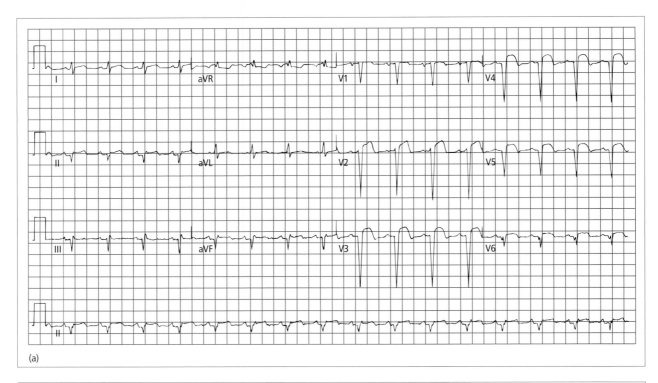

(a)

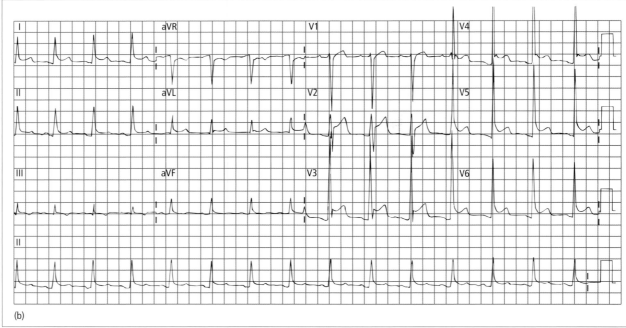

(b)

Fig. 23 ECGs: (a) anterior myocardial infarction and (b) acute pericarditis, where widespread ST segment elevation, concave upwards, is seen.

Approach to investigations and management

Investigations

ECG

Along with chest pain and pericardial rub, the ECG changes encountered in acute pericarditis form a triad of characteristic findings that can establish the diagnosis (Fig. 23).

Blood tests

Check FBC, electrolytes, renal and liver function, thyroid function, inflammatory markers (ESR and CRP) and cardiac enzymes. If clinically indicated, check blood cultures and serology for evidence of autoimmune rheumatic disorders. (See *Rheumatology and clinical immunology*, Section 3.2.) Checking 'viral titres' is not generally useful.

Chest radiograph

Look for cardiomegaly, suggesting an effusion, and for any areas of consolidation or pleural effusion (Fig. 24).

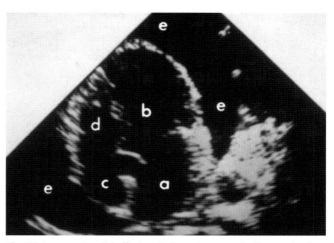

Fig. 25 Large pericardial effusion: the heart is surrounded by an echo-free space (e) formed by the effusion. a, left atrium; b, left ventricle; c, right atrium; d, right ventricle. (Courtesy of Dr J Chambers.)

Echocardiography

An echocardiogram that reveals a small amount of pericardial fluid can be very helpful in making the diagnosis of pericarditis. This is mandatory and urgent if the cardiac shadow is enlarged and you suspect cardiac tamponade (Fig. 25).

Other tests

Other tests, e.g. ventilation–perfusion scanning, should be performed if clinically indicated.

Management

This depends on the specific diagnosis:
- Acute pericarditis: see Section 2.6.1, p. 78
- Cardiac tamponade: see Section 2.6.2, p. 80
- Pneumonia: see *Infectious diseases*, Sections 1.2 and 1.4
- Pulmonary embolism: see Section 2.18, p. 115
- Connective tissue disease: see *Rheumatology and clinical immunology*, Sections 2.3.3 and 2.4.1
- Reflux oesophagitis: see *Gastroenterology*, Section 1.2.

In uncomplicated acute viral or idiopathic pericarditis, the illness is self-limiting. The patient should be reassured that they have not had a heart attack, and can be allowed home with simple analgesia, non-steroidal anti-inflammatory drugs (NSAIDs) often being particularly effective. Follow-up in a few weeks' time should be organized to ensure that the symptoms have settled. Admission will be warranted if the pain is severe, there is evidence of a large pericardial effusion or tamponade (which is a medical emergency), or if treatment of an underlying aetiology is indicated.

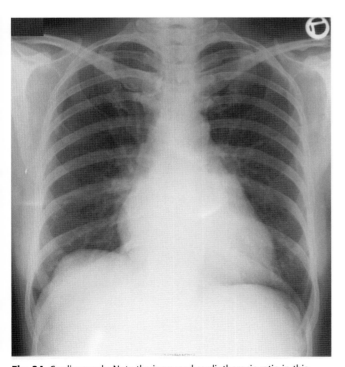

Fig. 24 Cardiomegaly. Note the increased cardiothoracic ratio in this posteroanterior film.

See *Infectious diseases*, Section 1.9.

Fowler NO. Cardiac tamponade. A clinical or an echocardiographic diagnosis? *Circulation* 1993; 87: 1738.

Shabetai R. Acute pericarditis. *Cardiol Clin* 1990; 8: 639–644.

Spodick DH. ECG in acute pericarditis. *Am J Cardiol* 1974; 40: 470.

Spodick DH. Pericarditis in systemic diseases. *Cardiol Clin* 1990; 8: 709–716.

1.15 Elevated blood pressure at routine screening

Case history

An obese 55-year-old publican is referred to your outpatient clinic for management of his blood pressure. He had attended his GP with pains in his legs and was found to have a blood pressure of 170/115 mmHg during the consultation. His father died of an MI at the age of 61. He takes no medication but smokes 20 cigarettes and drinks 4 pints of beer a day.

Clinical approach

This is an extremely common problem. The benefits of good control of elevated blood pressure are unassailable —this man already has several risk factors for vascular disease and failure to recognize and treat hypertension will add yet another. Your approach should be directed towards confirming an elevated blood pressure. By far the most likely diagnosis is essential hypertension, but do not fail to consider secondary causes (Table 12). Treatment

Table 12 Differential diagnosis of hypertension.

Comment	Diagnosis
Common	Essential hypertension
	False elevation as a result of inadequate blood pressure cuff size
	Isolated clinic ('white coat') hypertension
Must consider	Renal hypertension
	Renovascular hypertension
	Primary hyperaldosteronism (Conn's syndrome)
	Phaeochromocytoma
	Coarctation of the aorta
Other causes	Cushing's syndrome
	Acromegaly

offered must aim to reduce all modifiable cardiovascular risk factors.

History of the presenting problem

Hypertension is usually asymptomatic until organ damage intervenes. Some patients, on being given a diagnosis of hypertension, will ascribe many different and varied complaints to it. A multitude of symptoms, e.g. headache, epistaxis, tinnitus, dizziness, fainting, are often blamed on an elevated blood pressure, but probably occur with similar frequency in those whose blood pressure is normal.

Review of organ systems

Patients with chronic hypertension may present in cardiac failure, with breathlessnes and orthopnoea. Nocturia may suggest renal failure, which can be both a cause and a consequence of hypertension. In accelerated (malignant) phase hypertension (exceedingly unlikely in this case given the level of blood pressure) visual changes may result from retinal changes.

Could there be a secondary cause of hypertension?

A history of IHD, cerebrovascular disease or peripheral vascular disease would increase the likelihood of hypertension secondary to atheromatous renovascular disease. Are there any symptoms to support these diagnoses? His leg pains could be the result of intermittent claudication.

Is there any history of renal problems? Has he had medicals for work or insurance purposes? Have these been OK, or has he ever been told that he had protein in his urine? These questions might give a lead to the diagnosis of renal hypertension.

Episodes of palpitations, sweating or headaches might indicate a phaeochromocytoma, but would be much more likely to have a less exotic explanation (e.g. alcohol withdrawal).

Note that a strong family history of hypertension would support the diagnosis of essential hypertension.

Risk factors

In any patient presenting with hypertension it is very important to assess other cardiovascular risk factors, including the following:
- Smoking
- Diabetes
- Hyperlipidaemia
- Family history of cardiovascular events
- Alcohol consumption.

Examination

Examination and investigation of the patient with hypertension

Measurement of blood pressure—make sure that you take the time to do this properly:
- The patient should be recumbent for at least 3 min
- Use an adequate sized blood pressure cuff—a large cuff if the arm is large
- Measure blood pressure three times (at first visit it is recommended that the pressure is taken in both arms and the one with the higher value used thereafter)
- Record all readings, with the average of the second and third taken as the patient's value for consideration of treatment.

Unless the blood pressure is very high (diastolic BP >110 mmHg) measurements should be repeated on more than one occasion before deciding on whether or not to treat. A method similar to this has been used to measure blood pressure in most of the trials of treatment of hypertension, and to condemn someone to perhaps life-long drug treatment on the basis of a single reading taken casually is not good medicine.

The main objectives are to:
- assess for evidence of target organ damage
- uncover a secondary cause of hypertension.

General and cardiovascular

Perform a full examination, but take particular note of signs strongly suggesting secondary cause:
- Abdominal bruits
- Radiofemoral delay.

Look for signs indicating that there might be secondary cause. Is there peripheral vascular disease? Check for carotid or femoral bruits, abdominal aortic aneurysm and absent peripheral pulses.

Search for evidence of end-organ damage by hypertension:
- Cardiac: is there left ventricular hypertrophy or cardiac failure?
- Fundoscopy: are there hypertensive changes? (See Section 2.17, p. 110.)

When examining the patient with hypertension, consider the following:
- Essential hypertension: if elevated blood pressure, evidence of left ventricular hypertrophy or hypertensive retinopathy in the absence of a suspicion of a secondary cause.
- Isolated clinic hypertension: look for anxiety, e.g. tachycardia. Is the blood pressure lower when measured by the clinic nurse or the GP, or at place of work or at home? There must be no evidence of target organ damage.
- Renovascular disease: are there abdominal bruits, abdominal aortic aneurysm or other evidence of atherosclerosis?
- Coarctation: look for absent femoral pulses and radiofemoral delay, collaterals in the back muscles and a widespread systolic murmur heard best over the back.

Approach to investigations and management

Routine investigations

Urine

The way to detect renal disease causing hypertension is to test the urine with dipstix for proteinuria and haematuria. If this is positive for protein, quantification with a 24-h collection is required; if positive for blood, microscopy (to look particularly for red cells and casts) and culture are needed.

Blood tests

Check the FBC, electrolytes, renal and liver function, uric acid, fasting glucose and lipid profile. The most common cause of hypokalaemia is diuretic treatment, but low values are often found in untreated accelerated phase hypertension and in primary hyperaldosteronism. Is renal function normal? Is there glucose intolerance or frank diabetes? Is the cholesterol elevated?

ECG

Look particularly for evidence of left ventricular hypertrophy.

Chest radiograph

Assess heart size and look for pulmonary oedema and coarctation (Fig. 26).

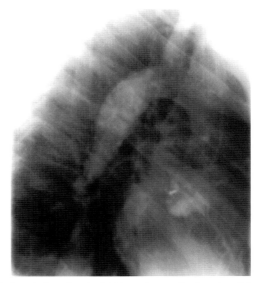

Fig. 26 Coarctation of aorta: in this angiogram the tapering of the aorta can be seen shortly after the arch on a plain radiograph the feature to look for is rib notching produced by collateral vessels (see Fig. 67, p. 92).

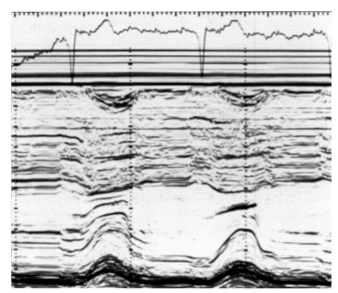

Fig. 27 Left ventricular hypertrophy: compare with the normal parasternal M-mode (see Fig. 112, p. 141). The interventricular septum is grossly thickened in this patient. (Courtesy of Dr J Chambers.)

Other investigations required in some cases

Echocardiography

This is more sensitive than the ECG at detecting left ventricular hypertrophy, especially if patients are of Afro-Caribbean descent (Fig. 27).

Twenty-four-hour ambulatory blood pressure monitoring

This may be needed to confirm a suspicion of 'white coat hypertension'.

Other tests

Specific tests to diagnose primary renal disease (serological tests, renal biopsy), renovascular disease (captopril renography, renal angiography), Conn's syndrome (plasma renin and aldosterone levels) or phaeochromocytoma (urinary catecholamines) will be required in some cases, but only where there is substantial clinical suspicion.

A number of other conditions, e.g. Cushing's syndrome or acromegaly, can be complicated by hypertension, but it is rare for hypertension to be the presenting feature.

Management

Management depends on the precise diagnosis:
• Essential hypertension: see Section 2.17, p. 110
• Isolated clinic hypertension: reassurance and avoidance of poisons (drugs)!
• Renal and renovascular disease: see *Nephrology*, Sections 1.11, 2.1.3 and 2.5.1

• Coarctation of the aorta: surgery to be considered
• Phaeochromocytoma: see *Endocrinology*, Section 2.2.5
• Primary hyperaldosteronism: see *Endocrinology*, Section 2.2.3
• Accelerated (malignant) hypertension: see Section 2.17.1, p. 113

Do not forget to offer advice and treatment (where possible) to reduce other cardiovascular risk factors. Decisions regarding the treatment of hypertension (or hypercholesterolaemia) should never be taken in isolation. It would be better for this man to stop smoking with some reduction in his blood pressure than to have 'perfect blood pressure' and a pack of cigarettes a day.

See *Endocrinology*, Sections 1.17 and 1.18.
See *Nephrology*, Section 1.11.
Devereux RB, Koren MJ, de Simone G, Okin PM, Kligfield P. Methods for detection of left ventricular hypertrophy: application to hypertensive heart disease. *Eur Heart J* 1993; 14(suppl D): 8–15.
McCrindle BW. Coarctation of the aorta. *Curr Opin Cardiol* 1999; 14: 448–452.
Mancia G, Parati G, Omboni S, Ulian L, Zanchetti A. Ambulatory blood pressure monitoring. *Clin Exp Hypertension* 1999; 21: 703–715.
Preston RA, Singer I, Epstein M. Renal parenchymal hypertension: current concepts of pathogenesis and management. *Arch Intern Med* 1996; 156: 602–611.
Ram CV. Renovascular hypertension. *Curr Opin Nephrol Hypertension* 1997; 6: 575–579.

1.16 Murmur in pregnancy

Case history

A 23-year-old woman is referred by her GP to the cardiology clinic after the discovery of a systolic murmur picked up during a routine antenatal visit. She is 29 weeks' pregnant with her first child.

Clinical approach

Your major concern will be to differentiate an innocent murmur from one that suggests underlying pathology (Table 13). Can you reassure the patient or, if there is a structural cardiac lesion, can you predict and prevent problems that might arise during the pregnancy? The most common diagnosis will be an innocent systolic murmur due to the hyperdynamic circulation, requiring no further intervention. Mitral or aortic valve disease, hypertrophic obstructive cardiomyopathy and congenital abnormalities, such as VSD, may require careful monitoring; at the very least they require antibiotic prophylaxis during vaginal delivery. Occasionally, rare and severe conditions such as cardiomyopathy of pregnancy can present in the third trimester.

Table 13 Differential diagnosis of a systolic murmur during pregnancy.

Comment	Diagnosis
Common	Innocent systolic murmur
	Venous hum
	Mammary soufflé
	Mitral valve prolapse
Must consider	Mitral valve disease (regurgitation/mixed/stenosis with tricuspid regurgitation)
	Aortic valve disease (stenosis/mixed/regurgitation with flow murmur)
	Hypertrophic cardiomyopathy
	Atrial or ventricular septal defect
Other causes	Peripartum cardiomyopathy

History of presenting problem

Most patients who present in this way will be asymptomatic. The presence of symptoms should raise the suspicion of significant pathology, but bear in mind that a degree of weakness, exertional dyspnoea, dizziness and peripheral oedema are quite common during pregnancy and are a result of physiological adaptation rather than intrinsic cardiac disease. Be sure to gauge the precise severity of the symptoms and relate it to the stage of the pregnancy.

Ask some general questions:
• Have you been getting out of breath more easily?
• How far can you walk?
• Have you woken up breathless at night?
• Any chest pains?
• Any palpitations? When do you get them?
• Any blackouts? What were you doing at the time?
• Do you ever feel as if you are going to pass out?

Relevant past history

Enquire about any previous cardiac history. Occasionally, a minor abnormality will have been documented in infancy or childhood and the patient may have been told that she has a murmur, 'hole' or 'sound' in her heart. Ask about any difficulties before the pregnancy that might also suggest a congenital abnormality; also ask about any heart problems in other family members. A history of sudden death at a young age might raise the possibility of a hereditary cardiomyopathy or Marfan's syndrome.

Examination

Examination of the pregnant patient with a systolic murmur:
• Do you think the patient looks unwell?
• Does the patient look Marfanoid?
• Is the carotid pulse slow rising or collapsing, suggesting severe aortic valve disease? Or is it jerky, suggesting hypertrophic cardiomyopathy (can be difficult to distinguish from the hyperdynamic circulation of pregnancy)?
• Does the murmur suggest valvular or structural abnormality or does it sound innocent?
• Is there any evidence of cardiac failure?
The bottom line is:
• Do you think that the heart is normal?

General

Be vigilant for evidence of systemic disease, which can present with valvular abnormalities. A complete examination is necessary. Most patients presenting with a murmur in pregnancy will look well: remember that if they do not, they are much more likely to have serious pathology.

Check temperature, and look carefully for any stigmata of endocarditis. (See Section 1.13, p. 38.)

Cardiovascular

A careful and thorough examination for signs of cardiac disease will form the main part of your assessment. Thinking all the time about the potential diagnoses, as listed in Table 13, take note of the following:
• Peripheral perfusion
• Pulse rate, rhythm and character
• Blood pressure
• JVP
• Apex
• Heart sounds
• Murmurs and radiation
• Lung bases
• Liver edge
• Peripheral oedema.

Approach to investigations and management

Investigations

ECG

Minor flattening of the T waves or axis shift are common in normal pregnancy, as are sinus tachycardia and ectopic beats. Look for evidence of atrial enlargement, left or right ventricular hypertrophy, or conduction abnormalities (Fig. 28).

Chest radiograph

This test is best avoided unless there are clear clinical indications.

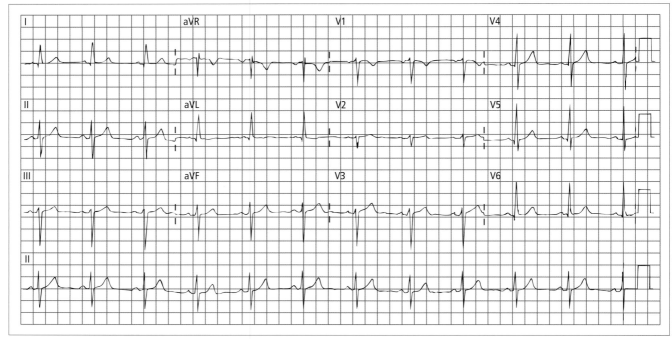

Fig. 28 ECG: axis shift in pregnant woman.

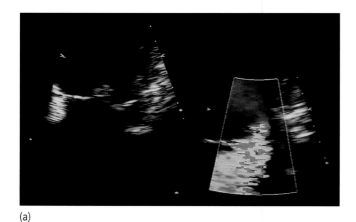

(a)

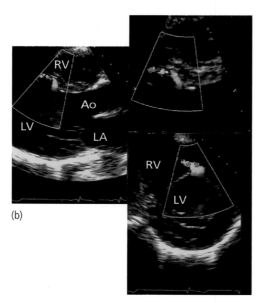

(b)

Echocardiography

This is the investigation of choice to confirm or rule out cardiac pathology (Fig. 29).

Management

- Innocent murmur, venous hum, mammary soufflé: no treatment required; reassure
- Aortic or mitral valve disease: see Section 2.5, p. 71
- ASD or VSD: see Section 2.7, p. 84
- Hypertrophic cardiomyopathy: see Section 2.4.1, p. 66
- Peripartum cardiomyopathy: see Section 2.15, p. 109.

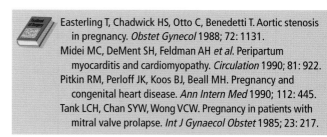

Easterling T, Chadwick HS, Otto C, Benedetti T. Aortic stenosis in pregnancy. *Obstet Gynecol* 1988; 72: 1131.

Midei MC, DeMent SH, Feldman AH *et al.* Peripartum myocarditis and cardiomyopathy. *Circulation* 1990; 81: 922.

Pitkin RM, Perloff JK, Koos BJ, Beall MH. Pregnancy and congenital heart disease. *Ann Intern Med* 1990; 112: 445.

Tank LCH, Chan SYW, Wong VCW. Pregnancy in patients with mitral valve prolapse. *Int J Gynaecol Obstet* 1985; 23: 217.

Fig. 29 (a) Mitral valve prolapse (MVP) and (b) ventricular septal defect (VSD). MVP: in the two-dimensional image on the left, the anterior mitral valve leaflet is seen to bow into the left atrium (arrow). The effect of this can be seen in the colour flow mapping on the right—a broad regurgitant jet can be seen. VSD: in these parasternal long and short axis views, a small jet of orange colour represents the abnormal blood flow across the septum from the left to right ventricle. LA, left atrium; LV, left ventricular; RV, right ventricle; Ao, aorta. (Courtesy of Dr J Chambers.)

2 Diseases and treatments

2.1 Coronary artery disease

2.1.1 STABLE ANGINA

Aetiology/pathophysiology/pathology

Chronic atheromatous plaques reduce coronary blood flow. Increased myocardial oxygen demand on exercise cannot be met, resulting in myocardial ischaemia and chest pain (angina pectoris).

Epidemiology

The estimated prevalence of this condition is 3–4% of the population.

Clinical presentation

Common

Common features include the following:
- Heavy central chest pain on exertion, relieved by rest
- Typically worse in cold weather, after meals
- Lower jaw or left arm pain.

Uncommon

- Exertional breathlessness ('angina equivalent').

Physical signs

Usually there are no physical signs in uncomplicated stable angina. Look for hypertension and signs of peripheral or cerebrovascular disease.

Investigations

An algorithm for investigation of the patient presenting with suspected angina is set out in Fig. 30:
- Resting ECG: often normal, but this does not rule out serious coronary disease.
- Exercise ECG: used to confirm the clinical diagnosis, assess exercise capacity objectively and determine prognosis. (See Section 3.1.1, p. 124.)
- Myocardial perfusion imaging (see Section 3.12.1, p. 143) or dobutamine stress echocardiography (see Section 3.11,

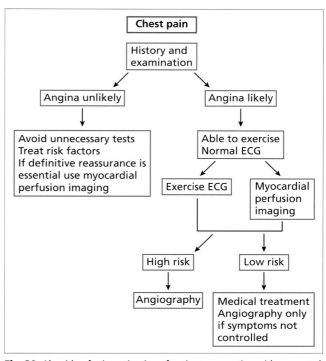

Fig. 30 Algorithm for investigation of patients presenting with suspected stable angina.

p. 141) may be used instead of exercise ECG in those unable to exercise or who have bundle-branch block.
- Lipid profile.
- FBC.
- Cardiac catheterization (see Section 3.8.1, p. 136).

Consider other causes of exertional chest pain:
- Syndrome X: typical exertional angina, positive exercise test and normal coronary angiogram. Usually in middle-aged women, possibly as an abnormality of coronary microvascular function; the treatment is medical
- Hypertrophic cardiomyopathy
- Severe anaemia
- Aortic stenosis.

Treatment

Short term

Aspirin, GTN and a β blocker are the first-line drugs.

Long term

Medical: other antianginal drugs (calcium antagonist, long-acting nitrate or nicorandil) may be added according to symptoms.

Percutaneous transluminal coronary angioplasty (PTCA) (see Section 3.8.2, p. 138) is generally indicated if there is symptomatic angina with suitable lesions in one or two coronary arteries. An improved life expectancy has not been demonstrated.

Coronary artery bypass grafting (CABG) improves life expectancy in patients with the following:
• Left main-stem stenosis
• Severe, proximal, three-vessel coronary disease, especially with impaired LV function (Fig. 31)
• Possibly proximal LAD lesion with one other vessel involved.

It is also indicated for symptomatic patients with less severe disease, in whom PTCA is not feasible or has failed.

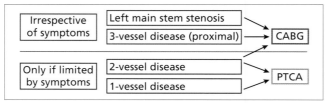

Fig. 31 Left coronary angiogram demonstrating proximal stenoses in two major vessels with retrograde filling of a blocked right coronary artery (arrow) via collaterals. This patient therefore has three-vessel coronary artery disease.

Non-medical (interventional) management of coronary artery disease is summarized in Fig. 32.

Complications

• Unstable angina
• MI
• Arrhythmia.

Prognosis

The prognosis is generally good; cardiac catheterization is the best means of risk stratification. The mortality rate ranges from 2% per year (single vessel disease) to 20% per year (left main-stem stenosis). Impairment of left ventricular function is an independent risk factor.

Prevention

Primary

• Stop smoking
• Treat hyperlipidaemia
• Treat hypertension
• Aggressive control of diabetes
• Hormone replacement therapy in women: controversial; observational studies suggest benefit but a large randomized trial did not confirm this
• Alcohol: observational studies suggest some benefit in moderation, but not proven to be effective.

Secondary

Continue with primary preventive measures (see above). Aspirin (plus a statin if indicated) reduces risk of MI. Clopidogrel is an alternative for those with aspirin allergy.

Disease associations

• Peripheral vascular disease
• Cerebrovascular disease.

```
┌─────────────┬──────────────────────────┐
│ Irrespective│ Left main stem stenosis  │──┐
│ of symptoms │ 3-vessel disease (proximal)│─┼─→ CABG
├─────────────┼──────────────────────────┤  │
│ Only if limited│ 2-vessel disease       │──┼
│ by symptoms │ 1-vessel disease         │──┴─→ PTCA
└─────────────┴──────────────────────────┘
```

Fig. 32 Interventional treatment of coronary artery disease. CABG, coronary artery bypass grafting; PTCA, percutaneous transluminal coronary angioplasty.

 Important information for patients:
• Explain that there are significant coronary narrowings but that the situation is stable
• Exertion within limits of symptoms is not dangerous, but avoid heavy lifting
• GTN may be used before exercise
• Gentle exercise (e.g. 30-min walk per day) is beneficial for the heart.

Antiplatelet Trialists' Collaboration. Collaborative overview of randomised trials of antiplatelet therapy. I: Prevention of death, myocardial infarction and stroke by prolonged antiplatelet therapy in various categories of patients. *BMJ* 1994; 308: 81–106.

Hillis LD, Rutherford JD. Coronary angioplasty compared with bypass grafting. *N Engl J Med* 1994; 331: 1086–1087.

Jackson R. Guidelines on preventing cardiovascular disease in clinical practice. *BMJ* 2000; 320: 659–661.

Swanton RH. Coronary artery disease. In: Swanton RH (ed.) *Cardiology* (Pocket Consultant). Oxford: Blackwell Science, 1998: 137–218.

Myers WO, Schaff HV, Gersh BJ *et al.* Improved survival of surgically treated patients with triple vessel coronary artery disease and severe angina pectoris. A report from the Coronary Artery Surgery Study (CASS) registry. *J Thorac Cardiovasc Surg* 1989; 97: 487–495.

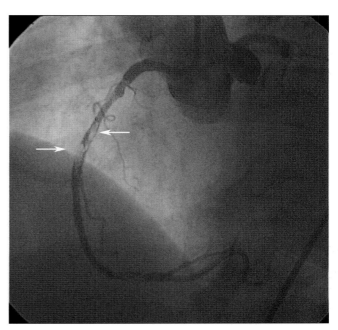

Fig. 34 Angiogram of right coronary artery in a patient with unstable angina. There is extensive thrombus present, seen as filling defects within the lumen (arrows).

2.1.2 UNSTABLE ANGINA

Aetiology/pathophysiology/pathology

An atheromatous coronary artery plaque erodes or splits, producing a thrombogenic surface that attracts platelets (Fig. 33). The resulting thrombus reduces (but does not completely block) coronary blood flow, producing acute ischaemia of the heart muscle (Fig. 34).

Epidemiology

There are over 230 000 admissions per year for this condition in the UK.

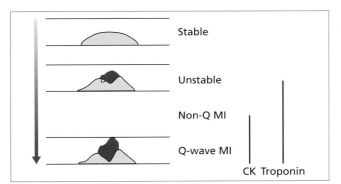

Fig. 33 Schematic diagram illustrating the sequence of events within a coronary artery during an acute coronary syndrome. Fissuring or erosion of an atherosclerotic plaque (yellow) leads to thrombosis (red), a rapid reduction in coronary blood flow and unstable angina. Transient complete occlusion leads to non-Q-wave (subendocardial) infarction, sustained occlusion to Q-wave (transmural) infarction. Highly sensitive troponin assays can detect microembolic heart muscle damage in unstable angina, allowing identification of those at higher risk of progression to infarction. CK, creatine kinase; MI, myocardial infarction.

Clinical presentation

Common

• Waxing and waning central chest pain at rest; partial relief from GTN
• Pain may be in the jaw or left arm
• Increasingly frequent and severe chest pain coming on with progressively less exertion (crescendo angina).

Uncommon

• Acute breathlessness (pulmonary oedema secondary to transient ischaemic LV dysfunction).

Physical signs

There are usually no specific signs in uncomplicated unstable angina.

Investigations

• ECG: may be normal; look for transient ST shift with pain; T-wave changes are less specific
• Cardiac biochemical markers: see Section 3.7, p. 136
• Stress testing may be useful if pain has settled but diagnosis in doubt, or to risk stratify once an unstable episode has settled
• Cardiac catheterization: see indications below.

Differential diagnosis

The differential diagnosis is as for MI (see Section 2.1.3, p. 55). Also consider coronary vasospasm.

Treatment

Myocardial infarction requiring thrombolysis must be excluded as soon as possible. The emphasis then switches to preventing progression to MI. Medical (antianginal and antithrombotic) treatment is the initial strategy, with cardiac catheterization reserved for persisting unstable symptoms or for certain high-risk subgroups.

Emergency

Emergency treatments include the following:
- Oxygen, analgesia, bedrest
- Aspirin, sublingual GTN, β blocker, low-molecular-weight heparin
- Consider heart-rate-lowering calcium antagonists (e.g. diltiazem) if a β blocker is contraindicated because of asthma, but avoid if there is significantly impaired LV function
- Glycoprotein IIb/IIIa inhibitors (e.g. tirofiban, eptifibatide, abciximab) are a new class of intravenous anti-platelet agents that improve outcome, particularly in patients undergoing urgent PTCA. Selective treatment of high-risk subgroups (e.g. troponin positive) may be the most effective way to use these expensive drugs (see recent NICE guidelines at www.nice.org.uk).

Short term

For continuing symptoms, use the following:
- Buccal nitrate or intravenous nitrate infusion
- Nicorandil.

If unstable symptoms do not resolve by 48 h, consider urgent cardiac catheterization with a view to revascularization (PTCA or CABG). This should also be considered in patients with the following:
- Post-infarct unstable angina
- Pulmonary oedema
- ST-segment shift with pain
- Recurrent unstable angina.

Long term

Once the acute episode has settled, the patient should be risk stratified in the same way as for stable angina (see Section 2.1.1, p. 51). This is done routinely in some hospitals before the patient is discharged.

Complications

Common

- Intractable or recurrent unstable angina
- MI.

Uncommon

- Pulmonary oedema
- Ventricular arrhythmias.

Prognosis

Morbidity

Fifteen per cent of patients with unstable angina progress to MI within 6 weeks.

Mortality

Ten per cent of patients die in the year after an episode of unstable angina.

Prevention

See Section 2.1.3, p. 55.

Important information for patients:
- Explain that the pain is a warning, not a heart attack
- Reassure that there is no significant heart muscle damage
- Explain that problems are best settled down with medication, if possible, but other treatments are available if they become necessary.

Braunwald E. Unstable angina: an aetiologic approach to management. *Circulation* 1998; 98: 2219–2222.
Heeschen C, Hamm CW, Goldmann B *et al.* Troponin concentrations for risk stratification of patients with acute coronary syndromes in relation to therapeutic efficacy of tirofiban. *Lancet* 1999; 354: 1757–1762.
Theroux P, Fuster V. Acute coronary syndromes. *Circulation* 1998; 97: 1195–1206.
Yeghiazarians Y, Braunstein JB, Askari A *et al.* Unstable angina pectoris. *N Engl J Med* 2000; 342: 101–114.

2.1.3 MYOCARDIAL INFARCTION

Aetiology/pathophysiology/pathology

Thrombus overlying an unstable plaque (see Fig. 33, p. 53) completely occludes the coronary artery, resulting in heart muscle necrosis. If the coronary occlusion is transient, only limited heart muscle death results (non-Q-wave infarction).

Epidemiology

- Each year there are 300 000 MIs in the UK.
- The mortality from coronary disease is in decline, but it remains the single most common cause of death in the UK (approximately 1 : 4 deaths).
- Death from an MI is almost three times higher in unskilled manual workers than in professional or managerial workers.

Clinical presentation

Common

- Acute onset with severe, crushing, central chest pain radiating to the jaw and/or left arm—unrelieved by nitrate
- Acute breathlessness (pulmonary oedema)
- Cardiac arrest (ventricular fibrillation).

Uncommon

- Pain in left arm alone, epigastrium or back
- Vomiting and sweating without pain
- Unexplained collapse
- Silent infarction (especially in people with diabetes and elderly people).

Physical signs

Common

There may be no abnormality on examination, but frequently the patient is pale, sweaty and obviously in pain. The patient may be hyper- or hypotensive. There may be pulmonary oedema.

Uncommon

The patient may present with only epigastric tenderness (inferior MI).

Investigations

Consider the following:
- ECG: ST-segment elevation and new bundle-branch block with an appropriate clinical history are both indications for thrombolysis (Fig. 35)
- Cardiac biochemical markers: see Section 3.7, p. 136
- Echocardiogram: indicated after an anterior MI or if there are haemodynamic complications (i.e. cardiogenic shock and/or pulmonary oedema)
- Serum cholesterol level is useful to guide initial statin therapy; sample <6 h after onset of pain because MI itself reduces cholesterol.

Differential diagnosis

The following may present in a similar way:
- Unstable angina
- Oesophagitis
- Musculoskeletal chest pain
- Thoracic aortic dissection.

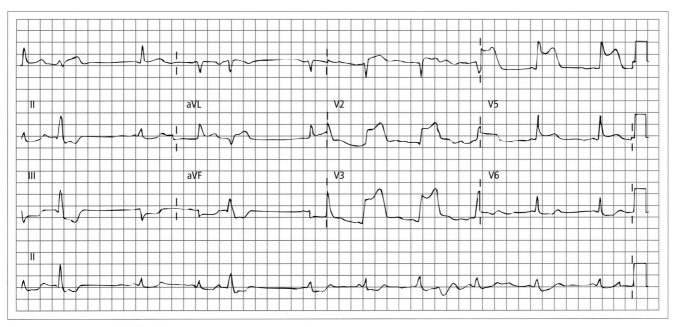

Fig. 35 Anterior myocardial infarction.

Treatment

Emergency

Indications for thrombolysis

- Typical chest pain at rest for >20 min
- ST elevation in two contiguous leads (≥1 mm inferiorly, ≥2 mm anteriorly) OR new bundle branch block
- Within 12 h of onset, but consider thrombolysis if 12–24 h with continuing pain

Act quickly; delay in thrombolysis increases mortality. A 'door-to-needle' time of 20 min should be achievable in most cases.

- Take history while obtaining intravenous access.
- Simultaneous recording of baseline observations and ECG by nurse.
- Oxygen, opiate analgesia and antiemetic.
- Aspirin 300 mg if no contraindication.
- Once diagnosis confirmed, quickly examine patient while nurse draws up thrombolytic agent. Ensure no contraindications to thrombolysis (Table 14).
- Thrombolysis.
- Transfer to cardiac care unit (CCU) for monitoring.

Emergency coronary angioplasty ('primary angioplasty') is an alternative to thrombolysis for MI. This may be a slightly better option if it can be performed by an experienced operator within 90 min of presentation, but most UK hospitals do not have these facilities.

Streptokinase (1.5 million units in 50 mL 0.9% saline over 1 h) is the first-line thrombolytic in the UK.
Consider recombinant tissue plasminogen activator (rTPA) if:
- Anterior MI; age <60 years; presenting within 6 h of onset
- Hypotension (streptokinase tends to lower blood pressure further)
- Streptokinase given ≥5 days before (neutralizing antibodies)
- Streptokinase allergy.

Table 14 Contraindications to thrombolysis.

Active internal bleeding
Active peptic ulcer
Bleeding tendency
Cerebrovascular accident in past 6 months (or at any time if haemorrhagic stroke)
Aortic dissection
Uncontrolled hypertension (>180/110 mmHg—bring down with nitrate infusion then thrombolyse)
Recent (<4 weeks) major trauma or surgery
Pregnancy

Note that anticoagulation in the therapeutic international normalized ratio (INR) range is a relative contraindication. Proliferative diabetic retinopathy is not a contraindication. Prior cardiopulmonary resuscitation is also not a contraindication unless prolonged or associated with obvious trauma.

Short term

The following have been shown to improve prognosis:
- β Blocker: orally within 24 h and continue indefinitely. Underused post-MI because of unfounded fears of side effects. Intravenous β blocker now controversial—may not confer added benefit. Oral diltiazem and verapamil are alternatives in patients with asthma, providing that LV function is not significantly impaired.
- ACE inhibitor: in patients with signs or echocardiographic evidence of LV dysfunction.
- Statin: year 2000 UK guidelines are to start if total cholesterol ≥5 mmol/L, which in practice is most patients post-MI.
- Warfarin: if there is persistent AF or large anterior MI with the risk of thromboembolism.
- Intensive insulin therapy (intravenous infusion for 24 h followed by insulin subcutaneously four times daily for 3 months) reduces mortality after MI in people with diabetes.
- Patients are usually kept in hospital for at least 5 days. Other antianginal drugs may be added to deal with residual stable angina (see Section 2.1.1, p. 51).

 NEVER SMOKE AGAIN.

Long term

When appropriate, stress testing (see Section 3.1.1, p. 124) is usually undertaken 4–6 weeks after MI to identify high-risk patients who should undergo cardiac catheterization. Many of these will have severe coronary disease, the prognosis of which is improved by CABG.

Complications

Common

- Haemorrhage induced by thrombolysis: transfuse as required. For life-threatening bleeds, consider reversal of streptokinase with fresh frozen plasma or cryoprecipitate.
- Ventricular fibrillation/tachycardia: promptly cardiovert; antiarrhythmic drugs rarely necessary if it occurs in the first 24 h.
- Atrial fibrillation: see Section 2.2.2, p. 59.
- Complete heart block: see Sections 2.2.1, p. 58 and 3.5, p. 132.
- Pulmonary oedema: see Section 2.3, p. 63.
- Cardiogenic shock: inotropic support, monitor pulmonary artery wedge pressure, consider intra-aortic balloon pumping and ventilation in patients with surgically correctable cause, e.g. VSD, acute mitral regurgitation.

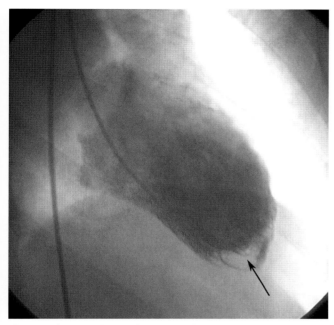

Fig. 36 Left ventriculogram showing apical mural thrombus (arrowed) after anterior myocardial infarction.

- Post-infarct unstable angina (16%).
- Reinfarction (3%).
- Pericarditis: usually benign; settles with NSAIDs.
- Stroke: consider reversing thrombolysis, request urgent CT scan of head.
- Arterial thromboembolism (AF or ventricular mural thrombus—Fig. 36).
- Deep venous thrombosis/pulmonary embolism.

Uncommon

- Left ventricular aneurysm
- Cardiac rupture: papillary muscle → acute mitral regurgitation (see Section 1.7, p. 23); septal → acquired VSD (see Section 1.7); free wall → tamponade (often sudden death).

Rare

- Dressler's syndrome: fever, pleuropericarditis, anaemia, raised ESR beginning 1–4 weeks after MI
- Frozen shoulder.

Prognosis

Morbidity

In the year after Q-wave MI:
- 25% develop unstable angina
- 10% have another infarction.
  The majority of patients admitted with an uncom-

plicated first MI will make a full recovery. Prognosis is determined by LV function at discharge and the results of stress tests (or cardiac catheterization if performed).

Non-Q-wave or subendocardial MI has a better prognosis than Q-wave MI over the first 6 weeks, but by 12 months the incidence of death is the same because of late reinfarction. Patients with non-Q-wave MI are therefore investigated more aggressively in the hope that prompt revascularization will prevent these late complications.

Mortality

- Of patients with a first MI, 30% do not reach hospital alive
- Of patients admitted to hospital, 10% die before discharge
- Of patients admitted to hospital, 10% die in the year after discharge.

Prevention

Primary

Prevention is via the control of the major risk factors for atherosclerosis (see Section 1.5, p. 15), usually managed in a primary care setting.

Secondary

- Aspirin, β blocker, ACE inhibitor
- Statin as indicated by cholesterol level.

Disease associations

Disease associations are cerebrovascular disease and peripheral vascular disease.

Important information for patients

On admission:
- Explain to the patient that he or she is having a heart attack, but that effective treatment is available
- The risk of haemorrhage following thrombolysis (3 per 1000) is outweighed by the benefits
- There is no net effect on stroke (increased haemorrhagic strokes offset by less ischaemic strokes).

On discharge:
- Good recovery is expected if there are no in-hospital complications
- Always carry GTN, even if free of angina
- Seek medical help if prolonged chest pain (>20 min) is not relieved by GTN
- You must give up smoking—reduces risk of reinfarction by 50%
- Gradually return to normal activities over the next 5 weeks. If available, a formal programme of cardiac rehabilitation is useful to reinforce these educational messages and restore patients' confidence.

Anon. Tackling myocardial infarction. *Drug and Therapeutics Bulletin* 2000; 38: 17–22.

Fibrinolytic Therapy Trialists Collaborative Group. Indications for fibrinolytic therapy in suspected acute myocardial infarction. *Lancet* 1994; 343: 311–322.

Faxon DP, Heger JW. Primary angioplasty—enduring the test of time. *N Engl J Med* 1999; 341: 1464–1465.

Freemantle N, Cleland J, Young P *et al*. β blockade after myocardial infarction: systematic review and meta regression. *BMJ* 1999: 318; 1730–1737.

The HOPE Study Investigators. Effects of an angiotensin converting-enzyme inhibitor, ramipril, on cardiovascular events in high-risk patients. *N Engl J Med* 2000; 342: 145–153.

http://www.dvla.gov.uk/at_a_glance/ch2_cardiovascular.htm

2.2 Cardiac arrhythmia

2.2.1 BRADYCARDIA

Aetiology

Virtually any condition that has a pathophysiological effect on the heart might affect normal electrophysiological properties and thus cause bradycardias. The more common conditions are listed in Table 15.

Pathology/pathophysiology

Sinoatrial dysfunction

- Abnormality of neurohormonal input to sinoatrial (SA) node, e.g. sympathetic/parasympathetic
- Abnormality of SA node leading to slow or failed conduction to atrial tissue.

Table 15 Possible causes of bradycardia.

Sinoatrial disease	Atrioventricular block
Ischaemic heart disease	Ischaemic heart disease
Idiopathic fibrosis	Aortic stenosis
Infective	Cardiomyopathy
Pericardial disease	Infection
Post-radiotherapy	Sarcoidosis
Post-cardiac surgery	Congenital
Trauma	Connective tissue disease
Amyloidosis	Antiarrhythmic drugs
	Post-radiotherapy
	Post-cardiac surgery
	Trauma
	Hypothermia

Table 16 Clinical classification of bradycardias.

Sinoatrial dysfunction	Atrioventricular block
Sinus bradycardia	First degree
Vasovagal syndrome	Second degree: Möbitz I (Wenckebach's)
Carotid sinus hypersensitivity	Second degree: Möbitz II
Junctional rhythm	Third degree: complete

Atrioventricular block

- Abnormality in conduction through AV node
- Failure to conduct rapidly throughout the ventricles.

Classification of bradycardias

Bradycardias can be divided clinically into SA dysfunction and AV block (Table 16).

Clinical presentation

Common

- Dizziness (presyncope)
- Syncope.

Uncommon

- Dyspnoea
- Exertional fatigue
- Heart failure.

Rare

Palpitations are unusual.

Physical signs

These include the following:
- Slow regular/irregular pulse
- Cannon waves in complete heart block
- Beat-to-beat variation in intensity of first heart sound in complete heart block
- Hypotension
- Pulmonary oedema

Consider carotid sinus massage to induce bradycardia.

 Do not perform carotid sinus massage on patients who have had a stroke or are known to have atherosclerotic carotid disease!

Investigations

In most cases the diagnosis will be made with one of the following:

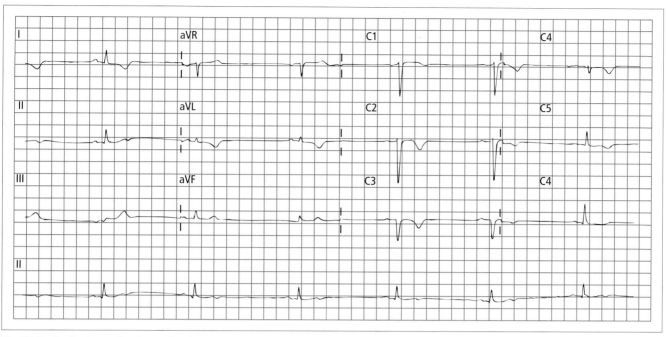

Fig. 37 Twelve-lead ECG of patient with ischaemic heart disease who presented with presyncope and was taking β blockers. Heart rate is <40/min.

- Twelve-lead ECG: see Section 3.1, p. 120
- Holter monitor: see Section 3.3, p. 127
- Patient-activated device
- Tilt-table testing.

Reversible causes of bradycardia:
- Hypothyroidism
- Drugs (Fig. 37)
- Hypothermia
- Electrolyte imbalance.

Treatment

Emergency/short term

In a patient with haemodynamic compromise consider the following:
- Intravenous atropine
- Temporary pacing: transvenous or transcutaneous (short-term measure).

Long term

Consider whether permanent pacemaker implantation is indicated. (See Section 3.5, p. 132.)

Zipes DP. Specific arrhythmias: diagnosis and treatment. In: Braumwald E (ed.) *Heart Disease: A textbook of cardiovascular medicine*, 5th edn. Philadelphia, PA: WB Saunders, Co., 1997: 863–876.

2.2.2 TACHYCARDIA

For practical purposes it is easiest to divide tachyarrhythmias into:
- Atrial fibrillation/flutter (AF)
- Atrioventricular nodal re-entry (AVNRT) and atrioventricular re-entry (AVRT) tachycardias
- Ventricular tachycardias (VT).

Aetiology/epidemiology

Atrial fibrillation/flutter

Atrial fibrillation affects 0.4% of the whole population affected, rising to 2–4% in people aged over 60 years and >11% in those over 75 years. Causes are numerous:
- IHD
- Congestive heart failure
- Valvular heart disease
- Hypertension
- Thyroid dysfunction
- Pulmonary abnormalities, e.g. pulmonary embolism
- Pericardial disease.

AVNRT/AVRT

This is the result of the presence of an additional conducting pathway, allowing a re-entry mechanism. In most cases, the electrical impulse is conducted antegradely (atrium to ventricle) via the AV node and retrogradely through the accessory pathway (concealed accessory pathway). If conduction is in an antegrade direction through the pathway, e.g. the Wolff–Parkinson–White syndrome, pre-excitation is seen on the surface ECG.

Ventricular tachycardias

Almost any pathological process affecting the ventricles may predispose to VT:
- MI (acute/chronic)
- Dilated cardiomyopathy
- Hypertrophic cardiomyopathy
- Valvular heart disease (especially aortic stenosis and mitral prolapse)
- Hypertension
- Congenital heart disease
- Long QT syndrome
- Cardiac tumours.

Pathophysiology/pathology

Tachyarrhythmias occur as a result of:
- Abnormal automaticity, e.g. VT after an MI
- Triggered activity, e.g. VT with long QT syndrome
- Re-entry, e.g. atrial fibrillation/flutter, AVRT/AVNRT, VT/ventricular fibrillation.

Clinical presentation

Common

- Palpitations
- Presyncope/syncope
- Breathlessness
- Chest pain.

Uncommon

Patients may complain only of lethargy.

Rare

Thromboembolism is unusual, except in AF.

Physical signs

Examination in sinus rhythm may be unremarkable. However, during tachycardia some physical signs may help to establish a diagnosis.

Atrial fibrillation/flutter

For the physical signs of AF, see Table 17.

Table 17 Clinical features distinguishing atrial fibrillation from atrial flutter.

	Atrial fibrillation	Atrial flutter
Pulse	Irregularly irregular	May be regular
JVP	Absence of 'a' waves	Rapid flutter waves
First heart sound	Variation in intensity	Constant intensity

JVP, jugular venous pressure.

AVNRT/AVRT

Physical signs are not especially helpful in making the diagnosis:
- Regular pulse
- JVP may be raised, but waveform is normal
- Constant intensity of first heart sound.

Ventricular tachycardias

Patients may or may not be significantly compromised:
- Hypotension
- Cannon waves.

Investigations

Investigations aim to exclude a structural thoracic/cardiac or metabolic cause: aside from an ECG, a chest radiograph, echocardiogram, thyroid function tests, renal function and electrolytes are appropriate in most cases.

Twelve-lead ECG

Documenting the arrhythmia with a 12-lead ECG will, in most cases, establish the diagnosis. In some cases where there is evidence of pre-excitation, the diagnosis can be relatively confidently made in sinus rhythm. Distinguishing some arrhythmias can be difficult:
- Atrial flutter versus atrial fibrillation: characteristic flutter waves (Figs 38 and 39)
- AVNRT versus AVRT: distinguishing these is rarely of clinical importance because, in most cases, the management is similar (Fig. 40)
- VT versus AVNRT/AVRT with aberrant conduction: see Section 3.1, p. 120.

Ambulatory monitoring

Documentation of an infrequent rhythm may be possible using 24-h Holter monitoring or patient-activated devices.

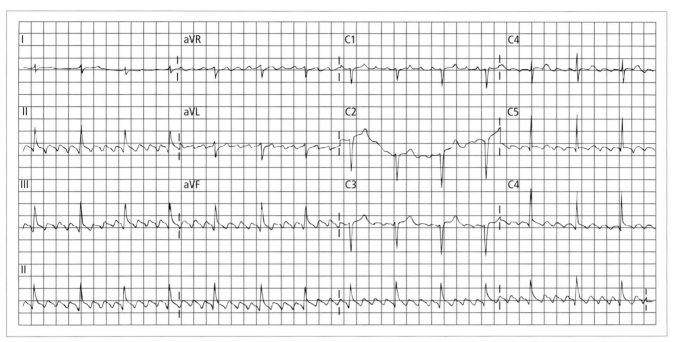

Fig. 38 ECG of atrial flutter: note the characteristic saw-tooth appearance of the baseline.

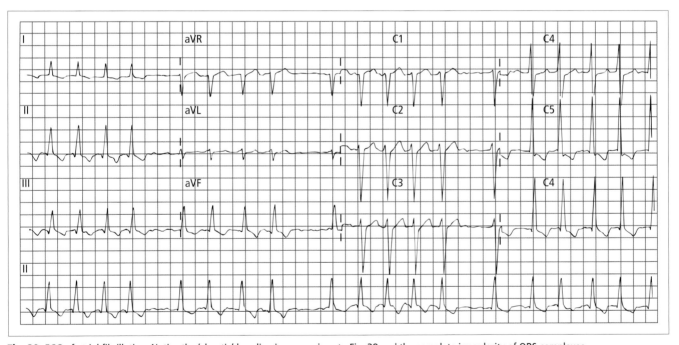

Fig. 39 ECG of atrial fibrillation. Notice the 'chaotic' baseline in comparison to Fig. 38 and the complete irregularity of QRS complexes.

Electrophysiological studies

See Section 3.2, p. 125.

Treatment

There are many different classifications of antiarrhythmic agents. The Vaughan–Williams classification is the most commonly used and is based on the cellular action of the drug (Table 18).

Emergency

Atrial fibrillation/flutter

If the patient is compromised, consider DC cardioversion or intravenous amiodarone.

AVNRT/AVRT

Most will respond to intravenous adenosine. Verapamil may be used if you are confident that the rhythm is not VT.

61

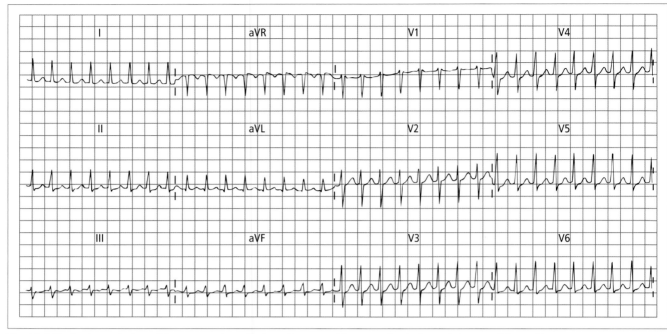

Fig. 40 ECG of atrioventricular nodal re-entry tachycardia. Note the very rapid rate, regular rhythm and absence of discernible P waves.

Table 18 Vaughan–Williams classification of antiarrhythmic drugs.

Category	Action		Example
1	A	Prolong action potential	Quinidine, procainamide, disopyramide
	B	Shorten action potential	Lidocaine, mexiletine
	C	Slow conduction	Propafenone
2	Block β-adrenergic receptors		Propranolol, atenolol, metoprolol
3	K⁺ channel blockers, prolong repolarization		Sotalol, amiodarone
4	Block slow calcium channels		Verapamil, diltiazem, nifedipine

Ventricular tachycardias

For resuscitation, see *Emergency medicine*, Section 1.1.

Short term

Atrial fibrillation/flutter

The main aim of treatment is the restoration of sinus rhythm. This may be achieved pharmacologically or electrically with DC cardioversion. In all cases, the risk of thromboembolism and the requirement to anticoagulate should be considered. Consider the following:
- Anticoagulation
- DC cardioversion
- Class III agent
- Digoxin (rate control only)
- Class I agent (if no coronary artery disease).

AVNRT/AVRT

- Class IA and IC agents
- Class II (β blockers)
- Class III (sotalol)
- Class IV (verapamil).

Ventricular tachycardias

- Class III agents
- Class I agents
- Class II agents
- Temporary pacing may prevent VT in patients with bradycardia-induced VT or long QT syndrome.

Long term

Most short-term drugs may be used long term, but more definitive therapies should be considered.

Atrial fibrillation/flutter

Consider the following:
- Anticoagulation
- Ablation for atrial flutter
- Ablation of AV node and permanent pacemaker for AF not controlled with drugs
- Implantable atrial defibrillator.

AVNRT/AVRT

Consider ablation (see Section 3.4.1, p. 130).

Ventricular tachycardias

Consider referral for ablation/ICD. (See Section 3.4, p. 130.)

DC cardioversion does the following:
• It terminates most arrhythmias secondary to re-entry mechanisms
• Depolarizing all excitable myocardium interrupts the re-entry circuit.

Cardioversion of atrial fibrillation/flutter

The following can be used as guidelines for anticoagulation:
• Duration <48 h: proceed without anticoagulation
• Duration >48 h: anticoagulation for 4–6 weeks before and 4 weeks after cardioversion
• Duration >48 h and no evidence of intracardiac thrombus on TOE: proceed without anticoagulation.

Sinus rhythm is achieved in approximately 85% of cases of atrial fibrillation/flutter, but recurrence rates may be high (up to 75% at 12 months).

Complications

Atrial fibrillation/flutter

Thromboembolism is the most significant and devastating condition.

AVNRT/AVRT

Complications are uncommon but, with the Wolff–Parkinson–White syndrome, rapid conduction of AF down an accessory pathway may precipitate ventricular fibrillation.

Ventricular tachycardias

Haemodynamic collapse and death is a potential risk in most cases of VT.

Prevention

Primary and secondary prevention of stroke/TIA. (See Section 2.14.1, p. 108.)

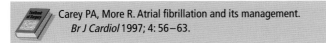
Carey PA, More R. Atrial fibrillation and its management. *Br J Cardiol* 1997; 4: 56–63.

2.3 Cardiac failure

Aetiology/pathophysiology/pathology

The common causes of heart failure are listed in Table 19.

After a single episode of cardiac damage, e.g. an MI, left ventricular dysfunction is often progressive even in the absence of further cardiac insults. This appears to result from the neurohumoral response to reduced cardiac output, which is initially compensatory but becomes detrimental in the long term (Fig. 41).

Epidemiology

The prevalence of heart failure is approximately 4 : 1000 (28 : 1000 at age >65). Heart failure is the primary diagnosis in about 4% of general medical admissions to hospital.

Increasing prevalence is the result of:
• an ageing population
• better survival after MI
• better survival with heart failure.

Clinical presentation

Heart failure commonly presents with the following:
• Exertional breathlessness
• Orthopnoea

Table 19 Causes of heart failure.

Cause	Relative frequency (%)
Ischaemic heart disease	40
Valve disease	9
Hypertension	6
Dilated cardiomyopathy/unknown	45

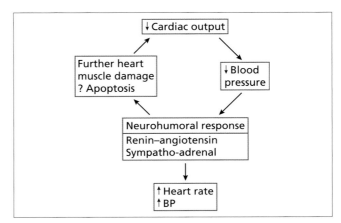

Fig. 41 The vicious cycle of progressive left ventricular damage.

- Paroxysmal nocturnal dyspnoea
- Cough productive of clear, frothy sputum
- Ankle swelling
- Fatigue.

 Severity of breathlessness in heart failure is graded according to the New York Heart Association (NYHA) class:
- NYHA I: impaired LV function but no symptoms
- NYHA II: breathless on vigorous exertion, e.g. walking briskly, walking uphill
- NYHA III: breathless during everyday activities, e.g. walking around the house
- NYHA IV: breathless at rest.

Physical signs

The physical signs include the following:
- Irregularly irregular pulse (AF)
- Elevated JVP (if up to angle of jaw suspect tricuspid regurgitation—check for systolic 'v' wave that coincides with contralateral carotid; check for pulsatile liver)
- Left parasternal heave (usually right ventricular hypertrophy, occasionally the result of greatly enlarged left atrium)
- Third heart sound (probably most sensitive and specific physical sign for LV dysfunction)
- Pansystolic murmur of functional mitral regurgitation
- Basal lung crackles
- Bilateral ankle oedema
- Ascites.

Investigations

Chest radiograph

Look for:
- heart size
- pulmonary oedema
- pleural effusions.

ECG

Look for:
- rhythm
- left atrial strain
- previous MI
- bundle-branch block.

Blood tests

- Urea and electrolytes: associated hyponatraemia, hypokalaemia (diuretic treatment), renal dysfunction
- Liver function tests: often mildly deranged in congestive cardiac failure.

Differential diagnosis

Consider the following:
- Cor pulmonale
- Nephrotic syndrome
- Liver failure.

Treatment

Emergency

In acute pulmonary oedema:
- sit up
- give oxygen (monitor blood gases)
- give intravenous diamorphine
- give intravenous furosemide (frusemide) 40–80 mg
- offload with intravenous infusion of nitrate titrated to maximum tolerated dose (but keep BP >90 mmHg systolic)
- check FBC, urea and electrolytes, cardiac enzymes
- consider pulmonary artery catheter, inotropic support or ventilation if these measures are unsuccessful.

Short term

Hospital treatment of congestive cardiac failure:
- Monitor fluid balance chart, daily weight (aim to lose 0.5–1 kg daily), and daily urea and electrolytes
- No-added-salt diet (but do not recommend a low-salt diet, which is extremely unpalatable)
- Intravenous loop diuretic, e.g. furosemide (frusemide) 80 mg once or twice daily
- ACE inhibitor (angiotensin II receptor blocker can be used if ACE inhibitor not tolerated)
- Consider anticoagulation (AF or grossly dilated left ventricle)
- Avoid calcium antagonists and NSAIDs.

If there is a good response, change to oral diuretics after 48 h. Aim to continue hospital treatment until the oedema is clearly improved, but in patients with impaired renal function it is better to accept some residual oedema than to precipitate acute-on-chronic renal failure. Do not use the JVP as the sole guide for treatment because this is often persistently elevated as a result of tricuspid regurgitation.

If weight loss is not satisfactory, add bendrofluazide 5 mg or metolazone 2.5–5 mg daily, but watch the renal function closely. If there is still no diuresis, consider higher doses of furosemide (frusemide) given by intravenous infusion over 2–6 h. Fluid restriction should be held in reserve for resistant cases. Rarely, inotropes (dopamine or dobutamine) are required for a few days to assist diuresis.

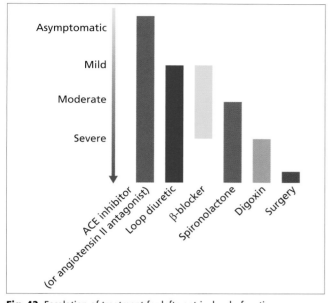

Fig. 42 Escalation of treatment for left ventricular dysfunction.

Long term

 You are a physician, doctor. You would promise life to a corpse if he could swallow pills. (Napolean Bonaparte)

Counselling the patient with heart failure can be very difficult as the prognosis is often poor. However, it is important to judge each case individually and not to give the patient unrealistic expectations.

Figure 42 shows long-term treatment options for those with heart failure. The following improve symptoms and life expectancy:
• ACE inhibitor in most patients.
• β Blocker, e.g. bisoprolol or carvedilol in patients with stable NYHA II or III symptoms. Start low, go slow. Hypotension should be dealt with by reducing the ACE inhibitor, fluid retention by increasing the loop diuretic. Try to continue the β blocker if at all possible, because these side effects are usually transient.
• Spironolactone in patients with NYHA III–IV and creatinine < 200 µmol/L, $K^+ < 5.5$ mmol/L. Check electrolytes weekly for 2 weeks and stop spironolactone if $K^+ > 6.0$ mmol/L.

Digoxin does not prolong life, but improves symptoms and reduces hospital admissions in more severe heart failure.

Cardiac transplantation is indicated for the following:
• Acute heart failure not responding to ventilation and inotropic support. A ventricular assist device (VAD—an artificial heart) may be used as a 'bridge to transplanta-

tion' if a suitable donor is not immediately available (Fig. 43). Heart function may improve (and transplantation be avoided) when 'rested' by one of these devices. However, use of a VAD is frequently complicated by thromboembolism and infection.
• Chronic progressive heart failure in patients with peak oxygen consumption (VO_{2max}) of <15 mL/kg/min during exercise (poor prognosis).

 … it is infinitely better to transplant a heart than to bury it so it can be devoured by worms. (Christiaan N. Barnard)

Complications

• AF
• VT
• Sudden death
• Progressive heart failure.

Prognosis

• Mortality related to ejection fraction and NYHA class
• Chronic stable heart failure: overall annual mortality rate = 10%
• Hospital series annual mortality rate = 30–50%
• Mortality rate of NYHA IV up to 60% in 1 year.

Prevention

Primary

• Prevention of MI (see Section 2.1, p. 51)
• Prompt reperfusion therapy for acute MI
• Avoid excess alcohol.

Secondary

ACE inhibitors, β blockers and spironolactone all reduce progression of heart failure and mortality.

Important information for patients:
• Advice about no-added-salt diet
• Moderate alcohol intake
• Avoid heavy lifting (potentially arrhythmogenic)
• May feel worse for a few days after starting β blocker
• Weigh daily and report to GP or increase diuretic if weight gain (>1 kg in 3 days or >2.5 kg in 2 weeks).

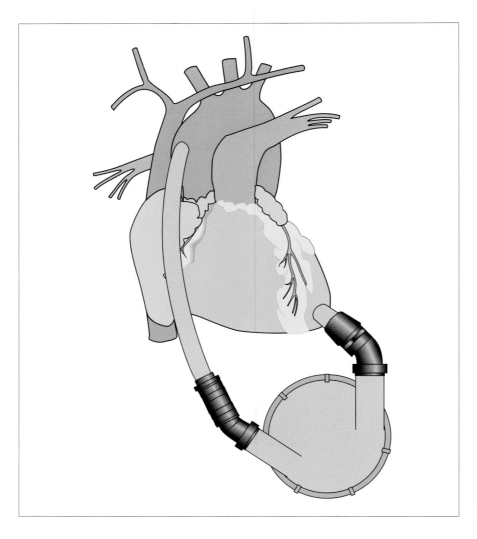

Fig. 43 Left ventricular assist device.

Houser SR, Lakatta EG. Function of the cardiac myocyte in the conundrum of end-stage, dilated human heart failure. *Circulation.* 1999; 99: 600–604.

Millane T, Jackson G, Gibbs CR *et al.* ABC of heart failure: acute and chronic management strategies. *BMJ* 2000; 320: 559–562.

Mann DL, Willerson JT. Left ventricular assist devices and the failing heart: a bridge to recovery, a permanent assist device, or a bridge too far? *Circulation* 1998; 98: 2367–2369.

Sharpe N. Benefit of beta-blockers for heart failure: proven in 1999. *Lancet* 1999; 353: 1988–1989.

2.4 Diseases of heart muscle

2.4.1 HYPERTROPHIC CARDIOMYOPATHY

Aetiology/pathophysiology/pathology

- Autosomal dominant
- Mutations found in at least eight genes (all encode contractile proteins, e.g. myosin β heavy chain, troponin T)
- Unexplained hypertrophy of the left (and occasionally the right) ventricle, which is usually focal, e.g. asymmetrical septal hypertrophy, apical hypertrophy
- Mechanism of hypertrophy unknown—possibly secondary to impaired function of contractile proteins (i.e. a compensatory phenomenon)
- Degree of hypertrophy variable even between individuals with the same mutation
- Left ventricular outflow tract obstruction may occur secondary to septal hypertrophy (Fig. 44)
- Mitral regurgitation may also be a feature, usually as a result of the Venturi effect in the presence of septal hypertrophy (Fig. 44).

Epidemiology

The prevalence of hypertrophic cardiomyopathy is 1 : 500 and it is the most common single-gene cardiac disorder.

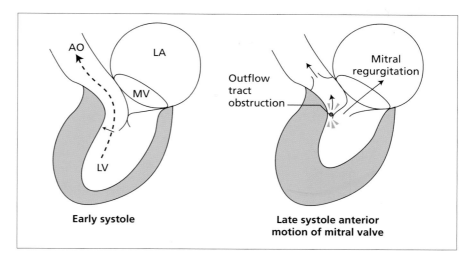

Fig. 44 Effect of asymmetrical septal hypertrophy in hypertrophic cardiomyopathy. In late systole, the septum contracts down on the outflow tract, obstructing flow and generating a gradient. This generates a negative pressure (Venturi effect) just proximal to the obstruction, sucking the mitral valve anteriorly (systolic anterior motion) and producing mitral regurgitation. AO, aorta; LA, left atrium; LV, left ventricle; MV, mitral valve.

Clinical presentation

Common

- Exertional chest pain
- Palpitations
- Asymptomatic murmur
- Abnormal ECG on screening.

Uncommon

- Syncope.

Rare

- Sudden death.

Physical signs

There may be no abnormal findings.

Common

- Jerky pulse
- Prominent apical impulse
- Systolic murmur at left lower sternal edge/apex.

Uncommon

- Fourth heart sound: often easier to feel (as a double apical impulse) than hear.

Investigations

The ECG and echocardiogram must be interpreted together because they provide complementary information.

ECG

The ECG is sensitive but not very specific. It varies from T-wave inversion to overt left ventricular hypertrophy.

Echocardiography

Echocardiography is specific but less sensitive than the ECG. Classically, there is asymmetrical septal hypertrophy with systolic anterior motion of the mitral valve leaflet, left ventricular outflow tract obstruction and secondary mitral regurgitation. Alternative patterns include apical, free wall or concentric LVH.

Twenty-four-h ECG

This is used to identify the cause of palpitations or detect asymptomatic arrhythmia.

Exercise ECG

This is used to provoke arrhythmia and assess the blood pressure response (important for prognosis or for vocational driving licence).

Magnetic resonance imaging

MRI may confirm the diagnosis if echocardiographic images are not clear (Fig. 45).

 It is possible to have hypertrophic cardiomyopathy without any hypertrophy. The diagnosis may be made on the family history plus an abnormal ECG.

Differential diagnosis

- Hypertensive cardiac hypertrophy: a concentric pattern of hypertrophy with documented hypertension.

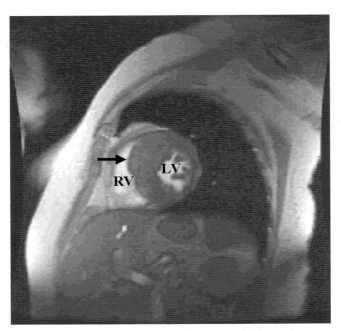

Fig. 45 Magnetic resonance imaging of the heart in the short axis, showing asymmetrical hypertrophy of the interventricular septum in hypertrophic cardiomyopathy (arrowed). LV, left ventricular cavity; RV, right ventricular cavity.

• Athlete's heart: differentiation may be difficult because some highly trained athletes, especially weight-lifters, rowers and cyclists, have an identical pattern of physiological hypertrophy. However, this will regress if training is discontinued. A septal thickness of >1.6 cm is likely to be pathological.

Treatment

No treatment is indicated in asymptomatic patients who do not have significant arrhythmia.

Antibiotic prophylaxis is generally recommended for dental and surgical procedures likely to produce a bacteraemia. Breathlessness and chest pain can be treated with β blockers or calcium antagonists, but often these only partially relieve symptoms. Severe breathlessness associated with an LV outflow tract gradient may be treated in a number of non-medical ways:

• Dual-chamber pacing: postulated to reduce gradient by activating the left ventricle from apex to base, so that the hypertrophied septum only contracts once most of the blood has been ejected from the left ventricle. Recent studies have been disappointing.

• Surgical myectomy: partial excision of the hypertrophied septum relieves gradient, but mortality rate is 1–2% at best.

• Percutaneous transluminal septal myocardial ablation is a promising new technique. A selected area of the obstructing septum is destroyed by alcohol injected into a carefully chosen septal artery (Fig. 46).

Complications

Common

• Atrial fibrillation: always anticoagulate because there is a high risk of thromboembolism. Often poorly tolerated, so consider cardioversion, with antiarrhythmic drugs to maintain sinus rhythm. Note that digoxin is contraindicated if there is significant LV outflow tract gradient (>50 mmHg), so use a β blocker or calcium antagonist for rate control.

Uncommon

• Ventricular tachycardia: give amiodarone—it may improve survival (although data from small retrospective studies). Consider ICD (see Section 3.4, p. 130).
• Progression to dilated cardiomyopathy: documented in up to 15% of early series, but certainly less common than this in modern practice.
• Sudden death.

Rare

• Endocarditis.

Prognosis

Risk of premature death associated with the following:
• Strong family history of sudden early death
• Diagnosis of hypertrophic cardiomyopathy in childhood
• Ventricular tachycardia on 24-h ECG monitoring
• Blood pressure drop on exercise
• Presence of certain high-risk mutations.

Disease associations

Friedreich's ataxia and the Wolff–Parkinson–White syndrome.

Important information for patients

Explain the following:
• It is an inherited condition
• There is a 50% chance of transmission to children
• It is benign in most cases, hence reassure low risk if appropriate
• Continue as far as possible with a normal life, but avoid competitive physical sports
• Seek medical advice in the event of palpitations, dizziness or blackouts
• Careful discussion before screening—no treatment is indicated in the absence of symptoms, and knowledge of the diagnosis will adversely affect life insurance, mortgages, etc.

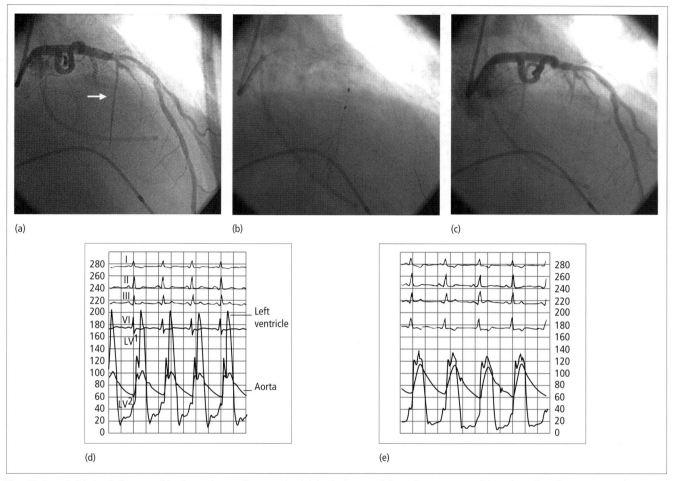

(a) (b) (c)

(d) (e)

Fig. 46 Septal ablation in hypertrophic obstructive cardiomyopathy. (a) A wire is passed through a coronary guide catheter into the target septal artery, indicated by arrow. A balloon catheter is passed, the wire is removed and the balloon inflated to occlude the artery. (b) Dye is injected down the lumen of the balloon catheter into the distal septal artery to confirm correct positioning. (c) Absolute alcohol is then injected to destroy selectively the septal artery, leaving a stump. Simultaneous pressure recordings reveal a left ventricular outflow tract gradient (peak ventricular minus peak aortic pressure) of approximately 100 mmHg (d) before the procedure, falling to (e) 15 mmHg afterwards.

Occupational aspects

Patients should not be professionals in sports requiring vigorous physical exertion. They may still hold vocational driving licences if they meet the DVLA criteria. (See Section 2.19, p. 118.)

McCully RB, Shen WK, Link MS *et al*. Extent of clinical improvement after surgical treatment of hypertrophic obstructive cardiomyopathy. *Circulation* 1996; 94: 467–471.

McKenna W, Oakley CM, Krikler DM *et al*. Improved survival with amiodarone in patients with hypertrophic cardiomyopathy and ventricular tachycardia. *Br Heart J* 1985; 53: 412–416.

Maron BJ, Nishimura RA, Tajik AJ *et al*. Efficacy of implantable cardioverter-defibrillators for the prevention of sudden death in patients with hypertrophic cardiomyopathy. *N Engl J Med* 2000; 342: 365–373.

Pelliccia A, Maron BJ, Spataro A *et al*. The upper limit of physiologic cardiac hypertrophy in highly trained élite athletes. *N Engl J Med* 1991; 324: 295–301.

Spirito P, Seidman CE, McKenna WJ *et al*. The management of hypertrophic cardiomyopathy. *N Engl J Med* 1997; 336: 775–785.

2.4.2 DILATED CARDIOMYOPATHY

Aetiology/pathophysiology/pathology

This is a chronic progressive disorder, of unknown aetiology, characterized by dilatation and systolic dysfunction of the left (and sometimes the right) ventricle. Some cases are probably the result of unrecognized alcohol abuse, 'burn-out' hypertension, or acute myocarditis. Familial dilated cardiomyo-pathy caused by mutations in cytoskeletal proteins has recently been described. Dilated cardiomyopathy also complicates muscular dystrophy.

Clinical presentation

This condition presents with congestive cardiac failure or arrhythmia (atrial or ventricular).

Investigations

The ECG often shows poor R-wave progression or LBBB. Echocardiography reveals a dilated left ventricle with globally impaired contraction. Focal areas of hypokinesia suggest ischaemic damage or prior myocarditis. Definitive diagnosis requires cardiac catheterization to ensure that there is no occult coronary disease.

Treatment/prognosis

See Section 2.3, p. 63.

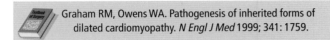

Graham RM, Owens WA. Pathogenesis of inherited forms of dilated cardiomyopathy. *N Engl J Med* 1999; 341: 1759.

2.4.3 RESTRICTIVE CARDIOMYOPATHY

Aetiology/pathophysiology/pathology

This is a chronic progressive condition characterized by excessively rigid ventricular walls that impair ventricular filling (diastolic dysfunction). Contractile (systolic) function is preserved. Causes are divided into the following:
• Myocardial, e.g. amyloid, sarcoid, storage diseases (often idiopathic)
• Endomyocardial, e.g. endomyocardial fibrosis, hypereosinophilic syndrome.

Epidemiology

This condition is rare in Western countries. Endomyocardial fibrosis is common in the tropics, particularly in Africa.

Clinical presentation

Symptoms

• Breathlessness, fatigue and ankle swelling.

Signs

• Elevated JVP, which rises on inspiration (Kussmaul's sign)
• Third and/or fourth heart sound

• Peripheral oedema
• Ascites.

Investigations

Chest radiograph

The heart size may be normal or increased. Pericardial calcification suggests constrictive pericarditis rather than restrictive cardiomyopathy. (See Section 2.6.3, p. 82.)

Echocardiography

Ventricular cavities are usually not dilated, but atrial cavities are often greatly enlarged. Rapid ventricular filling may be seen at the onset of diastole, which stops abruptly in early diastole.

Cardiac catheterization

Cardiac catheterization may be diagnostic in restrictive cardiomyopathy. Rapid ventricular filling in early diastole produces a 'square root sign' appearance of the LV diastolic pressure trace, which is also seen in pericardial constriction. However, other catheter data help differentiate the two conditions (Table 20).

Myocardial biopsy

This biopsy is sometimes useful to identify the cause of a restrictive cardiomyopathy.

Differential diagnosis

Restrictive cardiomyopathy must be distinguished from pericardial constriction, which is readily treated by surgery. Table 20 gives distinguishing features, but in up to 25% of patients it is not possible to tell and in these circumstances exploratory surgery may be justified.

Treatment

Response to medical treatment of heart failure is often poor. Successful combined heart and liver transplantation has been described in amyloid cardiomyopathy.

	Restrictive cardiomyopathy	Pericardial constriction
Third heart sound	Present	Absent
Pericardial calcification	Absent	In 50%
CT of the chest	Normal pericardium	Thickened pericardium
PA systolic pressure	Usually >50 mmHg	<50 mmHg
Diastolic pressure	LV > RV	LV = RV

Table 20 Differing features of restrictive cardiomyopathy and pericardial constriction.

LV, left ventricular; PA, pulmonary artery; RV, right ventricular.

Prognosis

The disease is generally relentlessly progressive with a high mortality.

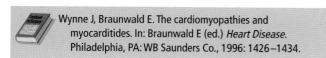

Wynne J, Braunwald E. The cardiomyopathies and myocarditides. In: Braunwald E (ed.) *Heart Disease.* Philadelphia, PA: WB Saunders Co., 1996: 1426–1434.

2.4.4 ACUTE MYOCARDITIS

See *Infectious diseases*, Section 1.9.

2.5 Valvular heart disease

2.5.1 AORTIC STENOSIS

Aetiology/pathophysiology/pathology

Senile: calcific/degenerative

This is the most common form of aortic stenosis, especially in those aged >65 years. Diabetes, hypercholesterolaemia and chronic renal failure are risk factors. Coexistent coronary artery disease is common.

Congenital bicuspid valve

Symptoms usually appear at the age of 40–50 years.

Rheumatic heart disease

This is an unusual cause of aortic stenosis.

Stenosis results from a combination of fibrosis and calcification, with additional commissural fusion in the case of rheumatic fever. The increased LV pressure load results in compensatory LV hypertrophy and a prolonged ejection time, with diastolic dysfunction, myocardial ischaemia and an increased risk of ventricular arrhythmias.

Clinical presentation

Common

Common symptoms are exertional angina, dyspnoea and syncope, and occasionally palpitations. There are symptoms of LV failure if presentation is late.

Uncommon

Embolic phenomena from calcific emboli. Gastrointestinal bleeding (idiopathic/angiodysplasia) may occur. May present with infective endocarditis.

Physical signs

 The murmur is not a guide to severity. Look for clinical signs that reflect the haemodynamic significance.

In mild aortic stenosis, there may be few signs aside from the classic ejection systolic murmur at the base of the heart, radiating to the carotids. When haemodynamically significant, other features include the following:
- Slow rising carotid pulse ± thrill
- Prominent 'a' wave in the JVP
- Undisplaced thrusting apex beat with LV heave
- Soft first heart sound with single (calcified valve) or reversed splitting of the second heart sound
- Fourth heart sound
- Soft early diastolic murmur may be heard.

In late presentation, classic signs may lessen and LV failure and secondary pulmonary hypertension dominate.

Investigations

ECG

- Look for LVH and, rarely, conduction disturbance.

Chest radiograph

- May be normal but suspect aortic regurgitation, LV dilatation or severe hypertrophy if cardiomegaly present.

Echocardiography

Two-dimensional echocardiography shows bicuspid valves, thickening and reduced mobility of leaflets and calcification (Fig. 47). Continuous wave Doppler allows quantification of the pressure drop across the aortic valve and the aortic valve area (Table 21).

Coronary angiography

Coronary angiography will be required in most cases to assess the coronary arteries before surgery.

 Consider the following in your differential diagnosis:
- Innocent systolic murmur: pregnancy, fever, anaemia, thyrotoxicosis
- Aortic sclerosis
- Hypertrophic obstructive cardiomyopathy
- Atrial or ventricular septal defect.

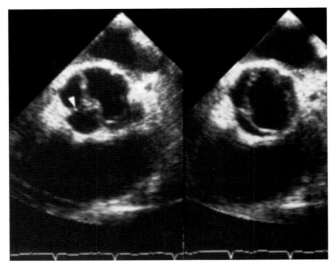

(a)

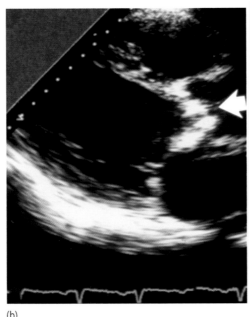

(b)

Fig. 47 (a) Bicuspid aortic valve with arrow indicating abnormal fusion of cusps. (b) Calcific aortic stenosis. In this parasternal long axis view, the aortic valve cusps (arrowed) appear markedly thickened and calcified. (Courtesy of Dr J Chambers.)

Table 21 Grading of aortic stenosis by aortic valve area.

Aortic stenosis	Aortic valve area (cm²)
Mild	>1.5
Moderate	1.1–1.5
Severe	≤0.8–1.0

Treatment

 Severe aortic stenosis is associated with a mean gradient of >70 mmHg. Note, however, that a lesser gradient can indicate critical stenosis if there is LV impairment.

Emergency

Admit the patient if there is heart failure and treat with diuretics. Exercise great caution with ACE inhibitors and other vasodilators, and never use them if the patient is hypotensive. Aim for early valve replacement as an emergency, if failure does not respond to treatment.

Long term

Follow moderate disease at yearly intervals with repeat echocardiography. Severe stenosis requires closer supervision to detect onset of symptoms. Antibiotic prophylaxis is required for dental procedures, etc. Valve replacement should be considered in all patients with severe aortic stenosis who become symptomatic. It is also indicated in asymptomatic patients who develop LV dysfunction.

Complications

The following are associated with aortic stenosis:
- Cardiac failure
- Sudden death
- Infective endocarditis
- Embolic disease
- Complete heart block.

Prognosis

Symptoms occur only after the stenosis has become severe. Mild aortic stenosis progresses to severe over 20 years in about 20% of cases, two-thirds remaining unchanged. Asymptomatic patients have an excellent prognosis. In symptomatic disease, the average survival with angina or syncope is 2–3 years, and with heart failure 1.5 years.

 Decena BF III, Tischler MD. Stress echocardiography in valvular heart disease. *Cardiol Clin* 1999; 17: 555–572.
Otto CM. Aortic stenosis: clinical evaluation and optimal timing of surgery. *Cardiol Clin* 1998; 16: 353–373.
Wierzbicki A, Shetty C. Aortic stenosis: an atherosclerotic disease? *J Heart Valve Dis* 1999; 8: 416–423.

2.5.2 AORTIC REGURGITATION

Aetiology/pathophysiology/pathology

Aortic regurgitation (AR) may result from primary disease of the valve leaflets, dilatation of the aortic root, loss of commissural support, failure of valve prosthesis, either alone or in combination. The result is the addition of a regurgitant volume to the normal inflow from the left atrium.

Aetiology of aortic regurgitation

Dilatation of the aortic root
- Degenerative (senile)
- Cystic medial necrosis: isolated/associated with Marfan's syndrome
- Aortic dissection
- Systemic hypertension
- Aortitis

Primary disease of valve leaflets
- Rheumatic heart disease
- Infective endocarditis
- Bicuspid valve
- Myxomatous degeneration
- Trauma

Loss of support of the aortic valve cusps
- High VSD
- Fallot's tetralogy

Failure of a prosthetic valve.

Clinical presentation

The patient may present with the following:
- Exertional dyspnoea
- Orthopnoea
- Paroxysmal nocturnal dyspnoea
- Palpitations and head pounding
- Angina.

Physical signs

Eponymous signs associated with aortic regurgitation:
- Quincke's: fingertip capillary bed pulsation
- de Musset's: head bobbing
- Corrigan's pulse: visible neck pulsations
- Müller's: uvular pulsations
- Duroziez's: systolic and diastolic murmurs heard over the femoral artery when compressed proximally or distally, respectively
- Traube's: pistol shot sounds over femoral arteries.

Examination in mild AR may be normal. More severe AR is associated with the following:
- Wide pulse pressure with a collapsing pulse
- Second heart sound single and loud; disappears in severe AR
- Displaced hyperdynamic apex beat ± systolic thrill
- Early diastolic murmur at left sternal edge: duration corresponds to severity
- Ejection systolic murmur ± third heart sound (increased flow)
- Austin Flint murmur: arising from mitral valve being struck by regurgitant blood.

Investigations

ECG

Look for the following:
- Normal/LVH
- Left atrial enlargement
- Prolongation of PR interval
- Non-specific ST segment and T-wave changes.

Chest radiograph

This is normal or shows cardiomegaly, which may be gross. There is pulmonary oedema in acute cases. Look out for evidence of aortic dissection.

Echocardiography

Two-dimensional echocardiography allows estimation of LV dimensions and ejection fraction, and determines the anatomy of the aortic valve and root. Dissection and endocarditis may be detected, but often require trans-oesophageal study. Continuous wave Doppler allows assessment of severity (Fig. 48).

Coronary angiography

Coronary angiography will be required before surgery to assess the coronary arteries in most cases.

Differential diagnosis

Consider pulmonary regurgitation and mitral stenosis with Graham Steell murmur.

Treatment

Emergency

In patients with acute severe AR or severe decompensated chronic AR, treat failure aggressively with diuretics

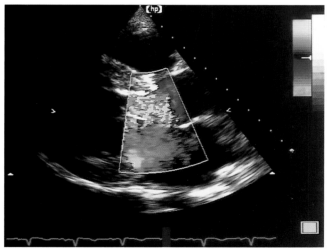

Fig. 48 Aortic regurgitation: in this parasternal long axis view, the broad regurgitant jet is seen mainly in blue. The diastolic timing can be seen from the lower velocity orange jet directly below, representing ventricular filling from the left atrium. (Courtesy of Dr J Chambers.)

± vasodilators ± inotropes. Look for the underlying cause and plan early or emergency valve replacement.

Short term

Treat heart failure with digitalis, diuretics and ACE inhibitors.

Long term

Patients with asymptomatic mild/moderate AR with normal ventricular function require regular monitoring only. Antibiotic prophylaxis is required.

Complications

Complications commonly encountered include the following:
- Progressive heart failure
- Mitral regurgitation
- AF
- Sudden death.

Prognosis

The risk of developing symptoms and/or LV dysfunction in severe AR with normal LV function is 4%/year. If there is LV dysfunction, the risk is >25%/year.

Prognosis is excellent in mild or moderate disease. In symptomatic severe AR the yearly mortality rate is >10%.

Carabello BA, Crawford FA Jr. Valvular heart disease. *N Engl J Med* 1997; 337: 32–41.
Bonow RO. Chronic aortic regurgitation: role of medical therapy and optimal timing for surgery. *Cardiol Clin* 1998; 16: 449–461.

2.5.3 MITRAL STENOSIS

Aetiology

Most mitral stenosis (MS) is acquired through rheumatic heart disease. It is more common in women, presenting in developed countries in the fourth or fifth decades of life.

Clinical presentation

Mitral stenosis commonly presents with the following:
- Exertional dyspnoea
- Orthopnoea
- Paroxysmal nocturnal dyspnoea
- Haemoptysis
- Palpitations
- Fatigue
- Weight loss
- Embolic phenomena in up to 15%.

Physical signs

Common

When MS becomes haemodynamically significant, common features include the following:
- Malar flush
- AF
- Undisplaced 'tapping' apex
- Left parasternal heave ± palpable opening snap and pulmonary second heart sound
- First heart sound may be loud
- Opening snap and mid-diastolic murmur, with presystolic murmur if in sinus rhythm
- Prominent 'v' waves and murmur suggestive of tricuspid regurgitation.

Uncommon

- Graham Steell murmur (pulmonary regurgitation)
- Presystolic murmur in AF
- Ascites, hepatomegaly, peripheral oedema.

Investigations

ECG

- Normal
- Left atrial enlargement or AF
- RVH.

Chest radiograph

- Normal
- Straightening of left cardiac border as a result of dilated left atrial appendage
- Pulmonary oedema
- Atrial double shadow along right cardiac border (Fig. 49).

Echocardiography

This provides a view of the valve and allows visualization of leaflet mobility, quantification of the valve area (Table 22), left atrial size and RV function. Doppler echocardiography allows assessment of the severity of the lesion, and estimation of the PAP. A transoesophageal study (TOE) is usually required to assess the suitability for valvuloplasty if this is being considered (Fig. 50).

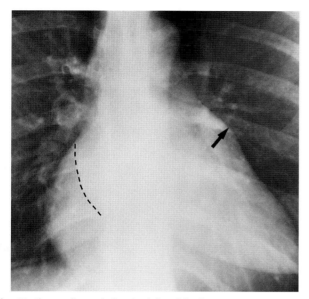

Fig. 49 Chest radiograph showing left atrial enlargement in a patient with mitral valve disease: note the double atrial shadow (left atrial border indicated by broken line) and dilatation of the left atrial appendage (arrow). Reproduced from Axford (ed.) *Medicine.* Oxford: Blackwell Science, 1996.

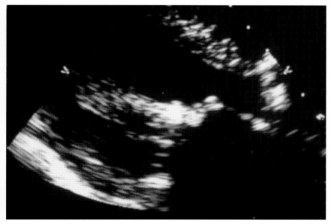

Fig. 50 Mitral stenosis: the tips of the valve leaflets and subvalvular apparatus have become thickened from rheumatic heart disease. (Courtesy of Dr J Chambers.)

Table 22 Severity of mitral stenosis assessed by mitral valve area.

Severity	Aortic valve area (cm²)
Mild	>1.5
Moderate	1.0–1.5
Severe	<1.0

Cardiac catheterization

This is used only if coexistent coronary artery disease is suspected.

Differential diagnosis

Consider the following:

- Austin Flint murmur
- Left atrial myxoma
- Tricuspid stenosis.

Treatment

Emergency

Treat acute pulmonary oedema with diuretics.

Short term

β Blockers or rate-limiting calcium antagonists may help symptoms. AF may require treatment (see Section 2.2.2, p. 59).

Long term

Formal anticoagulation with warfarin is required. Antibiotic prophylaxis is needed irrespective of severity. Surgical intervention is indicated if there is severe stenosis and > NYHA Class II symptoms: mitral valvuloplasty may be possible, alternatively open valvuloplasty or mitral valve replacement is required.

Complications

The following are possible:
- AF
- Pulmonary hypertension or infarction
- Chest infections
- Tricuspid regurgitation
- RV failure
- Thromboembolic disease.

Prognosis

In severe MS, 5-year survival rates range from 62% with NYHA Class III symptoms to 15% with Class IV. After valvotomy, 5-year survival rates are between 90 and 96%.

Lawrie GM. Mitral valve repair vs. replacement. Current recommendations and long-term results. *Cardiol Clin* 1998; 16: 437–448.
Bruce CJ, Nishimura RA. Newer advances in the diagnosis and treatment of mitral stenosis. *Curr Prob Cardiol* 1998; 23: 125–192.

2.5.4 MITRAL REGURGITATION

Aetiology/pathophysiology/pathology

Abnormalities of the mitral valve annulus, valve leaflets, chordae tendinae or papillary muscles may cause mitral regurgitation.

Common causes of mitral regurgitation in the adult

- Idiopathic mitral valve prolapse (MVP)—most common cause
- Papillary muscle dysfunction
- Ruptured chordae tendinae
- Annular dilatation
- Rheumatic heart disease
- Infective endocarditis
- ASD
- Failure of valve prosthesis/paraprosthetic leak.

Epidemiology

The prevalence of mitral valve prolapse varies from 1 to 6%, and is twice as common in women.

Clinical presentation

Common symptoms include exertional dyspnoea, orthopnoea, fatigue and lethargy. Occasionally, there are palpitations and, in severe acute mitral regurgitation, the patient may be very unwell with severe dyspnoea.

Physical signs

In mild disease, there are few signs apart from an apical pansystolic murmur radiating to the axilla. In more haemodynamically significant regurgitation, there can be the following:
- AF
- Laterally displaced, hyperdynamic apex beat with systolic thrill
- Left parasternal late systolic heave (atrial filling) in severe mitral regurgitation
- Soft first heart sound, wide splitting of second heart sound, third heart sound
- Late systolic murmur in association with a systolic click suggests MVP.

In acute severe mitral regurgitation, there is poor perfusion with pulmonary oedema.

Investigations

ECG

This may be normal, but look for AF, left atrial enlargement or LV hypertrophy.

Chest radiograph

This can be normal, or may show cardiomegaly with left atrial enlargement or mitral annular calcification (Fig. 51). There is pulmonary oedema in acute mitral regurgitation.

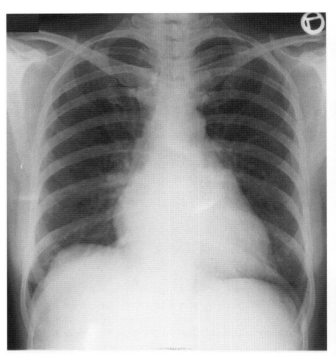

Fig. 51 Mitral annular calcification: a ring of calcification can be seen within the heart shadow.

Echocardiography

Assessment of severity is complex and the subject of some controversy. A transoesophageal study may be necessary to assess the feasibility of repair preoperatively, and in patients with acute mitral regurgitation (Fig. 52).

Coronary angiography

Coronary angiography may be required if there is a suspicion of coronary artery disease.

Treatment

Emergency

Treat acute pulmonary oedema and shock. Vasodilator therapy reduces the afterload and is of benefit. Intravenous nitroprusside may be life saving.

Short term

Symptomatic patients with severe mitral regurgitation who are awaiting surgery should receive diuretic and vasodilator therapy. Digitalis is of particular benefit in the treatment of AF, and anticoagulation will be required.

Long term

All patients must receive antibiotic prophylaxis. Mild-to-moderate disease requires monitoring only. Asymptomatic

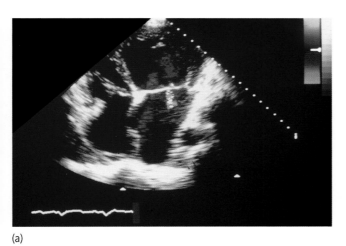

(a)

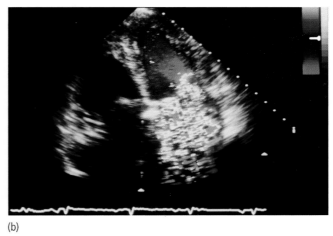

(b)

Fig. 52 (a) Mild and (b) severe mitral regurgitation. Note the difference in size of the regurgitant jets seen mainly as blue. (Courtesy of Dr J Chambers.)

patients with severe mitral regurgitation need closer follow-up to monitor LV function and symptom status.

Indications for surgery in severe mitral regurgitation:
- If surgical repair is possible, it should be considered in all patients aged <75 years who have a flail leaflet or persistent AF
- Deteriorating ventricular function (ejection fraction <60% or end-systolic diameter >45 mm)
- The presence of symptoms, although careful consideration of the aetiology and severity of LV dysfunction is needed in older patients.

Complications

The following are possible:
- LV failure
- AF
- Infective endocarditis
- Pulmonary hypertension
- RV failure
- Thromboembolism (more common in MVP)
- Sudden death (more common in flail leaflet).

Prognosis

Progression of mitral regurgitation depends on the aetiology, but develops in 15% of patients over a 10- to 15-year period with MVP. Without surgery, patients with severe mitral regurgitation have a 5-year survival rate as low as 45%. After surgery, the 5-year survival rates vary from 40% in mitral regurgitation caused by IHD to over 75% in rheumatic mitral valve disease.

Cooper HA, Gersh BJ. Treatment of chronic mitral regurgitation. *Am Heart J* 1998; 135(Pt 1): 925–936.
Quinones MA. Management of mitral regurgitation: optimal timing for surgery. *Cardiol Clin* 1998; 16: 421–435.

2.5.5 TRICUSPID VALVE DISEASE

Aetiology/pathophysiology/pathology

Tricuspid regurgitation (TR) is usually secondary to a combination of right ventricular dilatation and high pressure resulting from severe pulmonary hypertension. Tricuspid stenosis (TS) is almost invariably rheumatic in origin, and accompanies mitral stenosis. In both, right atrial enlargement and hypertrophy occur with the risk of AF.

Less common causes of tricuspid regurgitation:
- Infective endocarditis (especially drug addicts)
- Papillary muscle dysfunction
- Endocardial cushion defects
- Ebstein's anomaly
- Myxomatous degeneration causing prolapse
- Carcinoid syndrome.

Clinical presentation

This is usually asymptomatic, and in the case of TR usually discovered secondary to other more significant cardiac pathology. TR and TS may cause a sensation of neck pulsation, right upper quadrant discomfort and peripheral oedema. Occasionally, a low cardiac output syndrome comprising fatigue, weight loss and syncope may be present.

Physical signs

Tricuspid regurgitation causes prominent 'v' waves in the JVP, whereas TS causes prominent 'a' waves in sinus rhythm. In more severe cases, both cause pulsatile hepatomegaly, ascites and peripheral oedema. In TR, a pansystolic murmur which increases on inspiration and is heard best at the lower left sternal edge is usual. The corresponding murmur in TS is a presystolic murmur in sinus rhythm with mid-diastolic murmur.

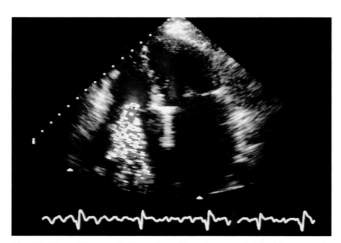

Fig. 53 Tricuspid regurgitation: a broad band seen mainly as blue extends back into the right atrium. (Courtesy of Dr J Chambers.)

Investigations

ECG

This is usually normal, but right atrial enlargement is a feature of tricuspid valve disease. There is evidence of RVH in TR.

Chest radiograph

- Often normal, but there may be an enlarged right atrium and superior vena cava in both TR and TS
- RV enlargement may be evident in TR.

Echocardiography

This gauges the severity and allows calculation of PAP from TR (Fig. 53).

Treatment

Both TR and TS are usually well tolerated irrespective of their severity. When TR is the result of a correctable left-sided cause, e.g. mitral valve disease, annuloplasty at the time of surgery is corrective. TS rarely requires valvotomy.

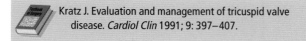 Kratz J. Evaluation and management of tricuspid valve disease. *Cardiol Clin* 1991; 9: 397–407.

2.5.6 PULMONARY VALVE DISEASE

Aetiology/pathophysiology/pathology

Pulmonary stenosis (PS) is usually congenital in origin, and may form part of Fallot's tetralogy. Rarely, it may be the result of rheumatic fever or the carcinoid syndrome. Pulmonary regurgitation (PR) invariably results from dilatation of the pulmonary annulus, which may occur with pulmonary hypertension. RVH and right atrial hypertrophy (RAH) result.

Clinical presentation

Both PR and mild PS are asymptomatic. More severe disease presents with a low cardiac output syndrome and right heart failure.

Physical signs

There is a characteristic harsh ejection systolic murmur at the left sternal edge in the second intercostal space, which is louder on inspiration. Other signs include the following:
- Prominent 'a' wave in JVP
- Thrill over pulmonary area, RV heave
- Soft pulmonary second heart sound
- RV fourth heart sound.

Pulmonary regurgitation is characterized by a decrescendo early diastolic murmur heard in the pulmonary area (Graham Steell murmur).

Investigations

ECG

This is normal, or there is RAH and RVH.

Chest radiograph

This is normal, or shows right atrial and ventricular enlargement.

Treatment

Pulmonary valvotomy may be necessary in severe PS. PR does not require treatment.

 Waller BF, Howard J, Fess S. Pathology of pulmonic valve stenosis and pure regurgitation. *Clin Cardiol* 1995; 18: 45–50.

2.6 Pericardial disease

2.6.1 ACUTE PERICARDITIS

Aetiology/pathophysiology/pathology

There are many causes of acute pericarditis (Table 23). In the developed world the cause of many cases is never established (idiopathic), but viral cause is often suspected,

Table 23 Causes of acute pericarditis.

Acute idiopathic pericarditis	
Infectious	Viral
	TB
	Other bacteria
	Fungi
Inflammatory	Post myocardial infarction/cardiotomy
	Autoimmune rheumatic disorder
Other	Neoplastic
	Uraemia
	Trauma
	Aortic dissection
	Hypothyroidism
	Irradiation
	Drugs, e.g. hydralazine

coxsackie B being most often incriminated. TB is a major cause in the developing world.

There is inflammation of the pericardium with infiltration of polymorphonuclear leucocytes, increased pericardial vascularity and deposition of fibrin. Inflammation can involve the superficial myocardium and fibrinous adhesions may form between the pericardium and epicardium, and between the pericardium and adjacent sternum and pleura. The visceral pleura may exude fluid, leading to pericardial effusion.

Clinical presentation

Common

- Chest pain: usually retrosternal or left precordial in location, radiating to the trapezius ridge and neck. The pain is aggravated by supine posture, coughing, deep inspiration and swallowing, and eased by sitting up and leaning forward. It may be preceded by a few days of malaise.
- Fever.

Uncommon

- Dyspnoea.
- Symptoms of any underlying cause.
- Acute epigastric pain mimicking an acute abdomen.
- Anginal type pain.
- Cardiac tamponade.

Physical signs

The patient may present with the following:
- Pericardial friction rub
- Fever
- Evidence of an underlying disease
- Signs associated with tamponade.

Investigations

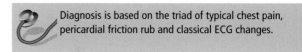

Diagnosis is based on the triad of typical chest pain, pericardial friction rub and classical ECG changes.

ECG

The ECG may be normal. There is an initial, widespread (not V1 or aVr), upwardly concave ST elevation, followed by return of the ST segments to baseline and flattened T waves. T waves then become inverted before returning to normal over 1 week. It is necessary to distinguish these changes from those of acute MI, in which ST elevation is convex and regional, R waves are lost, Q waves form, and conduction abnormalities may develop (Fig. 54).

Blood tests

Look for the following:
- Elevated white cell count, ESR, CRP
- Renal function to exclude uraemia
- Serial cardiac enzymes which may show a modest rise
- As directed by suspicion of underlying cause (Table 23).

Chest radiograph

This is often normal, but look for evidence of pericardial effusion, malignancy, TB or aortic dissection.

Echocardiography

Echocardiography is useful to exclude pericardial effusion or suspicion of aortic dissection.

Differential diagnosis

Consider the following:
- Acute coronary syndrome
- Aortic dissection
- Pulmonary embolism
- Musculoskeletal pain.

Treatment

Emergency

Pericardiocentesis if there is cardiac tamponade.

Short term

Admit if there is severe pain or large effusion, or for treatment of underlying condition. There should be bedrest,

79

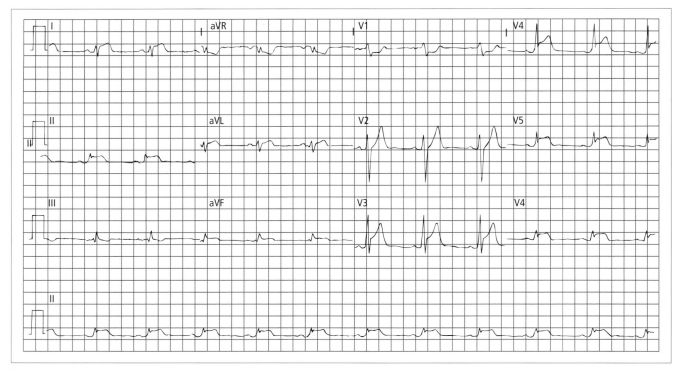

Fig. 54 ECG showing changes of acute pericarditis.

with oral NSAIDs given for symptomatic relief. Consider corticosteroids if there is severe pain not responding to NSAIDs after 48 h.

> Stop any oral anticoagulants because of the risk of intrapericardial haemorrhage and tamponade.

Long term

If idiopathic relapsing pericarditis develops, corticosteroids are traditionally used. More recently, colchicine has been gaining favour.

Complications

Beware of the following:
- Pericardial effusion
- Idiopathic relapsing pericarditis
- Cardiac tamponade
- Constrictive pericarditis.

Prognosis

There is complete resolution within 3 months in 80% of patients; 20% develop idiopathic relapsing pericarditis with chronic symptoms of pericardial inflammation. Cardiac tamponade may cause death if untreated, as may some of the precipitating conditions.

 Adler Y, Finkelstein Y, Guindo J *et al*. Colchicine treatment for recurrent pericarditis: a decade of experience. *Circulation* 1998; 97: 2183–2185.

Fowler NO. Recurrent pericarditis. *Cardiol Clin* 1990; 8: 621–626.

Maisch B. Pericardial diseases, with a focus on aetiology, pathogenesis, pathophysiology, new diagnostic imaging methods, and treatment. *Curr Opin Cardiol* 1994; 9: 379–388.

2.6.2 PERICARDIAL EFFUSION

Aetiology/pathophysiology/pathology

Pericardial effusion may develop in acute pericarditis from any cause. The normal pericardial space contains 15–50 mL fluid and can only accommodate a rapid increase in pericardial volume to 150–200 mL before the intrapericardial pressure (IPP) starts to rise. When accumulation of fluid occurs more gradually, volumes of up to 2 L may be present.

Acute cardiac tamponade typically follows cardiac trauma (which may be iatrogenic), aortic dissection, spontaneous bleeding or cardiac rupture after an MI. Chronic tamponade usually results from malignancy, idiopathic pericarditis or uraemia, although almost any cause of acute pericarditis may be responsible.

Clinical presentation

Common

In most cases, the IPP does not rise significantly and the

patient is asymptomatic, although a mild oppressive chest ache is occasionally present.

Uncommon

In a large pericardial effusion without tamponade, compression of adjacent structures may lead to the following:
- Dysphagia (oesophagus)
- Cough (bronchus/trachea)
- Hiccups (phrenic nerve)
- Hoarseness (laryngeal nerve)
- Abdominal bloating and nausea (abdominal viscera).

Physical signs

In most patients, the examination will be normal. In large effusions without tamponade, there may be muffled heart sounds, crackles (compression of lung parenchyma) or Ewart's sign (patch of dullness below the angle of the left scapula caused by compression of the base of the left lung). There may also be pericardial friction rub or signs of cardiac tamponade.

Cardiac tamponade may present in three ways:
1 Cardiac arrest
2 A severely ill patient who is stuporous or agitated and restless (survivor of acute tamponade)
3 With dyspnoea, chest pain, weight loss, anorexia and weakness (more slowly developing tamponade).

Rapid recognition of the clinical signs of tamponade is essential:
- Tachypnoea and tachycardia
- Pulsus paradoxus (pulse becomes impalpable on inspiration in severe cases)
- Elevated jugular venous pressure with prominent systolic *x* descent and absence of diastolic *y* descent
- Rarely, normal JVP in severe dehydration.

If you suspect the diagnosis—organize an urgent echocardiogram.

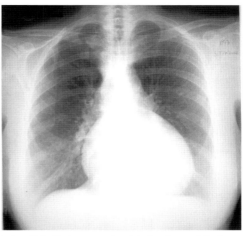

Fig. 55 Pericardial effusion: note the globular shape of the heart shadow.

Investigations

ECG

This is usually normal, although changes of acute pericarditis may be present. There may be a non-specific reduction in QRS voltage and T-wave flattening. Electrical alternans is suggestive of a large effusion.

Chest radiograph

This is often normal; a large effusion may cause an enlarged globular cardiac silhouette with clear lung fields. Look for separation of the pericardial fat lines and a left-sided pleural effusion (Fig. 55).

Echocardiography

Echocardiography is the most sensitive test for detection of pericardial fluid (as little as 20 mL). Diastolic left and right heart collapse suggest tamponade (Fig. 56).

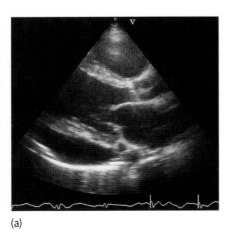
(a)

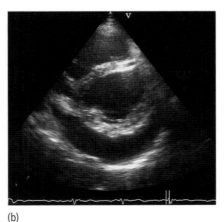
(b)

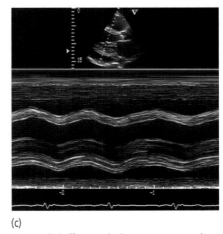
(c)

Fig. 56 Large pericardial effusion. (a) Parasternal long axis, (b) short axis and (c) M-mode views of a large pericardial effusion which appears as an echo-free space immediately adjacent to the heart. (Courtesy of J Harris.)

Pericardiocentesis

Pericardiocentesis is essential and urgent in cardiac tamponade. It is also needed for diagnosis if there is a suspicion of purulent or tuberculous pericarditis or prolonged and otherwise unexplained illness. Details are beyond the scope of this text.

Differential diagnosis

In chronic cases consider the following:
- Constrictive pericarditis
- Restrictive cardiomyopathy.

In those with tamponade, consider causes of circulatory collapse (see *Emergency medicine*, Sections 1.1 and 1.2), in particular massive PE and severe asthma.

Treatment

Consider the following:
- Urgent pericardiocentesis in tamponade
- Symptom relief as for acute pericarditis (see Section 2.6.1, p. 78)
- Recurrent or persistent symptomatic effusions may require balloon pericardiostomy or surgical pericardiectomy.

Complications

Common

Complications arise more commonly from the underlying conditions than from the effusion, although chronic pericardial effusion lasting more than 6 months may be seen. This is more likely after idiopathic, uraemic, myxoedematous or malignant pericarditis.

Uncommon

Uncommon complications are cardiac tamponade and constrictive pericarditis.

 Chong HH, Plotnick GD. Pericardial effusion and tamponade: evaluation, imaging modalities, and management. *Compr Ther* 1995; 21: 378–385.
Devlin GP, Smyth D, Charleson HA, Heaven DJ, McAlister HF. Balloon pericardiostomy: a new therapeutic option for malignant pericardial effusion. *Aust NZ Med* 1996; 26: 556–558.
Tsang TS, Oh JK, Seward JB. Diagnosis and management of cardiac tamponade in the era of echocardiography. *Clin Cardiol* 1999; 22: 446–452.

2.6.3 CONSTRICTIVE PERICARDITIS

Aetiology/pathophysiology/pathology

Constrictive pericarditis is characterized by an abnormally thickened and non-compliant pericardium, which limits ventricular filling in mid- to late diastole. This results in elevated cardiac filling pressures and the equalization of end-diastolic pressures of all four chambers. The clinical features are secondary to systemic venous congestion.

Before the 1960s, tuberculous constrictive pericarditis was the most common cause of pericardial constriction worldwide. In the developed world, its importance has declined, and the aetiology is usually idiopathic, post-radiotherapy or postsurgical.

Clinical presentation

Common

Oedema, abdominal swelling and discomfort caused by ascites or hepatic congestion are most frequent. Vague abdominal symptoms such as postprandial fullness, dyspepsia, flatulence and anorexia may also be present. Cachexia and fatigue suggest a reduced cardiac output.

Uncommon

Exertional dyspnoea and orthopnoea may occur when ventricular pressures become severely elevated, as may platypnoea (dyspnoea in upright position).

Physical signs

Common

Elevation of the JVP with prominent x and y descents is the most important clinical sign, plus the following:
- AF
- Kussmaul's sign (inspiratory rise in JVP)
- Pericardial knock (third heart sound)
- Hepatosplenomegaly, ascites and peripheral oedema
- Cachexia.

Uncommon

Uncommon complications are pulsus paradoxus and signs of severe liver failure.

Investigations

ECG

This may be normal or show non-specific generalized T-wave changes, low-voltage complexes or AF.

Chest radiograph

This is usually normal, but the cardiac silhouette may be either reduced or enlarged. Left atrial enlargement, pleural effusions and pericardial calcification are non-specific findings.

Echocardiography

Echocardiography shows pericardial thickening and abnormal diastolic filling.

Cardiac catheterization

This is usually needed to confirm the diagnosis, with characteristic equalization of end-diastolic pressures in the two ventricles, persisting with respiration and fluid challenge (Fig. 57).

CT/MRI

These imaging techniques may be used to demonstrate the extent and distribution of pericardial thickening (Fig. 58).

Others

As dictated by clinical suspicion of underlying cause. (See Section 2.6.1, p. 78.)

Differential diagnosis

Consider the following:
- Chronic pericardial effusion
- Restrictive cardiomyopathy: see Section 2.4.3, p. 70
- Superior vena caval obstruction: excluded if there is a pulsatile waveform in JVP
- Congestive cardiac failure
- Nephrotic syndrome
- Malignant hepatic or intra-abdominal disease.

Treatment

A minority of patients may be managed medically with diet and diuretic therapy. Most will require pericardiectomy: early operation is recommended.

Complications

Severe venous congestion with chronic hepatic impairment is common. Death results from the consequences of an inadequate cardiac output.

Prognosis

Morbidity

Without treatment, most patients deteriorate progressively

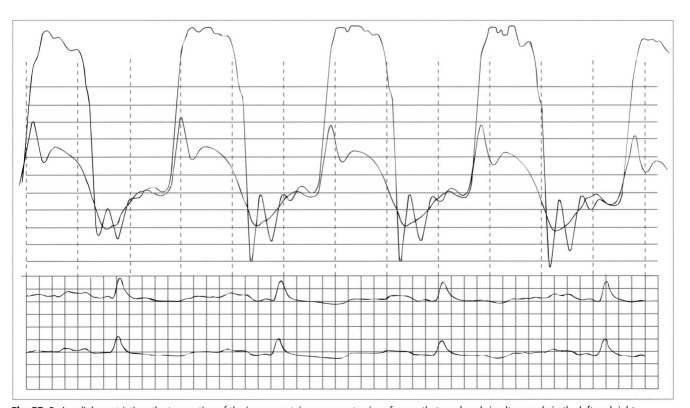

Fig. 57 Pericardial constriction: the top section of the image contains pressure tracings from catheters placed simultaneously in the left and right ventricles. The pressures from the two chambers are seen to equalize at the end of diastole. (Courtesy of E Tomsett.)

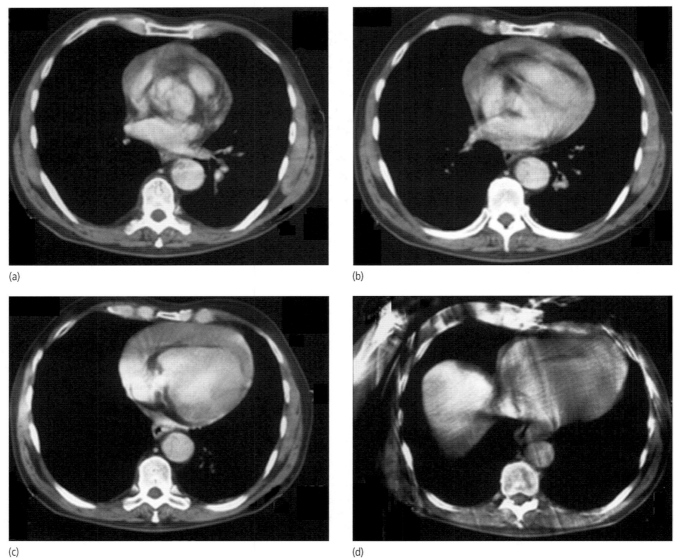

(a)

(b)

(c)

(d)

Fig. 58 Pericardial thickening: these sections (a, b, c and d) through the heart show a markedly thickened pericardium.

with severely limiting symptoms. With pericardiectomy, 90% improve and 50% may gain complete relief of symptoms.

Mortality

The outlook in untreated cases is poor. Hospital mortality rate after pericardiectomy is between 5 and 16%, and 5-year survival rate after surgery is between 74 and 87%.

Mehta A, Mehta M, Jain AC. Constrictive pericarditis. *Clin Cardiol* 1999; 22: 334–344.

Tuna IC, Danielson GK. Surgical management of pericardial diseases. *Cardiol Clin* 1990; 8: 683–696.

Vaitkus PT, Kussmaul WG. Constrictive pericarditis vs. restrictive cardiomyopathy: a reappraisal and update of diagnostic criteria. *Am Heart J* 1991; 122: 1431–1441.

2.7 Congenital heart disease

With advances in paediatric treatment a large number of individuals with congenital heart disease have now survived into adulthood (1 million in the USA). Conditions can be divided into cyanotic and acyanotic (see Table 24).

 Particular care should be taken to prevent infective endocarditis associated with dental or surgical procedures using appropriate prophylactic antibiotics. The highest risk is associated with high-pressure jets of blood:
- Tetralogy of Fallot
- Ebstein's anomaly
- VSD
- Patent ductus arteriosus
- Coarctation of the aorta.

Table 24 Congenital heart lesions.

Cyanotic	Acyanotic
Tetralogy of Fallot	Atrial septal defect (ASD)
Eisenmenger's	Ventricular septal defect (VSD)
Transposition of the great arteries	Patent ductus arteriosus
Ebstein's anomaly	Coarctation of the aorta

All lesions require echocardiography to determine anatomy and direction of shunts. MRI also gives detailed anatomical information. Most lesions require cardiac catheterization for calculation of the magnitude of the shunt and pulmonary vascular resistance. These investigations are not listed again under each individual section, unless there is a particular point to note.

The following are the complications of chronic cyanosis (right-to-left shunting causing hypoxaemia):

• Polycythaemia, causing hyperviscosity (symptoms—visual disturbance, headache, dizziness and paraesthesiae) and increased thrombotic risk
• Abnormal haemostasis and thus haemorrhagic risk
• Paradoxical embolism causing cerebral abscess or stroke.

Venesection and isovolumic replacement should be carried out only in patients with symptoms of hyperviscosity, not based on the haematocrit.

Some particular genetic conditions are associated with specific cardiac abnormalities (Table 25).

2.7.1 TETRALOGY OF FALLOT

Aetiology/pathophysiology/pathology

This consists of a large VSD, overriding of the aorta, right ventricular outflow tract obstruction (RVOTO) and RVH (Fig. 59). Left and right ventricular pressures are equal (large VSD) and so RVOTO causes right-to-left

Table 25 Examples of genetic diseases affecting the cardiovascular system.

Syndrome	Inheritance	Gene/chromosome	Cardiac manifestations	Management
Marfan's	AD	Fibrillin/15q	Aortic root dilatation/rupture	Echo surveillance, β blockade, elective aortic root repair when >5.5 cm diameter
Turner's		45 X0	Coarctation of the aorta, bicuspid aortic valve	Echo surveillance of valve, surgery for coarctation
Noonan's	AD	12q24	Pulmonary stenosis most common	
Down's		Trisomy 21	AV canal defects	Surgical
Di George	AD or sporadic	22q deletion	Conotruncal	Surgical
Williams		7 deletion	Supravalvar aortic stenosis	Echo surveillance
Holt–Oram	AD	TBX5/12q	Septal defects (hand–heart)	See Sections 2.7.5, p. 89, and 2.7.6, p. 90
Muscular dystrophies	Various	Various	Conduction defects, cardiomyopathy—may also be seen in female carriers of X-linked	Pacing for heart block, standard treatment for LV dysfunction, echo and ECG screening of carriers

See also cardiomyopathy (see Section 2.4, p. 66 and muscular dystrophies (see *Neurology*, Section 2.2.3). AD, autosomal dominant; LV, left ventricular.

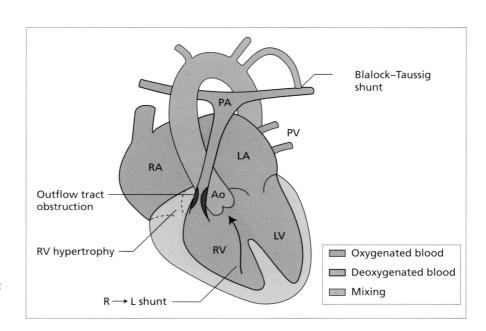

Fig. 59 Tetralogy of Fallot with left Blalock–Taussig shunt. Ao, aorta; LA, left atrium; LV, left ventricle; PA, pulmonary artery; PV, pulmonary veins; RA, right atrium; RV, right ventricle.

shunting (cyanosis), which increases with any decrease in systemic vascular resistance.

Epidemiology

This is the most common cyanotic congenital heart defect after infancy.

Clinical presentation

Presentation is with cyanosis from birth or early infancy; adults have limiting exertional dyspnoea and complications of chronic cyanosis.

Physical signs

Look for the following:
- Cyanosis
- Clubbing (Fig. 60)
- RV heave
- Normal S1, inaudible P2, RV outflow ejection systolic murmur ± thrill.

Investigations

- ECG: R-axis deviation and RVH
- Chest radiograph: boot-shaped heart.

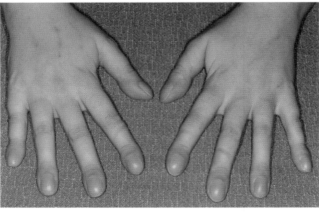

(a)

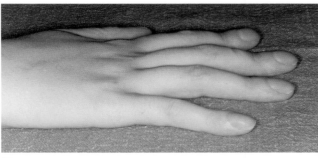

(b)

Fig. 60 Example of digital clubbing in a patient with cyanotic heart disease.

Treatment

Previously, treatment was with systemic-to-pulmonary artery shunts (e.g. Blalock–Taussig shunt—see Fig. 59) to increase pulmonary blood flow; older adult patients will therefore have these shunts. Currently, complete surgical correction is standard.

Complications

- Ventricular arrhythmias
- AF or atrial flutter
- Pulmonary regurgitation with RV dilatation and failure
- Recurrent RVOTO.

Prognosis

Without surgical repair, the survival rate is 66% at age 1 and 10% at age 20 years.

With complete surgical correction, the mortality rate is <3% in children, slightly higher in adults, with a small excess late mortality as a result of ventricular arrhythmias.

2.7.2 EISENMENGER'S SYNDROME

Aetiology/pathophysiology/pathology

A large left-to-right shunt causes increased pulmonary blood flow, resulting in vascular obstructive disease, pulmonary hypertension and RVH. As the pulmonary vascular resistance exceeds the systemic resistance the shunt is reversed, causing cyanosis (Fig. 61). This usually occurs during or after adolescence.

Clinical presentation

- Cyanosis
- Limiting exertional dyspnoea
- Palpitations (AF or atrial flutter)
- Haemoptysis
- Syncope and sudden death
- RV failure in advanced disease.

Physical signs

Look for the following:
- Cyanosis
- Clubbing
- RV heave and loud P2 (contrast with Fallot's tetralogy), right-sided S4
- Signs of tricuspid or pulmonary regurgitation.

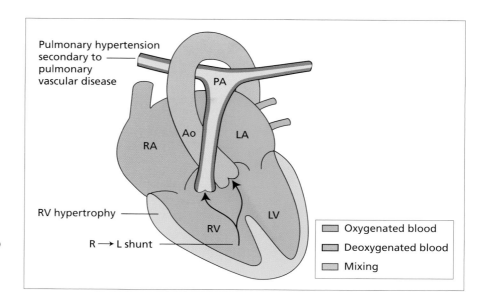

Fig. 61 Eisenmenger's syndrome secondary to ventricular septal defect. Ao, aorta; LA, left atrium; LV, left ventricle; PA, pulmonary artery; RA, right atrium; RV, right ventricle.

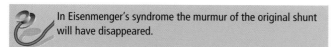
In Eisenmenger's syndrome the murmur of the original shunt will have disappeared.

Investigations

- Look for RVH ± atrial arrhythmias on the ECG.
- The chest radiograph may demonstrate prominent central pulmonary arteries and peripheral pruning.
- The response to pulmonary vasodilators on cardiac catheterization should be tested.

Treatment

See Section 2.12.1, p. 101. Avoid anticoagulants (existing coagulation abnormality) unless there is a very compelling indication for them.

Complications

Atrial arrhythmias and the complications of chronic cyanosis.

Prognosis

After diagnosis, the 10-year survival is 80% and the 25-year survival 40%. A poor prognosis is associated with the following:
- Syncope
- Signs of RV failure
- Low cardiac output
- Severe hypoxaemia.

Prevention

By closure of haemodynamically significant left-to-right shunts or protective pulmonary artery banding to reduce pulmonary flow before the development of pulmonary vascular disease.

Important information for patients

Avoid volume depletion, systemic vasodilators, altitude, heavy exertion and pregnancy.

2.7.3 TRANSPOSITION OF THE GREAT ARTERIES

Aetiology/pathophysiology/pathology

The aorta arises anteriorly from the right ventricle (the systemic ventricle) and the pulmonary artery from the left, so the two circulations are completely separate. A communication (foramen ovale, patent ductus arteriosus or septal defect) between them is necessary for survival (Fig. 62).

Clinical presentation

Clinical presentation is with cyanosis from birth, and LVF in infancy if the left-to-right shunt is large.

Physical signs

Signs are of cyanosis and a single loud S2 (anterior aorta).

Investigations

- The ECG may show right axis deviation and RVH.
- Look for cardiomegaly with increased pulmonary vascularity on the chest radiograph.

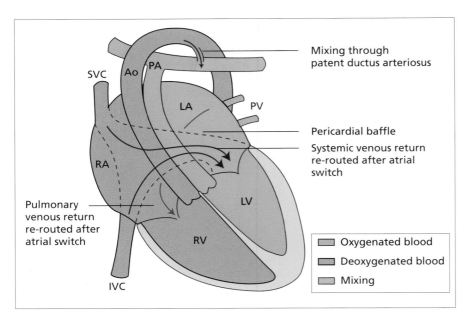

Fig. 62 Transposition of the great arteries with the circulations mixing through a patent ductus arteriosus. The effect of an atrial switch operation is shown in dashed lines, re-routing the venous return to the correct great vessel. In the arterial switch, the great vessels are transected above the valves and switched, with reimplantation of the coronaries. Ao, aorta; IVC, inferior vena cava; LA, left atrium; LV, left ventricle; PA, pulmonary artery; PV, pulmonary veins; RA, right atrium; RV, right ventricle; SVC, superior vena cava.

Treatment

Emergency

The need is to create or increase intracardiac mixing—prostaglandin E to maintain a patent ductus arteriosus and/or atrial septostomy.

Surgery

The treatment was previously by atrial switch (Mustard or Senning) in which the venous returns were re-routed through the atria (Fig. 62), so the physiological circulation was restored, but the right ventricle remained systemic and eventually failed. Currently, treatment is by arterial switch in neonates.

Prognosis

There is a mortality rate of 90% by 6 months without intervention.

2.7.4 EBSTEIN'S ANOMALY

Aetiology/pathophysiology/pathology

The tricuspid valve (regurgitant or stenotic) is displaced down into the right ventricle, leaving a small functional ventricle. Eighty per cent of these patients have an ASD or patent foramen ovale (PFO) and right-to-left shunting occurs if the right atrial pressure rises (Fig. 63).

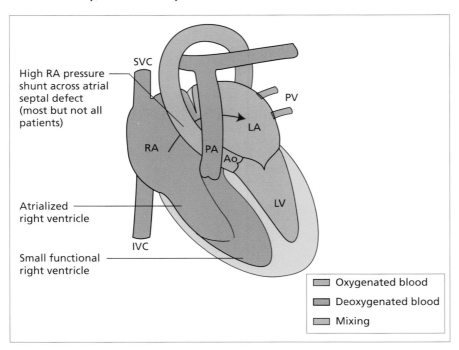

Fig. 63 Ebstein's anomaly with shunting across an associated atrial septal defect. Ao, aorta; IVC, inferior vena cava; LA, left atrium; LV, left ventricle; PA, pulmonary artery; PV, pulmonary veins; RA, right atrium; SVC, superior vena cava.

Clinical presentation

There is a wide spectrum of presentation, from an incidental finding to severe venous congestion and cyanosis.

Physical signs

Signs may include the following:
- Cyanosis
- Tricuspid regurgitation
- Hepatomegaly.

Investigations

Look for the following on the ECG:
- Tall/broad P waves
- RBBB
- First-degree heart block
- δ wave.

Treatment

- Diuretics and digoxin for LV failure
- Antiarrhythmics or ablation for arrhythmias
- Tricuspid repair/replacement and surgical closure of ASD.

Complications

Complications are atrial arrhythmias and/or accessory pathways (the Wolff–Parkinson–White syndrome).

2.7.5 ATRIAL SEPTAL DEFECT

Aetiology/pathophysiology/pathology

Atrial septal defects may be ostium primum, secundum or sinus venosus in type (Fig. 64). The haemodynamic consequences depend on the size of the defect; generally, blood shunts from the left atrium to the right because the right ventricle is more compliant than the left. The right ventricle may dilate and fail, or pulmonary hypertension and possibly Eisenmenger's syndrome develop.

 A patent foramen ovale is common in young people. It does not permit left-to-right shunting but allows right-to-left shunting when right atrial pressure exceeds left (e.g. Valsalva manoeuvre); opinion is divided about whether this represents an increased risk of stroke as a result of paradoxical embolism.

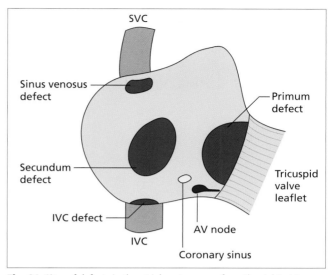

Fig. 64 Sites of defects in the atrial septum seen from the right atrium. AV, atrioventricular; IVC, inferior vena cava; SVC, superior vena cava.

Epidemiology

Atrial septal defects make up 30% of congenital heart disease detected in adults. Female : male = 2 : 1; 75% are ostium secundum.

Clinical presentation

The following are the most common presentations:
- Incidental finding
- Atrial arrhythmias
- Exertional fatigue or dyspnoea
- Right heart failure
- Paradoxical embolism.

Physical signs

Wide fixed splitting of S2 (equalization of RV and LV stroke volumes throughout the respiratory cycle). Pulmonary flow murmur (soft) and RV heave if there is a large shunt.

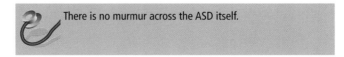 There is no murmur across the ASD itself.

Investigations

ECG

Look for the following:
- Right axis deviation and RBBB
- Left axis deviation in ostium primum defects
- Atrial arrhythmias.

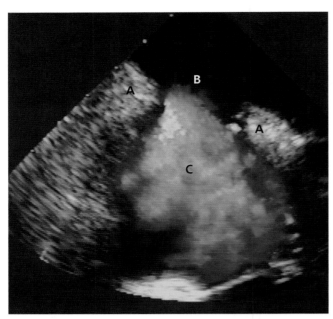

Fig. 65 Transoesophageal echo image of left-to-right flow across a large atrial septal defect. A denotes the atrial septum, B the left atrium and C the flow into the right atrium. (Courtesy of Dr LM Shapiro.)

Chest radiograph

Prominent pulmonary vasculature.

Echocardiography

Transoesophageal echocardiography is ideal with micro-bubble contrast to visualize shunting (Fig. 65).

Treatment

This consists of closure (surgical or percutaneous device) if the pulmonary : systemic flow ratio (shunt) is >1.5 : 1 and management of the complications, e.g. arrhythmias.

Prognosis

Shunt <1.5 : 1: excellent
Shunt >1.5 : 1: untreated—life expectancy 5th decade (RV failure, rarely Eisenmenger's syndrome).

2.7.6 VENTRICULAR SEPTAL DEFECT

Aetiology/pathophysiology/pathology

A small defect causes a high-pressure left-to-right jet but no haemodynamic abnormality, whereas a large shunt can eventually result in Eisenmenger's syndrome.

Epidemiology

This is the most common congenital heart lesion in children; one-third close by the age of 2 years.

Clinical presentation

Presentation is usually as an asymptomatic pansystolic murmur. If later, it presents with dyspnoea or cyanosis.

Physical signs

- Pansystolic murmur ± thrill at the lower left sternal edge
- Signs of pulmonary hypertension
- Clubbing and cyanosis of Eisenmenger's syndrome.

Treatment

The surgical closure of haemodynamically significant shunts, if the pulmonary hypertension is not already too severe.

2.7.7 PATENT DUCTUS ARTERIOSUS

Aetiology/pathophysiology/pathology

The ductus arteriosus is part of the lung bypass circuit in the fetal circulation, connecting the descending aorta to the left pulmonary artery (see Fig. 62). If it does not close as normal after birth, left-to-right shunting results.

Epidemiology

Patent ductus arteriosus (PDA) accounts for 10% of PDA in cases of congenital heart disease, with a higher incidence in maternal rubella or pre-term infants.

Clinical presentation

Patients present with the following:
- Small PDA: asymptomatic murmur
- Moderate or large shunt: fatigue, dyspnoea, palpitations or eventually Eisenmenger's syndrome.

Physical signs

Signs include the following:
- Continuous machinery murmur in the second left intercostal space
- Significant shunt: wide pulse pressure and hyperdynamic apex or (large shunt) signs of LV failure
- Pulmonary hypertension: machinery murmur shortens (as proportion of cardiac cycle during which pulmonary pressure < systemic reduces) and eventually disappears.

Investigations

ECG

This is abnormal only if there is a large shunt—left atrial (LA) and LV hypertrophy.

Chest radiograph

This is abnormal only if there is a large shunt—prominent proximal pulmonary arteries and ascending aorta, pulmonary plethora.

Treatment

Because of the ongoing risk of endocarditis, closure (surgical or percutaneous) is recommended in all cases except where pulmonary hypertension has already developed.

Complications

Infective pulmonary artery endarteritis and consequent septic pulmonary emboli. Ductal aneurysm and calcification can also occur with risk of rupture.

Prognosis

Without closure, one-third of patients will be dead by the age of 40 and two-thirds by 60.

Surgery generally does not require cardiopulmonary bypass and the mortality rate is very low (<0.5%).

2.7.8 COARCTATION OF THE AORTA

Aetiology/pathophysiology/pathology

A flow-limiting ridge extends into the lumen of the aorta at the site of the fetal ductus arteriosus (see Section 2.7.7, p. 90), usually just distal to the left subclavian artery (Fig. 66). An arterial supply to the lower body is achieved by extensive collateralization.

Epidemiology

This condition is more common in males than in females.

Clinical presentation

Common

• Asymptomatic: incidental finding of murmur or systolic hypertension in the arms.

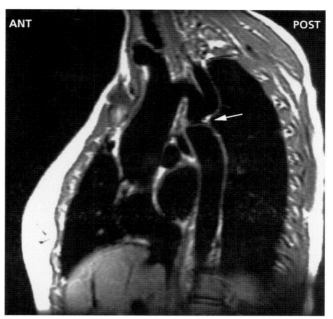

Fig. 66 Magnetic resonance imaging scan of coarctation of the aorta (arrowed).

Uncommon

• Symptoms of hypertension (epistaxis, headache)
• Palpitations
• Claudication in the legs.

Physical signs

The systolic pressure is usually greater in the arms than in the legs with weak and delayed femoral pulses. A harsh ejection systolic murmur (± thrill in suprasternal notch) may be heard along the left sternal edge and in the back.

Investigations

• Chest radiograph: notching of posterior third to eighth ribs (enlarged intercostal arteries because of collateral flow—Fig. 67), the site of the coarctation with pre- and poststenotic dilatation.
• CT, MRI or angiography to define lesion.

Treatment

• Surgical repair if the transcoarct gradient >30 mmHg
• Balloon dilatation carries a higher risk of aneurysm formation and is not established as a first-line treatment.

Complications

These may include the following:
• LV failure
• Aortic dissection
• Premature coronary disease.

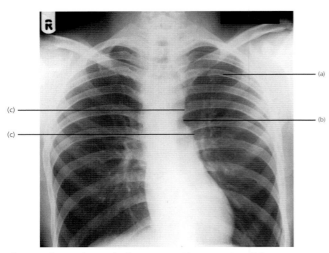

Fig. 67 Chest radiograph of a patient with coarctation of the aorta, showing rib notching (a), the site of the coarct (b) and pre and post stenotic dilatation (c). (Reproduced from Ray, Ryder, Wellings *An Aid to Radiology for the MRCP.* Oxford: Blackwell Science, 1999.)

Prognosis

- Uncorrected: 75% mortality rate by the age of 50 years
- Corrected: survival depends on the age at surgery—the younger the better.

Disease associations

- Turner's syndrome
- Bicuspid aortic valve.

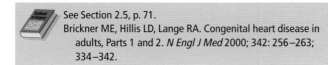

See Section 2.5, p. 71.
Brickner ME, Hillis LD, Lange RA. Congenital heart disease in adults, Parts 1 and 2. *N Engl J Med* 2000; 342: 256–263; 334–342.

2.8 Infective diseases of the heart

2.8.1 INFECTIVE ENDOCARDITIS

Aetiology/pathophysiology/pathology

Microbial infection of the endocardium usually affects the heart valves, less often at the site of a septal defect, chordae tendinae or mural endocardium. Prosthetic valves may also be infected. Infective endocarditis (IE) develops as a result of a two-stage process:

1 Non-bacterial thrombotic endocarditis (NBTE): a sterile mass arises from the deposition of platelets and fibrin on areas of endocardium injured from exposure to high-velocity jets, flow from a high- to low-pressure chamber or across a narrow orifice.

2 Trauma to the skin or mucosa, especially the oral mucosa,

precipitates a bacteraemia with organisms that have the capacity to adhere to the NBTE, leading to an infected vegetation. Bacteraemia rates are higher in the presence of diseased mucosa, especially if infected.

The consequences of IE vary from trivial to catastrophic valvular and paravalvular tissue destruction.

Epidemiology

The incidence of IE has declined in recent decades to 2 : 100 000 per year with an increase in average age to 47–64 years. Risk increases with age and IE is more common in men.

Clinical presentation

- Acute IE: rapid onset of high fever, rigors and prostration over days
- Subacute IE: insidious onset over weeks with fever, weight loss, myalgias/arthralgias and malaise.

Infective endocarditis may mimic a broad range of medical conditions that can obscure the diagnosis:

- New or worsening heart failure
- Neurological presentation secondary to cerebral abscess or embolus
- Pneumonia and pulmonary infarction in right-sided IE, or left-sided if a septal defect.

Physical signs

The main sign is fever, which is high grade in acute IE and low grade in subacute infections. Conjunctival, buccal or palatal petechial haemorrhages are quite common, unlike skin petechiae affecting the extremities. A new or changing heart murmur is characteristic. A fluctuating confusional state is frequent, especially in elderly people, and signs of embolization are only too common. The classic skin and nail signs of splinter haemorrhages, finger clubbing, Osler's nodes and Janeway's lesions are quite rare, as are Roth's spots. There may be heart block from the involvement of conducting tissue.

 Infective endocarditis must always be considered in a patient presenting with chronic fever, weight loss and malaise, irrespective of the presence of a murmur. Elderly patients may present with little apart from confusion. The absence of the much over-emphasized 'classic' signs of Janeway's lesions etc. does not exclude the diagnosis.

Investigations

Definite pathological diagnosis can be achieved only via isolation or culture of the bacteria from material obtained from a vegetation or abscess. This is not possible in most patients, and diagnosis depends on clinical criteria.

Table 26 Frequency of various organisms in infective endocarditis.

Organism	NVE (%)	IV drug abuse (%)	Early PVE (%)	Late PVE (%)
Viridans streptococci	35	5	<5	25
Enterococci	25	10	<5	<5
Staphylococcus aureus	23	50	20	10
Coagulase-negative staphylococci	<5	<5	30	20
Gram-negative bacteria	<5	5	20	10
Fungi, e.g. *Candida*	<5	5	10	5
Polymicrobial	<1	5	5	5
Other bacteria	<5	5	5	5
Culture negative	5–10	<5	<5	<5

IV, intravenous; NVE, native valve endocarditis; PVE, prosthetic valve endocarditis.

Blood tests

- Mild-to-moderate normochromic/normocytic anaemia
- Leucocytosis is usual in acute IE, but may be absent in the subacute infection
- CRP and ESR are usually elevated
- Positive rheumatoid factor and elevated γ-globulins are common.

Blood cultures

Three sets at least 1 h apart from three sites must be taken as a minimum in all patients (Table 26).

Urinalysis

Microscopic haematuria ± proteinuria are common, with heavy proteinuria and red cell casts an occasional finding, indicating glomerulonephritis.

Echocardiography

For suspected NVE, a transthoracic study is the investigation of choice. If inadequate, negative or non-diagnostic in a patient with a high suspicion of IE, TOE should be performed. TOE is the investigation of choice in suspected PVE (Fig. 68).

 Negative blood cultures may indicate suppression as a result of previous antibiotic therapy, fastidious organisms or an alternative diagnosis.

Treatment

Emergency

Treat embolic sequelae, heart failure (see Section 2.3) and septic shock (see *Emergency medicine*, Section 1.28). In an ill patient, antibiotics will need to be started before the culture results are available.

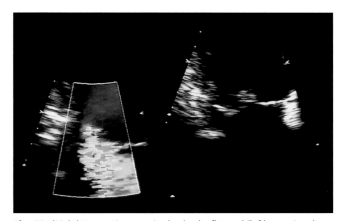

Fig. 68 (Right) Vegetation on mitral valve leaflet and (left) associated mitral regurgitation. (Courtesy of Dr J Chambers.)

Short term

Antibiotic treatment should be determined by the antibacterial sensitivities of the isolated organism with close liaison with your microbiologist (Table 27). Monitor for signs of continued infection—repeating cultures if necessary—changing murmurs, cardiac failure and embolic phenomena, and change venous access sites every 3–4 days. Carry out regular urinalysis and testing of renal and liver function, CRP and ESR, FBC and ECG. Weekly echocardiography should be performed. Check antibiotic levels regularly. Duration of therapy varies according to the severity of infection and organism. A total antibiotic course lasting 4–6 weeks is usually given, the first 2 weeks intravenously. Early valve replacement may be required if there has been severe damage, a compromise having to be made between adequate sterilization of the valve and the haemodynamic compromise secondary to valve destruction.

Long term

Follow-up of valve lesions will be required and patients must be made aware of the need for antibiotic prophylaxis.

Presentation	Antibiotic regimen
Gradual onset	Benzylpenillin 2.4 g 4-hourly i.v. + gentamicin 3 mg/kg/d in one to three divided doses guided by levels
Acute onset	Flucloxacillin 2 g 6-hourly i.v. + gentamicin 3 mg/kg/d in one to three divided doses guided by levels
Recent prosthetic valve	Vancomycin 15 mg/kg 12-hourly i.v. over 60 min guided by levels + gentamicin 3 mg/kg/d in one to three divided doses guided by levels + rifampicin 300 mg 12-hourly p.o.
Intravenous drug abuser	Vancomycin 15 mg/kg 12 hourly i.v. over 60 min guided by levels

Table 27 Antibiotic treatment for infective endocarditis. Modify when microbiological sensitivities are known.

Prognosis

In uncomplicated streptococcal NVE, the mortality rate is <10%, whereas aspergillus PVE is associated with virtually a 100% rate.

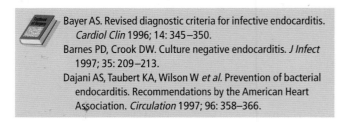

Bayer AS. Revised diagnostic criteria for infective endocarditis. *Cardiol Clin* 1996; 14: 345–350.
Barnes PD, Crook DW. Culture negative endocarditis. *J Infect* 1997; 35: 209–213.
Dajani AS, Taubert KA, Wilson W *et al.* Prevention of bacterial endocarditis. Recommendations by the American Heart Association. *Circulation* 1997; 96: 358–366.

2.8.2 RHEUMATIC FEVER

Aetiology/pathophysiology/pathology

Rheumatic fever results from an abnormal immune response to pharyngeal infection with group A β-haemolytic streptococci (GAS). There is evidence of a genetic predisposition with specific B-cell antibody D8/17 in >90%, and linkage with HLA-DR1, -2, -3 and -4.

Characteristic perivascular Aschoff's nodules have a widespread distribution in the connective tissues of joints, tendons and blood vessels. A pancarditis may develop, with endocardial inflammation affecting valve leaflets, chordae tendinae and papillary muscles. Fusion of leaflets and chordae leads most commonly to mitral stenosis, which is worsened further by the progressive fibrosis and eventual calcification that occur after the acute episode. Mitral regurgitation may occur and tricuspid involvement is seen in 10%. Aortic valve involvement more commonly leads to aortic regurgitation (Fig. 69).

Epidemiology

Rheumatic fever is rare in developed countries, with an incidence of <5 per 100 000 per year, usually between the ages of 4 and 18.

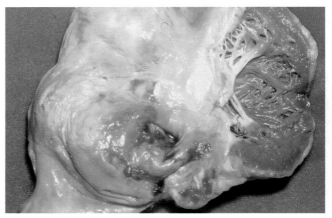

Fig. 69 Rheumatic mitral valve disease. The thickened and contracted mitral valve leaflets with the fish-mouth valve orifice can be seen in this postmortem specimen.

Table 28 Duckett–Jones criteria for diagnosis of rheumatic fever.

Major	Minor
Carditis	Fever
Migrating polyarthritis	Previous rheumatic fever
Chorea	Raised CRP or ESR
Erythema marginatum	Arthralgia
Subcutaneous nodules	Long PR interval

Diagnosis is based on evidence of antecedent streptococcal infection, e.g. positive throat swab for group A β-haemolytic streptococci (GAS), elevated streptococcal antibodies or a history of recent scarlet fever, together with either two or more major criteria or one major plus two minor criteria. CRP, C-reactive protein; ESR, erythrocyte sedimentation rate.

Clinical presentation/physical signs/investigations

See Table 28.

Blood cultures

These help to exclude infective endocarditis.

Blood tests

Look for the following:
• Anaemia and leucocytosis

- Elevated ESR and CRP
- Streptococcal serology.

ECG

- Normal
- May show prolonged PR interval.

Chest radiograph

This is either normal or shows cardiomegaly, pericardial effusion, pulmonary oedema or increased pulmonary vascularity.

Echocardiography

Echocardiography helps to exclude infective endocarditis, valvular abnormalities, myocardial dysfunction, pericarditis and pericardial effusion.

Consider the following in your differential diagnosis:
- Infective endocarditis
- Viral infection ± congenital cardiac abnormality
- Non-rheumatic acute streptococcal infections
- Juvenile chronic arthritis
- SLE
- Traumatic or septic arthritis
- Gout.

Treatment

Emergency

Treat heart failure (see Section 2.3, p. 63). Severe valve lesions with deteriorating cardiac function may rarely require valve replacement.

Short term

Bedrest eases joint pains. A 10-day course of oral/intramuscular penicillin (erythromycin in allergic patients) will eradicate the organism. Treatment with salicylates or steroids is symptomatic and does not affect the outcome.

Long term

Duration of anti-inflammatory therapy varies from 1 month in mild cases to 2–3 months in more severe ones. Taper steroid therapy at the end of the course with the substitution of aspirin to reduce rebound inflammation.

Prognosis

Joint pain and fever usually settle within 2 weeks. The risk of residual heart disease increases with the severity of the initial carditis, as does the risk of further damage during any rheumatic recurrence.

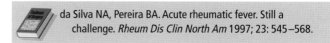

da Silva NA, Pereira BA. Acute rheumatic fever. Still a challenge. *Rheum Dis Clin North Am* 1997; 23: 545–568.

2.9 Cardiac tumours

Aetiology/pathophysiology/pathology

The only clinically important cardiac tumours in adults are malignant secondary deposits and myxoma. Cardiac metastases occur most commonly with lung and breast carcinomas and melanosarcomas. Of myxomas, 75% occur in the left atrium, with the remainder being mainly in the right atrium and rarely in the ventricles. They commonly arise from the endocardium at the border of the fossa ovalis as a pedunculated mass that may prolapse through the mitral orifice, mimicking mitral stenosis.

Epidemiology

Remember that myxomas are very rare tumours; they cause left atrial obstruction 200–400 times less commonly than mitral stenosis. It should therefore appear low down on any list of differential diagnoses, particularly as the typical presentation is relatively non-specific.

Prevalence of myxoma is estimated at 2 per 100 000 in the general population, most commonly at age 30–60 years, and with a female : male sex ratio of 2 : 1.

Clinical presentation

Non-specific symptoms such as exertional dyspnoea with fever and weight loss are the most common features of myxoma. Paroxysmal nocturnal dyspnoea, haemoptysis, dizziness and syncope may also occur. Embolic phenomena may lead to an erroneous diagnosis of endocarditis.

Malignant tumours usually present more acutely with the sudden development of heart failure or haemorrhagic pericardial effusion, various arrhythmias or heart block.

Physical signs

Fever, finger clubbing or anaemia reflects the chronic nature of myxoma. Auscultatory findings that mimic

(a)

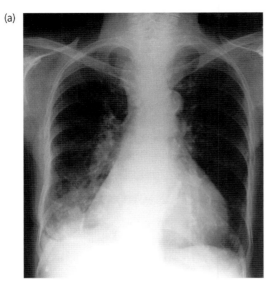

(b)

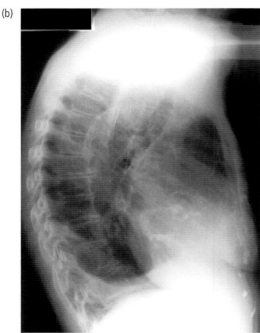

Fig. 70 Intracardiac calcification: (a) posteroanterior and (b) lateral views illustrating visible deposition of calcium within the heart.

mitral stenosis, with or without mitral regurgitation, may be present. These characteristically vary with posture, unlike primary valve disease. A friction rub or 'tumour plop' may also help to distinguish myxomas clinically. Clinical findings in malignant tumour deposits are dominated by the manner of acute deterioration.

Investigations

Blood tests

In myxoma these typically show anaemia of chronic disease, elevated white cell count, decreased platelet count,

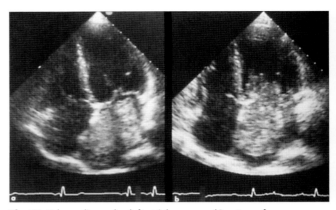

Fig. 71 Echocardiography: left atrial myxoma. (Courtesy of Dr J Chambers.)

elevated inflammatory markers (ESR/CRP) and increased γ-globulins.

Chest radiograph

A bizarre cardiac contour suggests a tumour. Sudden cardiac or pericardial enlargement, mediastinal lympadenopathy or irregular/indistinct cardiac border indicates malignancy. Intracardiac calcification may be seen in myxoma (Fig. 70).

Echocardiography

Echocardiography is usually diagnostic; occasionally a transoesophageal study may be required (Fig. 71).

Others

Cardiac catheterization and endomyocardial biopsy are occasionally helpful, as are other imaging techniques such as CT or MRI.

Differential diagnosis

Consider endocarditis and mitral valve disease.

Treatment

Palliative therapy is indicated for malignant cardiac deposits, with specific management of cardiac complications. The surgical removal of myxoma is curative.

Complications

Complications are thromboembolic disease and cardiac failure in myxoma. There can also be pericardial disease, heart failure, arrhythmias, or sudden death and heart block in malignant disease.

Prognosis

With complete removal of a myxoma, a normal lifespan should be expected. Recurrences are more likely with 'syndrome myxoma'.

Disease associations

Myxomas are familial, with autosomal dominant transmission in 10%—termed 'syndrome myxoma'.

 McAllister HA Jr, Hall RJ, Cooley DA. Tumors of the heart and pericardium. *Curr Prob Cardiol* 1999; 24: 57–116.

2.10 Traumatic heart disease

Traumatic heart disease is often fatal. Rapid diagnosis and intervention are vital in reducing both mortality and morbidity.

Aetiology

- Road traffic accident
- Assault
- Sports injuries
- Falls
- Kicks from animals.

Pathophysiology/pathology

Virtually all cardiac components may be affected by thoracic trauma. Trauma may cause the following:

Myocardium

Contusion (approximately 20% of patients after blunt trauma), laceration/pericardial tamponade or rupture (ventricles > atria).

Pericardium

Pericarditis, laceration or post-pericardiotomy syndrome.

Endocardium

Ruptured chordae/papillary muscles or valves.

Coronary arteries

Injury/rupture/thrombosis (the LAD artery most commonly).

Conduction system

Bundle-branch block, AV block or atrial/ventricular arrhythmias.

Clinical presentation

The initial insult is usually obvious and leads directly to presentation. Occasionally apparent minor trauma causes significant mediastinal injury, leading to a more insidious presentation:
- Chest pain (including angina)
- Presyncope/syncope.

Physical signs

Look for the following:
- Pulsus paradoxus
- Quiet heart sounds
- Pulmonary oedema
- Murmur/thrill of mitral regurgitation
- Diastolic murmur of aortic regurgitation if ascending aorta involved.

Investigations

ECG

Look specifically for the following:
- ST/T changes (usually non-specific)
- ST elevation secondary to pericarditis
- Acute MI
- Arrhythmias (AF, sinus tachycardia).

Cardiac enzymes

- Elevated CK-MB fraction (may be elevated if huge musculoskeletal trauma)
- Elevated troponin (T/I) (see Section 3.7, p. 136).

Chest radiograph

- Widened mediastinum (Fig. 72)
- Ribs/sternal fracture
- Haemothorax.

Echocardiography (transthoracic and transoesophageal)

- Pericardial effusion
- Abnormal wall motion (contusion)
- TOE best for identifying myocardial injury and valvular involvement.

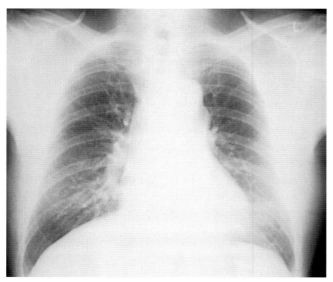

Fig. 72 Chest radiograph of patient with traumatic aortic rupture. Note the widened mediastinum and abnormal descending aortic outline.

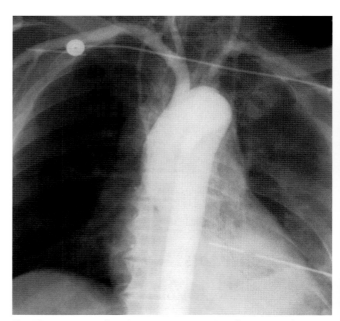

Fig. 73 Aortogram of aortic rupture/trans-section. The aortic outline is clearly irregular, representing aortic rupture.

 TOE is contraindicated in the following:
- Severe facial trauma
- Cervical spinal injury
- Possible oesophageal injury.

Aortography

Aortography is usually considered the 'gold standard' for diagnosing aortic trauma (Fig. 73). Damage is most commonly seen in the upper descending aorta—the site of the ligamentum arteriosum.

Computed tomography

Computed tomography may identify surrounding haematoma, but will not always establish the integrity of the aorta.

Radionuclide imaging

Reduced myocardial perfusion with contusion or ischaemia secondary to coronary thrombosis may be demonstrated.

Treatment

Emergency

If there is haemodynamic compromise, consider urgent pericardiocentesis/operative intervention for pericardial tamponade. If there is any doubt, seek immediate contact with a cardiothoracic surgical centre.

Short term

High risk

Monitor initially and mobilize gently.

Low risk

Early gentle mobilization.

Long term

Long-term treatment may require further cardiac evaluation with radionuclide imaging/cardiac catheterization.

 Risk stratification after chest trauma
- Minor trauma and normal/abnormal ECG: relatively low risk
- Major trauma with associated thoracic or extrathoracic injuries and normal/abnormal ECG: relatively high risk.

 Always consider aortic rupture when serious thoracic injuries have occurred

- 80% mortality rate
- often have back pain as well as chest pain
- high risk group: head-on collision at speed, ejection from vehicle, death of other person involved, fall from great height
- >50% have the following triad: increased arterial pressure/pulse amplitude in upper limbs; reduced arterial pressure/pulse amplitude in lower limbs; widened mediastinum on chest radiograph
- definitive investigation is aortography
- immediate surgical repair required
- intravenous β blockers reduce aortic wall stresses as interim measure before surgery.

Banning AP, Pillai R. Non-penetrating cardiac and aortic trauma. *Heart* 1997; 78: 226–229.

Olsovsky MR, Wechsler AS, Topaz O. Cardiac trauma diagnosis, management, and current therapy. *Angiology* 1997; 48: 423–432.

Pretre R, Chilcott M. Blunt trauma to the heart and great vessels. *N Engl J Med* 1997; 336: 626–632.

2.11 Diseases of systemic arteries

2.11.1 AORTIC DISSECTION

Aetiology/pathophysiology/pathology

The aortic intima tears, exposing a diseased media that is split in two longitudinally by the force of blood flow. This dissection usually progresses distally for a variable distance. Medial degeneration is often idiopathic but may be the result of cystic medial necrosis, especially in Marfan's syndrome. There is also an association with the following:

- Hypertension (history of hypertension in 80% of cases)
- Pregnancy
- Trauma.

Aortic dissection is classified according to whether or not there is involvement of the ascending aorta (Stanford classification—Fig. 74). This has practical and prognostic implications.

Epidemiology

- Peak age >60 years
- Male : female = 2 : 1.

Clinical presentation

Common

There is central chest pain in 90%—classically a tearing pain that migrates to the back (interscapular) as dissection proceeds. A dissected aorta found incidentally in a patient without pain is usually chronic and therefore low risk. Thoracic back pain of sudden onset is also common.

Uncommon

- Syncope
- Stroke
- Acute pulmonary oedema
- Electromechanical dissociation (EMD) arrest.

Physical signs

Common

- Hypotension
- Unequal radial pulses or brachial blood pressures (found in 50% of proximal dissections)
- Aortic regurgitation
- Pericardial rub
- Pleural effusion

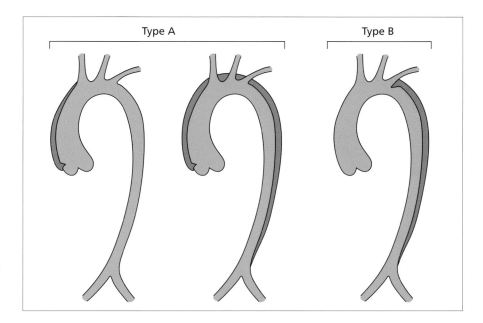

Fig. 74 Stanford classification of aortic dissection. Type A refers to dissection of the ascending aorta, with or without involvement of the descending aorta. In type B, dissection is confined to the descending aorta. This classification has implications for prognosis and treatment.

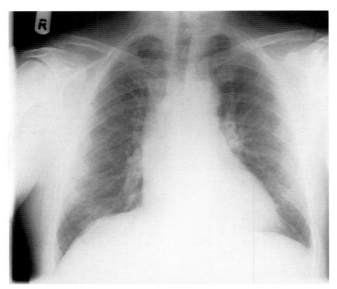

Fig. 75 Chest radiograph showing widened mediastinum. Blood in the pleural space from a leaking aorta may show as an effusion.

- Tamponade (see Section 2.6.2, p. 80)
- Hemiplegia.

Investigations

ECG

The ECG may reveal inferior MI (if dissection extends to the right coronary artery). Anterior infarction is rarely seen, perhaps because occlusion of the left main coronary artery results in such a big infarct that the patient does not reach hospital alive.

Chest radiograph

This may show widened mediastinum (Fig. 75), but an absence of this does not rule out aortic dissection. Blood in the pleural space from a leaking aorta may show as an effusion.

Echocardiography

The diagnosis is suggested by the following:
- Dilated aortic root
- Aortic regurgitation
- Pericardial effusion
- Dissection flap in the ascending aorta (unusual).

Other investigations

Consider the following:
- CT scan of the chest with contrast
- Aortography
- MRI
- TOE (Fig. 76).

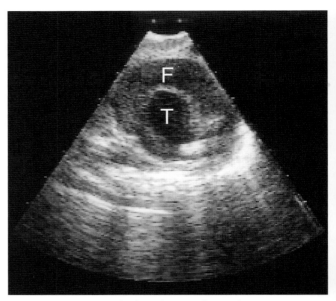

Fig. 76 Transoesophageal echocardiogram of aortic dissection demonstrating the true (T) and false (F) lumina in the descending aorta. (From Armstrong P, Wastie ML. *Diagnostic Imaging* (4th edn). Oxford: Blackwell Science, 1998.)

The differential diagnosis of aortic dissection should include the following:
- MI/unstable angina
- Thoracic vertebral pathology, e.g. fracture, discitis
- Pulmonary embolism.

Treatment

Emergency

- Do not await confirmation of diagnosis before starting medical treatment
- Transfer to the CCU
- Lower systolic blood pressure to <120 mmHg with intravenous labetolol or sodium nitroprusside
- If confirmatory imaging cannot be obtained quickly, arrange urgent transfer to cardiothoracic centre
- Type A dissection requires emergency repair unless chronic (>2 weeks)
- Type B dissection is generally managed medically because risks of surgery outweigh benefits. Consider surgery if there is a rupture or vital organ/limb ischaemia.

Short term

After 24 h, begin transfer of blood pressure control to oral agents, e.g. β blocker, ACE inhibitor or calcium antagonist.

Complications

Death caused by aortic rupture or tamponade is common. Occlusion of any of the major aortic branches may occur, producing the following:
- Hemiplegia
- Acute renal failure
- Mesenteric ischaemia
- Lower limb ischaemia.

Prognosis

There is an early mortality rate of 1% per hour if left untreated. The mortality rate in the first 2 weeks is about 80%, after which a dissection would be classed as chronic.

 Treasure T, Raphael MJ. Investigation of suspected dissection of the thoracic aorta. *Lancet* 1991; 338: 490–495.

2.12 Diseases of pulmonary arteries

2.12.1 PRIMARY PULMONARY HYPERTENSION

Primary pulmonary hypertension is defined as a sustained elevation of pulmonary artery pressure (PAP) to a mean of more than 25 mmHg at rest or 30 mmHg with exercise, in the absence of a demonstrable cause.

Aetiology/pathophysiology/pathology

The aetiology is unknown. The following have been suggested:
- Genetic: 10% of cases are familial (localized to chromosome 2) with autosomal dominant inheritance and genetic anticipation (a feature of trinucleotide repeat sequence disorders).
- Autoimmune.
- Pulmonary vascular endothelial dysfunction: this may be cause or effect.

Similar pulmonary vascular disease is seen in patients with portal hypertension, HIV infection or a history of cocaine or appetite-suppressant use.

Increased pulmonary vascular resistance is produced by:
- Vasoconstriction (increased thromboxane and endothelin, decreased prostacyclin and nitric oxide)
- Vascular wall remodelling (medial hypertrophy and smooth muscle proliferation)
- Thrombosis *in situ*.

This results in right ventricular hypertrophy (RVH), then failure, as a result of increased afterload.

Epidemiology

Incidence is about 1 per million per year, with use of appetite suppressants associated with a greater than 20-fold increased risk. Female : male is 2 : 1, with most diagnoses made in the fourth decade.

Clinical presentation

 Early symptoms of primary pulmonary hypertension (PPH) are non-specific.

Common
- Exertional dyspnoea
- Fatigue
- Angina (right ventricular ischaemia)
- Syncope/near syncope, especially exertional.

Uncommon
- Peripheral oedema
- Raynaud's phenomenon—mostly in women
- Haemoptysis.

Physical signs
- Loud P2 (pulmonary component of second heart sound)
- S4 originating from the right ventricle (pressure overload)
- Left parasternal heave
- Pansystolic murmur, prominent jugular 'v' waves and pulsatile liver of tricuspid regurgitation
- Peripheral oedema and elevated JVP of RV failure (RVF).

 Clubbing is not a feature of PPH and, if present, may indicate lung disease or cyanotic congenital heart disease as the underlying cause of the pulmonary hypertension.

Investigations

To confirm pulmonary hypertension, determine prognosis and guide therapy.

Echocardiogram
- Dilated and/or hypertrophied right heart
- Measurement of PAP

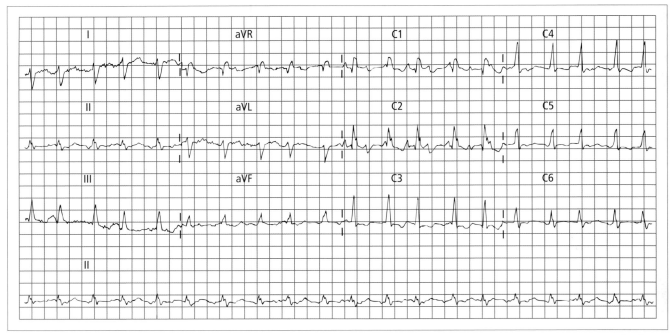

Fig. 77 ECG of patient with pulmonary hypertension, showing right ventricular hypertrophy and right axis deviation. The patient is also in atrial fibrillation. (Courtesy of the Pulmonary Vascular Disease Unit at Papworth Hospital.)

• Exclusion of shunts, valvular and left ventricular abnormalities

• A transoesophageal study may be necessary to see an ASD.

ECG

Look for (Fig. 77):
• Tall P waves
• Right axis deviation
• RV hypertrophy.

Chest radiograph

Look for prominent pulmonary arteries with peripheral pruning, and for features of underlying lung disease (Fig. 78).

Left and right heart catheterization

Measure pressures and saturations (prognosis and shunt calculation) and assess response to acute vasodilators such as prostacyclin, adenosine or inhaled nitric oxide.

To exclude secondary causes

• Blood: FBC (for secondary polycythaemia), liver function tests, ESR, rheumatoid factor and autoantibody screen, and consider HIV test

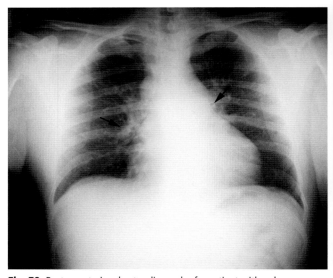

Fig. 78 Posteroanterior chest radiograph of a patient with pulmonary hypertension, showing prominent pulmonary arteries (arrowed) and cardiomegaly. (Courtesy of the Pulmonary Vascular Disease Unit at Papworth Hospital.)

• Pulmonary function tests to exclude obstructive or restrictive lung disease
• Sleep study if there is a suspicion of obstructive sleep apnoea
• Exclusion of pulmonary thromboembolism by: ventilation–perfusion ($\dot{V}/\dot{Q}$) scan, spiral CT scan of the chest with contrast, or pulmonary angiography (Fig. 79).

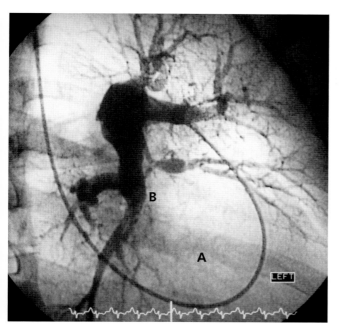

Fig. 79 Left pulmonary angiogram of a patient with thromboembolic pulmonary hypertension, showing (B) the characteristic bands and cut-offs of vessel occlusion and (A) lack of perfusion in the left lower lobe. (Courtesy of the Pulmonary Vascular Disease Unit at Papworth Hospital.)

Primary pulmonary hypertension—consider the following in your differential diagnosis:
- Secondary pulmonary hypertension
- LV outflow tract obstruction
- IHD.

Treatment

- Anticoagulation
- Diuretics with daily weight avoiding excessive fluid depletion
- Oxygen for hypoxaemia
- High-dose calcium channel blockers in those who have a significant fall in pulmonary vascular resistance on acute vasodilator testing
- Consideration of intravenous/nebulized prostacyclin therapy in those of poor functional class who fail to respond to acute vasodilator testing
- Consideration of atrial septostomy to decompress the right ventricle and improve left-sided filling pressures
- Lung or heart–lung transplantation in those who fail to respond to any other treatment.

Prognosis

Survival depends on right ventricular function and can be predicted by:
- Mixed venous oxygen saturation (adverse if <60%)
- Right atrial pressure (adverse if >15 mmHg)

- Cardiac index (adverse if <2 L/min/m²)
- Exercise tolerance (6-min walk test)
- Response to vasodilators.

Overall 5-year survival is 20%, but the subgroup with adverse haemodynamics have a 20% 3-year survival. Responders to chronic calcium channel blocker therapy have a 95% 5-year survival.

Anticoagulation, prostacyclin and heart–lung transplantation (5-year survival of 50–60%) all confer a survival benefit.

Important information for patients

Strongly advise against pregnancy. Avoid the oral contraceptive pill if possible—it may exacerbate pulmonary hypertension.

Gaine SP, Rubin LJ. Primary pulmonary hypertension. *Lancet* 1998; 352: 719–725.

2.12.2 SECONDARY PULMONARY HYPERTENSION

Secondary pulmonary hypertension is defined as sustained elevation of the mean PAP to >25 mmHg at rest or 30 mmHg on exercise, with an identified cause.

Aetiology/pathophysiology

Causes of secondary pulmonary hypertension are shown in Table 29.

Vascular wall remodelling and vasoconstriction increase pulmonary vascular resistance and therefore PAP, with resulting RVH and right ventricular failure (RVF). When the primary cause is respiratory, this is known as cor pulmonale.

Table 29 Causes of secondary pulmonary hypertension.

Mechanism	Cause
Increased left atrial pressure	Aortic/mitral valve disease
	Left ventricular dysfunction
Left-to-right shunts	ASD, VSD, PDA
Chronic pulmonary disease	COAD
	Bronchiectasis
	Pulmonary fibrosis
Chronic venous thromboembolism	–
Chronic hypoventilation/hypoxia	Kyphoscoliosis
	Respiratory muscle weakness
	Obstructive sleep apnoea

ASD, atrial septal defect; COPD, chronic obstructive pulmonary disease; PDA, patent ductus arteriosus; VSD, ventricular septal defect.

Clinical presentation

- Ankle oedema
- Dyspnoea (may be associated with the underlying primary condition)
- The primary condition.

Physical signs

The signs of the primary condition, including cyanosis if present, and then of pulmonary hypertension, RVH, dilatation and failure:
- Left parasternal heave
- Loud P2
- Elevated JVP with prominent 'v' wave
- Pansystolic murmur of tricuspid regurgitation
- Pulsatile liver
- Ankle oedema.

Investigations

See Section 2.12.1, p. 101.

Differential diagnosis

Consider left ventricular dysfunction and primary pulmonary hypertension.

Treatment

General

- Optimize treatment of the underlying condition
- Diuretics
- Calcium channel blockers
- Consideration of prostacyclin therapy
- Lung or heart–lung transplantation.

Specific

Shunts

Consideration of defect closure or pulmonary artery banding (some protection of pulmonary vasculature against high right-sided flow), if pulmonary hypertension not already too severe.

Chronic obstructive pulmonary disease

Long-term oxygen therapy benefits selected patients with chronic obstructive pulmonary disease. (See *Respiratory medicine*, Section 2.12.1.)

Thromboembolism

Anticoagulation and consideration of IVC filter or pulmonary thromboendarterectomy.

Ventilatory disorders

Consideration of nocturnal continuous positive airway pressure (CPAP) or nasal positive pressure ventilation. (See *Respiratory medicine*, Section 2.12.2.)

Prognosis

The prognosis is related to the underlying condition and the severity of the pulmonary hypertension. The 5-year survival rate of COPD with oedema is 30%.

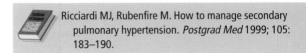
Ricciardi MJ, Rubenfire M. How to manage secondary pulmonary hypertension. *Postgrad Med* 1999; 105: 183–190.

2.13 Cardiac complications of systemic disease

2.13.1 THYROID DISEASE

Clinical presentation

Hyperthyroidism

A patient with hyperthyroidism may have:
- Sinus tachycardia
- Sustained or paroxysmal AF
- Hyperdynamic left ventricle.

Hypothyroidism

A patient with hypothyroidism may have:
- Bradycardia with prolonged QT interval
- Cardiac enlargement
- Pericardial effusion.

Treatment

Hyperthyroidism

Short term

- β Blockers for symptomatic relief until rendered euthyroid

- AF generally reverts to sinus rhythm with treatment of thyroid disease.

Long term

- Cardioversion after anticoagulation if AF persists.

Hypothyroidism

Treat with thyroxine, starting in very small doses to avoid precipitation of myocardial ischaemia. The effusion resolves and drainage is hardly ever required.

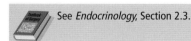 See *Endocrinology*, Section 2.3.

2.13.2 DIABETES

Aetiology/pathophysiology/pathology

Accelerated atherogenesis

This is the result of the following:
- Dyslipidaemia: enhanced atherogenicity of low-density lipoprotein (LDL), increased triglyceride and decreased high-density lipoprotein (HDL)
- Hypercoagulable state and increased platelet aggregation
- Hyperinsulinaemia (in type 2 diabetes) promoting vascular smooth muscle proliferation
- Glycosylated proteins promoting the production of oxidants.

Autonomic neuropathy

This causes impairment of the protective sensation of angina (silent ischaemia) and thus causes prolonged ischaemia, arrhythmias and sudden death.

Diabetic cardiomyopathy

There is impairment of systolic and diastolic function independent of macroscopic coronary artery disease, possibly secondary to microvascular disease.

Epidemiology

In people with diabetes the risk of acute MI is increased by 50% for a man and 150% for a woman. Mortality and the rate of all major complications are also increased.

Clinical presentation

Silent ischaemia may lead to atypical presentations, e.g. acute MI as ketoacidosis.

Treatment

Acute MI

Standard treatment plus an insulin infusion ('sliding scale'). The absolute benefit of all standard interventions is greater in people with diabetes.

Coronary revascularization

Diabetic coronary disease is more diffuse and distal, so that both CABG and angioplasty have poorer outcomes than in people without diabetes, although recent work suggests that coronary stenting plus the use of a glycoprotein IIb/IIIa receptor blocker (antiplatelet) may improve results.

Prevention

Primary

Good glycaemic and blood pressure control, and avoidance of smoking.

Secondary

Treatment with a statin and an ACE inhibitor, though most of this high-risk group should now be on these drugs as primary prevention.

2.13.3 AUTOIMMUNE RHEUMATIC DISEASES

Clinical presentation

The autoimmune rheumatic diseases have the following cardiac associations.

Systemic lupus erythematosus (SLE)

- Premature atherosclerosis: important to differentiate, if possible, from coronary vasculitis (also in SLE) because the latter needs steroids
- Pericarditis ± effusion: clinically in 30%; at post-mortem examination in 60%
- Sterile valvular vegetations (Libman–Sachs) in 60%, rarely clinically significant
- Myocarditis
- Conduction defects.

Primary antiphospholipid syndrome

- Pulmonary thromboembolism (also in SLE if anticardiolipin antibody positive)
- Degenerative mitral valve disease.

Rheumatoid arthritis

- Pericarditis: often clinically silent but may lead to symptomatic effusion or constriction
- Rheumatoid nodules causing valvular regurgitation and AV block
- Coronary vasculitis (rare).

Systemic sclerosis

- Pulmonary hypertension: the major cause of death in systemic sclerosis
- Pericarditis and chronic effusions
- Myocardial fibrosis causing ventricular dysfunction and conduction abnormalities.

Investigations

Coronary angiography

Coronary angiography may help to distinguish between vasculitis and atheromatous disease.

Echocardiography

Transoesophageal echocardiography should be used if necessary for close inspection of valve abnormalities.

Treatment

Pericarditis

Non-steroidal anti-inflammatory drugs (NSAIDs) and steroids are used if necessary for symptomatic relief. Tamponade requires immediate pericardiocentesis followed by steroids.

Myocarditis

The standard management of LV dysfunction and consideration of anticoagulation (see Section 2.3, p. 63).

Pulmonary hypertension

The standard management (see Section 2.12, p. 101).

2.13.4 RENAL DISEASE

Aetiology/pathophysiology/pathology

Features of end-stage renal failure/renal replacement include:
- Uraemia
- Elevated serum phosphate and calcium phosphate product
- Anaemia
- Electrolyte imbalance
- Hypertension
- Dyslipidaemia
- Amyloidosis (β_2 microglobulin).

These result in the following cardiovascular complications via the mechanisms shown in Fig. 80:
- Myocardial ischaemia
- Ventricular arrhythmias and sudden death
- Impaired ventricular function
- LV hypertrophy
- Valvular calcification, aortic > mitral, with rapidly progressive stenosis in a small proportion and the risk of endocarditis.

The heart in renal failure

Do not confuse fluid overload with LV dysfunction, although the two often coexist. LV function is impaired by uraemia and improves with dialysis, not just with the removal of fluid.

Epidemiology

Cardiovascular disease is much commoner in patients receiving renal replacement than the general population and is the most common cause of death (40–50%). Those in whom renal failure is associated with diabetes are at particularly high risk.

Investigations

- Myocardial ischaemia: coronary angiography if intervention or renal transplantation is being considered; nuclear perfusion imaging has a poor predictive value in these patients.
- Consider echocardiography for assessment of valves, LV function and pericardial effusion.

Treatment

Aim to normalize the haemoglobin and blood pressure and, if possible, to dialyse as well. If coronary artery disease is present, bypass grafting is the treatment of choice

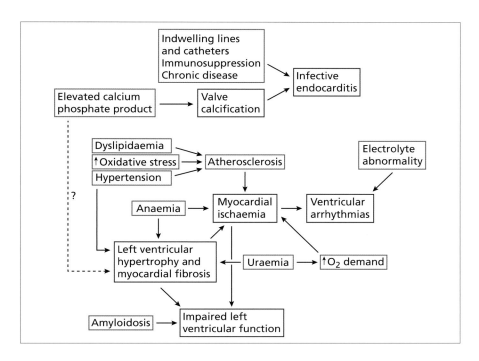

Fig. 80 The pathogenesis of cardiac complications of renal failure.

because the post-angioplasty re-stenosis and coronary event rate are very high. The indications for surgery in calcific valve disease and endocarditis are the same as in a patient without renal disease. Uraemic pericarditis is an absolute indication for dialysis; cardiac tamponade (of any cause) requires immediate pericardiocentesis. Recurrent effusions may warrant pericardiectomy (a 'window' to allow drainage into the pleural space).

 Prescribing in renal failure: see *Clinical pharmacology*, Section 5.6.

Be aware that a patient on dialysis may have large fluctuations in serum potassium, with effects on antiarrhythmic therapy.

Prognosis

The presence of LV dysfunction in a dialysis patient reduces the 2-year survival rate from 80 to 33%. Acute MI and cardiac surgery have a higher mortality than in the general population, but CABG and valve surgery are still an acceptable risk when indicated.

Prevention

Careful control of phosphate and calcium phosphate product reduces valve calcification. Good aseptic technique is essential when inserting and using dialysis catheters to minimize the risk of infective endocarditis. Aim for good control of blood pressure and serum cholesterol and maintenance of haematocrit at about 35%. Stop smoking!

 Hussain S, Isenberg DA. Autoimmune rheumatic diseases and the heart. *Hosp Med* 1999; 60: 95–99.

Hyde T, Timmis AD. Diabetes and the heart. *Hosp Med* 1999; 60: 90–94.

Staffeld CG, Pastan SO. Cardiac disease in patients with end-stage renal disease. *Cardiol Clin* 1995; 13: 209–223.

Woolfson RG. Renal disease and the heart. *Hosp Med* 1999; 60: 85–89.

2.14 Systemic complications of cardiac disease

2.14.1 STROKE

Aetiology

There are many cardiac causes of stroke:
- AF
- MI (acute/chronic)
- Dilated cardiomyopathy
- Infective endocarditis
- Valvular disease
- Prosthetic mechanical valve
- Intracardiac mass
- Hypertension
- Aortic dissection.

Physical signs

Common

- AF (up to 25%)
- Murmurs (particularly mitral predisposing to AF).

Uncommon

- Pulmonary oedema
- Added hearts sounds.

Investigations

ECG

There is a significant chance that, if there is underlying cardiac pathology resulting in thromboembolism, the ECG will be abnormal.

Examination of the ECG for cardiac cause of stroke:
- AF
- Previous MI (in 90% of cases the MI is anterior)
- Persistent ST elevation suggestive of LV aneurysm
- LVH suggestive of hypertension or aortic stenosis.

Chest radiograph

Look for abnormal cardiac shape/size, pulmonary oedema and wide mediastinum suggestive of enlarged aorta.

Echocardiography

If any possible cardiac cause has been identified from the history, examination or ECG/chest radiograph, it is reasonable to examine the structure and function of the heart for the following:
- Structural abnormalities
- Intracardiac thrombus
- TOE: particularly suited for examination of the left atrial appendage
- Consider paradoxical embolus: look for intracardiac shunts, if necessary using contrast.

Treatment

In general, correct the underlying abnormality and aim for restoration of sinus rhythm where possible. (See Section 2.2.2, p. 59.)

Complications

The risk of haemorrhage into an ischaemic stroke if anticoagulated usually outweighs the benefit of secondary prevention.

Prevention

Anticoagulation in atrial fibrillation/flutter should be considered in all patients as follows.

Primary prevention of stroke/TIA

In patients who do not have a history of stroke/TIA:
- Structurally abnormal heart—warfarin
- Structurally normal heart, age <65 years, no hypertension, no previous stroke/TIA, no diabetes—aspirin
- Structurally normal heart, age >65 years—warfarin.

Secondary prevention after stroke/TIA

In patients who have had a previous stroke/TIA:
- Exclude haemorrhagic stroke—warfarin
- If warfarin contraindicated—aspirin
- Warfarin therapy—aim for an international normalized ratio (INR) of 2.0–3.0. This will give satisfactory protection while minimizing the risks of haemorrhage. A number of near patient monitoring devices are now available, so specifically selected patients may be able to monitor the level of anticoagulation themselves.

Barnett HJM, Eliasziw M, Meldrum HE. Evidence based cardiology: prevention of ischaemic stroke. *BMJ* 1999; 318: 1539–1543.

2.15 Pregnancy and the heart

Aetiology

Normal physiological changes in pregnancy include the following:
- Decrease in systemic and pulmonary vascular resistance
- Increase in heart rate, blood volume (large shifts after delivery) and cardiac output
- No significant change in blood pressure
- Anaemia (caused by increased blood volume and/or haematinic deficiency).

These can all cause problems in women with cardiovascular disease.

Clinical presentation

Fatigue, mild dyspnoea, ankle oedema, palpitations (usually ectopics) and postural dizziness are all common in normal pregnancy, but likely to be more severe in those with cardiac disease.

Physical signs

An S3, a soft systolic murmur at the lower left sternal edge and mild ankle oedema are all common in normal pregnancy. Look for signs of worsening cardiac failure and/or exacerbation of the physical signs of particular cardiac lesions.

Investigations

Exclude cardiac disease:
• Echocardiography for ventricular function and murmurs
• ECG/24-h tape for palpitation
• Chest radiograph rarely clinically indicated, but should be performed if it is, because the dose to a screened fetus is negligible.

Prognosis/treatment

In a patient with pre-existing cardiac disease the ability to tolerate pregnancy is related to the following:
• Cyanosis
• Pulmonary hypertension
• Haemodynamic significance of the lesion
• Pre-pregnancy functional status.

High risk

Primary pulmonary hypertension/Eisenmenger's syndrome

There is a 50% maternal mortality rate and patients should be strongly advised to undergo sterilization.

Mitral stenosis

Mitral stenosis may present for the first time in pregnancy with pulmonary oedema secondary to increased cardiac output or an episode of AF. Treatment consists of diuretics to clear the pulmonary oedema and digoxin or β blockers to control heart rate and thereby improve atrial emptying. Mitral valvuloplasty may be necessary.

Aortic/pulmonary stenosis

Gradients are exacerbated by decreased vascular resistance and there is no effective medical therapy.

Marfan's syndrome

There is an increased risk of aortic dissection; those who already have echocardiographic evidence of aortic root dilatation >4.5 cm should be advised against pregnancy.

Intermediate risk

• Coarctation of the aorta (risk of aortic dissection)
• Hypertrophic cardiomyopathy
• Cyanotic congenital heart disease without pulmonary hypertension—note increased risk (40%) of fetal death if mother is cyanotic.

Low risk

• Well-tolerated valvular regurgitation
• Septal defects without pulmonary hypertension
• Totally corrected congenital heart disease
• Prosthetic valves: bioprostheses do not require anticoagulation but pregnancy reduces their lifespan. There is no consensus of opinion on the optimum management of anticoagulation in pregnant women with mechanical valves. In addition to the issues discussed in *Clinical pharmacology*, Section 5.3, there is the concern that heparin is not as effective as warfarin in preventing valve thrombosis.

Antibiotic prophylaxis is recommended for vaginal delivery in cases at high risk of endocarditis (prosthetic valves, prior subacute bacterial endocarditis [SBE], complex cyanotic congenital heart disease and surgical shunts) and for instrumented delivery in any cardiac lesion, but not for caesarean section.

New cardiac disease in pregnancy

Thromboembolic disease

Thrombolysis should be used for a massive life-threatening PE, as in the non-pregnant patient.

Peripartum cardiomyopathy

This presents as dilatated cardiomyopathy in the third trimester or in the first 6 months postpartum.

Hypertension

Hypertension may be chronic (i.e. predates the pregnancy or develops before 20 weeks) or pregnancy induced (part of a spectrum that includes pre-eclampsia).

Important information for patients

Recurrence risk of non-syndromic congenital heart disease in the baby is 3–5%

Magee LA, Ornstein MP, von Dadelszen P. Management of hypertension in pregnancy. *BMJ* 1999; 318: 1332–1336.

Oakley GDG. Pregnancy and heart disease. In: Julian DG, Camm AJ (eds) *Diseases of the Heart*, 2nd edn. Philadelphia, PA: WB Saunders Co., 1996: 1331–1337.

Williams D. Pregnancy and the heart. *Hosp Med* 1999; 60: 100–104.

2.16 General anaesthesia in heart disease

Pathophysiology

General anaesthesia produces a number of significant changes in cardiovascular physiology. The key to management and assessment of patients with cardiovascular disease undergoing general anaesthesia lies in understanding these changes, also the direct effects of anaesthetic agents and of inadequate ventilation, including the following:

- Changes in arterial pressure
- Changes in central venous pressure
- Hypoxaemia
- Hypercapnia
- Acidosis.

Epidemiology

The following are the risks of reinfarction during an anaesthetic after MI:

- Within 3 months: 6%
- Between 3 and 6 months: 2%.

Clinical presentation

The risk of general anaesthesia in patients who have had a previous MI is considerably higher than in those who have not. It is important to identify those patients at particular risk so that their management can be optimized before surgery and their anaesthetic particularly tailored to their medical condition. Key factors in assessment are to establish the exercise tolerance of the patient and to identify whether symptoms are stable or unstable.

Investigations

The following tests may help to determine anaesthetic risk.

Exercise testing

This will give an indication of exercise tolerance and possible IHD.

Ambulatory monitoring

Only appropriate in those patients who give a history suggestive of arrhythmias.

Echocardiography

Routine echocardiography is of little value, but may be helpful in those with a history of IHD or suspected structural abnormalities.

Coronary angiography

If there is doubt about the stability of coronary symptoms, documentation of the coronary anatomy before surgery should be considered.

The following place patients in a higher-risk group when undergoing surgery under general anaesthesia:

- MI within 6 months
- Congestive heart failure (pulmonary oedema or gallop rhythm)
- Rhythm other than sinus rhythm
- Aortic stenosis
- Metabolic abnormality (hypoxia, acidosis, renal insufficiency, liver disease)
- Age >70 years
- Emergency operation.

Larsen SF, Olesen KH, Jacobsen E *et al.* Prediction of cardiac risk in non-cardiac surgery. *Eur Heart J* 1987; 8: 179.

Lee TH. Reducing cardiac risk in non-cardiac surgery. *N Engl J Med* 1999; 341: 1838–1840.

2.17 Hypertension

Aetiology/pathophysiology/pathology

Most cases of hypertension are of unknown aetiology (essential hypertension) reflecting the interaction of multiple genetic and environmental factors on control systems such as the renin–angiotensin and autonomic

Table 30 Secondary causes of hypertension.

Commonly present with hypertension
  Renal disease
  Renal artery stenosis—atherosclerotic or fibromuscular dysplasia
  Coarctation of the aorta
  Phaeochromocytoma
  Primary hyperaldosteronism (Conn's syndrome)

Rarely present with hypertension as the dominant feature, but may be associated with it
  Cushing's syndrome
  Exogenous steroids
  Hyperthyroidism
  Myxoedema
  Acromegaly
  Excessive liquorice consumption

nervous systems. The impact of any single factor is small. Although responsible for only a minority of cases, secondary causes must not be neglected because treatment may cure the hypertension and reduce morbidity associated with the primary disease (Table 30).

Epidemiology

Blood pressure is a continuous variable, so hypertension is difficult to define. Up to one-quarter of adults in Western populations are found to have a blood pressure of >140/90 mmHg at screening, the proportion increasing with age, rising from 4% in those aged 18–29 years to 65% in those >80 years.

Clinical presentation

Common

Essential hypertension is usually asymptomatic until complications, e.g. cardiac failure, intervene. Headache (occipital and present on waking, settling gradually during the day), epistaxis and nocturia are frequently described, but are non-specific. Hypertension is commonly detected 'opportunistically' when a patient attends with some complaint and the doctor or nurse takes the opportunity to measure the blood pressure. It may also be detected at routine health screening, or as part of a deliberate assessment of a patient's cardiovascular risk, e.g. when presenting with symptoms that might indicate cardiovascular disease, e.g. IHD, stroke/TIA, peripheral vascular disease.

Uncommon

Presentation with symptoms suggestive of a secondary cause.

Physical signs

Apart from elevated blood pressure, commonly there are no other abnormal signs. In moderate or severe hypertension, a loud aortic second sound may be heard. Look for evidence of the following:
• LVH.
• Hypertensive retinopathy: grade I—light reflex from the arterial wall is increased as a result of thickening; grade II—the arterial light reflex is wider, giving rise to a 'silver wire' appearance. Nipping of the veins is an optical illusion caused by the inability to see the blood within the vein through the thickened arterial wall. There is a generalized reduction in the diameter of arteries compared with veins. Focal arterial narrowing may be seen.
• Signs of associated vascular disease: vascular bruits, absent pulses.

Investigations

All patients should have the tests shown below.

Blood tests

FBC, electrolytes, renal function, fasting glucose and lipids.

Urine

A clean mid-stream urine should be tested for blood, protein and glucose. In the presence of haematuria or proteinuria, the sample should be sent for microscopy and culture.

ECG

The ECG may be normal; look for signs of LVH and/or coronary artery disease.

Chest radiograph

Normal, cardiomegaly, pulmonary oedema, coarctation (Fig. 82).

Other

Other tests may be required in some cases.

To determine whether hypertension is present in patients with no evidence of end-organ damage—check the 24-h ambulatory blood pressure or arrange for measurement of the blood pressure at home or work to diagnose the presence of isolated clinic ('white coat') hypertension.

To assess for end-organ damage—echocardiography, look for LVH, systolic and/or diastolic failure.

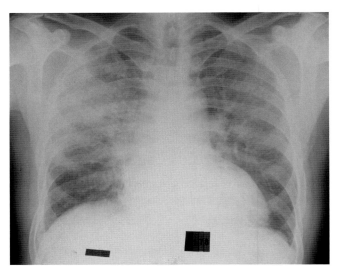

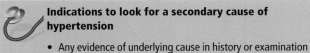

Fig. 81 Pulmonary oedema.

Indications to look for a secondary cause of hypertension

- Any evidence of underlying cause in history or examination (Table 30).
- Accelerated (malignant) hypertension.
- Hypokalaemia (not diuretic induced).
- Young age (<35 yr).
- Resistant hypertension (uncontrolled by 3 drugs).

To pursue the possibility of secondary causes, do the following:
- 24-h urine collection: may require creatinine clearance, urinary protein excretion, catecholamines.
- Renal ultrasonography: the presence of two small kidneys indicates chronic renal disease; marked asymmetry of renal size (more than 2 cm difference in length) increases the probability of renal artery stenosis.
- Doppler ultrasonography of renal arteries, captopril renography or renal angiography (conventional, digital subtraction, MRI) to look for renal artery stenosis.
- Test of plasma renin and aldosterone.
- Other investigations as led by clinical suspicion.

Differential diagnosis

Consider the following:
- Essential hypertension
- Secondary hypertension
- Erroneous reading of elevated blood pressure as a result of an inadequate cuff size
- Isolated clinic hypertension ('white coat hypertension').

Treatment

Secondary causes of hypertension may require specific treatment. In essential hypertension, advise lifestyle modi-

fication (see key point below) and monitor blood pressure. In mild hypertension (diastolic BP <105 mmHg), check blood pressure on another occasion before initiating treatment; in moderate (diastolic BP >105 mmHg) or severe (diastolic BP >115 mmHg) hypertension, commence drug therapy. Tailor the choice of initial drug according to associated medical conditions. Review every 4–6 weeks. Aim for blood pressure of <140/85 mmHg.

Advice regarding lifestyle modifications for patients with hypertension

- Stop smoking
- Appropriate weight loss
- Moderation of alcohol intake (<14 units/week for women, <21 units for men)
- Dietary changes: lower saturated fat, increase oily fish, fruit and vegetable intake
- Limit salt intake
- Sensible exercise.

Drug treatment of hypertension

Points to remember:
- Tailor initial therapy, based on coexistent medical conditions, e.g. ACE inhibitor in heart failure, β blocker in IHD
- Remember evidence of variation in response with age and some races, e.g. thiazide and calcium antagonists tend to be more effective than β blockers and ACE inhibitors in elderly and Afro-Caribbean individuals
- Be prepared to use combination therapy to allow low dosages, reducing the side effects.

Complications

- Retinopathy, LVH, proteinuria
- Vascular events: stroke, MI, peripheral arterial disease
- Cardiac failure, worsening of pre-existing renal failure
- Worsening hypertension (especially if poorly treated).

Prognosis

Morbidity

Essential hypertension increases the risk of stroke sixfold, of coronary artery disease and heart failure threefold, and doubles the risk of peripheral vascular disease. Renal failure usually occurs only in malignant hypertension, but elevated blood pressure increases the progression of renal failure from other causes. Treatment of hypertension is well established to reduce the incidence of cardiovascular disease.

Mortality

- At an age <50 years, both diastolic and systolic hypertension are risk factors for cardiovascular death. A reduction of 5–6 mmHg in diastolic pressure is associated with a 12% reduction in mortality rate over 5 years.

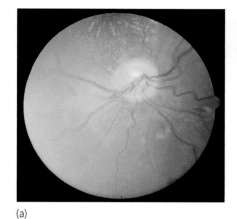 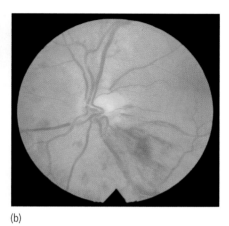

(a)   (b)

Fig. 82 Hypertensive retinopathy: (a) grade IV showing mild papilloedema, hard exudates (12 o'clock), cottonwool spots and flame haemorrhages (4 o'clock); (b) grade III showing extensive flame-shaped haemorrhages. (Courtesy of Professor J Ritter.)

• At an age >50 years, evidence suggests that the systolic blood pressure is the important determinant of risk, with an inverse relationship with diastolic blood pressure, i.e. the greater the pulse pressure for a given value of systolic pressure, the higher the risk.

Anonymous. Tight blood pressure control and risk of macrovascular and microvascular complications in type 2 diabetes: UKPDS 38. UK Prospective Diabetes Study Group. *BMJ* 1998; 317: 703–713.

Franklin SS, Khan SA, Wong ND, Larson MG, Levy D. Is pulse pressure useful in predicting risk for coronary heart disease? The Framingham heart study. *Circulation* 1999; 100: 354–360.

Hansson L, Zanchetti A, Carruthers SG *et al*. Effects of intensive blood-pressure lowering and low-dose aspirin in patients with hypertension: principal results of the Hypertension Optimal Treatment (HOT) randomised trial. HOT Study Group. *Lancet* 1998; 351: 1755–1762.

Ramsay LE, Williams B, Johnston GD *et al*. British Hypertension Society guidelines for hypertension management 1999: summary. *BMJ* 1999; 319: 630–635.

2.17.1 ACCELERATED PHASE HYPERTENSION

Aetiology/pathology

The aetiology is unknown, but patients with accelerated phase hypertension are more likely than those with 'benign' (not accelerated phase) hypertension to have a secondary cause. Pathological hallmark is the presence of fibrinoid necrosis in the arterioles.

Epidemiology

The incidence is around 1–2 : 100 000 per year.

Clinical presentation

• Hypertensive encephalopathy: visual disturbance, headaches, drowsiness, epileptic fits

• Other hypertensive emergencies: pulmonary oedema, acute renal failure, aortic dissection, pre-eclampsia.

Physical signs

Common

The diagnosis cannot be made without high blood pressure and evidence of fibrinoid necrosis of the vessels, which can be viewed directly only in the fundi:

• Grade III retinopathy: flame-shaped superficial haemorrhages or 'dot-and-blot' haemorrhages deeper within the retina, cottonwool spots (retinal microinfarcts); hard exudates (Fig. 82).

• Grade IV retinopathy: haemorrhages and exudates with papilloedema (Figs 82 and 83).

Attempts used to be made to distinguish between accelerated (grade III) and malignant (grade IV) hypertension because prognosis used to be worse in grade IV. This is no longer the case, and the term 'malignant hypertension' (originally coined because of the dire prognosis before effective antihypertensive treatment was

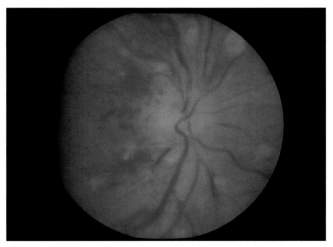

Fig. 83 Hypertensive retinopathy: grade IV showing florid papilloedema, haemorrhages and cottonwool spots. (Courtesy of Mr H Towler.)

113

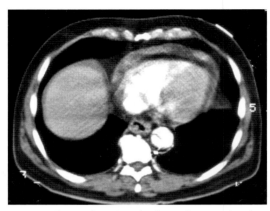

Fig. 84 CT scan of aortic dissection. The descending aorta is enlarged and contrast shows a double lumen.

available) should be avoided—it makes patients think that they have cancer.

Uncommon

Drowsiness, coma, epileptic fitting, stroke, pulmonary oedema, aortic dissection.

Investigations

Immediate

Check urine for blood, protein and red cell casts. Perform ECG, chest radiograph, FBC, electrolytes, renal and liver function tests. If there is a clinical suspicion of aortic dissection (Fig. 84), urgent CT scan of the chest or TOE is needed. If there is a clinical suspicion of renal inflammatory condition, e.g. SLE, vasculitis or scleroderma, specific serological tests will be needed.

Elective

When blood pressure has been controlled, all patients with accelerated phase hypertension require a thorough work-up for secondary causes of hypertension. Renal biopsy may be required.

Differential diagnosis

The differential diagnosis is of acute glomerulonephritis or renal vasculitis, or scleroderma renal crisis.

Treatment

All patients with accelerated phase hypertension should be admitted to hospital for blood pressure control. General management consists of the following:
- Bedrest.

- No smoking: cigarettes cause an acute rise in blood pressure in accelerated hypertension!
- Monitor blood pressure regularly: every hour to start with, then less frequently.
- Monitor fluid input/output, daily weight and renal function (serum creatinine).
- Intravenous furosemide (frusemide) if there is pulmonary oedema.
- Aim to lower diastolic pressure by 15–20 mmHg over 24 h with oral atenolol 50–100 mg daily or nifedipine 10–20 mg 8-hourly (tablets, not sublingual formulation). Alternatively, intravenous therapy may be required: labetolol or nitroprusside. Most would avoid ACE inhibitors in the acute setting in case the patient had renal artery stenosis.
- Avoid rapid reduction in blood pressure—cerebral autoregulation is impaired and there is a substantial risk of causing ischaemic 'watershed' stroke. In most cases, aim to reduce the diastolic blood pressure to 100–105 mmHg over 2–3 days.
- Consult renal team if there is renal impairment or other suspicion of primary renal condition: patients with presenting creatinine <300 µmol/L are likely to recover renal function; those with creatinine >300 µmol/L are likely to progress to end-stage renal failure and require long-term renal replacement therapy.

Complications will require specific management:
- Hypertensive encephalopathy: coma—check airway, breathing, circulation; protect airway; give high-flow oxygen. Epileptic fits—anticonvulsants.
- Aortic dissection: use intravenous β blockade to slow heart rate; urgent imaging; urgent cardiothoracic surgical consultation.
- Renal failure: may require urgent dialysis/ultrafiltration to remove fluid if pulmonary oedema present.
- Pre-eclampsia: delivery of child.

Complications

Stroke, aortic dissection, chronic renal failure.

Prognosis

If untreated, 80% will die within 2 years. One recent series reported a 69% survival rate at 12 years.

Ahmed MEK, Walker JM, Beevers DG, Beevers M. Lack of difference between malignant and accelerated hypertension. *BMJ* 1986; 292: 235–237.

McGregor E, Isles CG, Jay JL, Lever AF, Murray GD. Retinal changes in malignant hypertension. *BMJ* 1986; 292: 233–234.

Webster J, Petrie JC, Jeffers TA, Lovell HG. Accelerated hypertension—patterns of mortality and clinical factors affecting outcome in treated patients. *Q J Med* 1993; 86: 485–493.

2.18 Venous thromboembolism

2.18.1 PULMONARY EMBOLISM

Embolism can be from any source (e.g. tumour, air, amniotic fluid), but this section will consider only thrombotic venous thromboembolism.

Aetiology/pathophysiology/pathology

Virchow's triad (local trauma to the vessel wall, hypercoagulability and venous stasis) causes thrombosis in the deep veins of the legs, pelvis or (more rarely) arms, which may propagate and extend proximally. Thrombus may dislodge and embolize to the pulmonary arterial tree, causing physical obstruction and the release of vasoactive substances, elevating pulmonary vascular resistance and resulting in the following:
• Redistribution of blood flow, causing ventilation–perfusion mismatch and impairment of gas exchange
• Increased RV afterload, causing dilatation and dysfunction of the right ventricle.

Epidemiology

The incidence of venous thromboembolism in the general population (in the USA) is 0.1% per year. Pulmonary embolism is the cause of 10% of all deaths in hospital.

The following are risk factors (found in 80–90% of patients with PE):
• Thrombophilia: factor V Leiden; deficiencies of antithrombin III, protein C and protein S; hyperhomocysteinaemia; antiphospholipid antibodies or lupus anticoagulant. (See *Haematology*, Section 1.20.) Ask about personal and family history of thromboembolism.
• Surgery/trauma/fractures (especially lower limb).
• Immobilization of any cause.
• Obesity.
• Smoking.
• Hypertension.
• Old age.
• Pregnancy/postpartum.
• Current (not prior) use of combined oral contraceptive or HRT—minor risk only.
• Malignancy.
• Chronic cardiorespiratory disease.

> PE is rare if aged <40 with no risk factors.

Clinical presentation

Common

• Isolated dyspnoea
• Pulmonary infarction: pleuritic pain, cough or haemoptysis
• Massive PE: severe dyspnoea, syncope and haemodynamic collapse
• Deep venous thrombosis (DVT): swollen, firm, tender calf.

> A young woman with isolated pleuritic chest pain and no risk factors except the oral contraceptive pill is extremely unlikely to have a PE if she has a respiratory rate of <20/min and a normal chest radiograph. But the risk of missing a life-threatening condition means that you should pursue investigation unless you can make a confident alternative diagnosis.

Uncommon

• Progressive ankle oedema and dyspnoea (secondary pulmonary hypertension)
• Pyrexia of unknown origin
• AF.

Physical signs

Common

• Tachypnoea
• Tachycardia
• Crackles on auscultation
• Pleural rub.

Uncommon

• Cyanosis
• Raised JVP, left parasternal heave, loud P2, pansystolic murmur of tricuspid regurgitation
• Swollen, firm calf of DVT.

Investigations

Investigations must be used in conjunction with an assessment of the clinical probability of PE.

ECG

Most commonly the ECG shows sinus tachycardia, sometimes anterior T-wave inversion. Atrial fibrillation, new RBBB, right axis deviation, RVH and S1Q3T3 are rare.

Chest radiograph

This may be normal, but common findings in PE include focal infiltrate, segmental collapse, raised diaphragm and pleural effusion. Wedge-shaped infarct and focal oligaemia are less common. A useful investigation in exclusion of differential diagnoses.

Arterial blood gases

Hypoxaemia and hypocapnia increase the suspicion, but normal gases do not exclude a diagnosis of PE.

Venous ultrasonography

This is used if there is clinical suspicion of a current DVT, although normal results do not exclude a PE.

Ventilation–perfusion lung scanning

This is useful if it is normal, or indicates a high probability of PE, correlated with clinical suspicion. Other results are difficult to interpret, especially in the presence of pre-existing cardiorespiratory disease. Perfusion scanning alone gives comparable diagnostic yield (Fig. 85).

Spiral chest CT with contrast

Increasingly used in the diagnosis of pulmonary emboli (Fig. 86). Clearly the imaging technique of choice when there is pre-existing cardiorespiratory disease.

Pulmonary angiography

Pulmonary angiography remains the 'gold standard', but with spiral chest CT, indications are diminishing.

Echocardiography

Echocardiography identifies RV pressure overload and dysfunction, as well as excluding other causes of haemodynamic collapse. It is useful as a quick source of information in a critically ill patient.

Plasma D-dimer enzyme-linked immunosorbent assay (ELISA)

This test is sensitive but not specific, i.e. it helps to exclude the diagnosis.

Consider the following in the differential diagnosis of PE:
- Pleurisy/breathlessness
- Pneumothorax
- Pneumonia
- Musculoskeletal pain
- Rib fracture
- Asthma/chronic airflow obstruction

Circulatory collapse
- MI
- Cardiac tamponade.

Treatment

Emergency

For massive PE with hypotension, treatment should be one of the following:
- Thrombolysis: different protocol from MI, via a peripheral vein or pulmonary artery catheter—as successful as embolectomy
- Embolectomy: transvenous catheter or open surgical—only if thrombolysis contraindicated or patient fails to respond
- Colloid to maintain right-sided filling in hypotension.

Short term

- Analgesia.
- Heparin: unfractionated or low molecular weight. Prevents further thrombus formation and permits endogenous fibrinolysis. Continue until INR >2.0.
- Oxygen.
- Warfarin, once heparinized.

Paradoxically, warfarin without heparin may initially increase hypercoagulability.

Long term

Continue warfarin for 6 weeks to 3 months if the risk factor is temporary; consider long term for recurrent embolism and persisting risk factors such as thrombophilia. Consider thrombophilia screening—especially if there is a family history. (See *Haematology*, Section 1.20.) Inferior vena caval (IVC) filters are indicated for recurrent PE in the presence of adequate anticoagulation or if anticoagulation is contraindicated.

Complications

The most significant complication is secondary pulmonary hypertension.

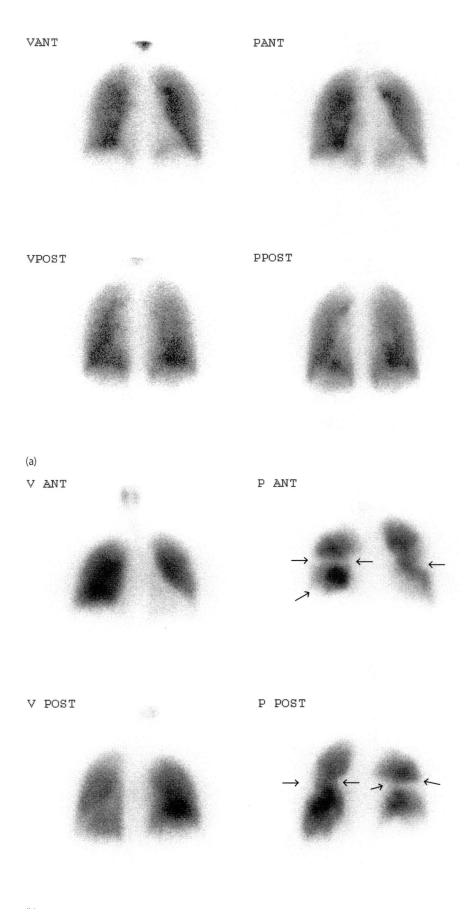

(a)

Fig. 85 (a) Normal ventilation–perfusion ($\dot{V}/\dot{Q}$) scan. Anterior and posterior views are shown. (b) Multiple perfusion defects (arrowed) which are not matched by ventilation defects and therefore indicate a high probability of pulmonary embolism.

(b)

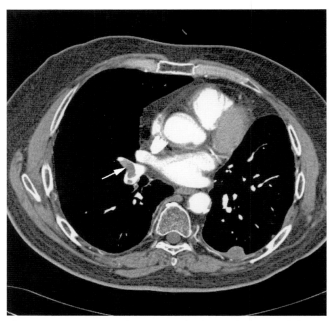

Fig. 86 Contrast CT scan of a patient with a large pulmonary embolus visible as a grey filling defect (arrowed) against the white contrast in the pulmonary artery.

Prognosis

Overall mortality rate at 3 months is 15.0–17.5%, reflecting in large part the underlying conditions. Right ventricular dysfunction on echocardiography predicts an adverse outcome. Note that the mortality associated with anticoagulation (following established guidelines) is very low at 0.1% of cases.

Prevention

Primary

- Consideration of compression stockings and prophylactic heparin in hospitalized patients, especially those with trauma, the critically ill and general and orthopaedic surgery
- Discourage smoking

Secondary

- Thrombophilia screening and consideration of the duration of anticoagulation
- Discourage smoking and advise alternatives to the oral contraceptive pill
- Weight loss and blood pressure control if necessary
- Consideration of IVC filter in selected cases.

Disease associations

- Thrombophilia
- Malignancy

- Antiphospholipid syndromes
- Hypertension.

Goldhaber SZ. Pulmonary embolism. *N Engl J Med* 1998; 339: 93–104.

2.19 Driving restrictions in cardiology

Group 1 entitlement (normal driving)

Angina

Patients may drive providing that there are no symptoms at rest or at the wheel.

Angioplasty

Patients must not drive for 1 week.

MI/CABG

Patients must not drive for 1 month.

Arrhythmia

Patients must not drive if the arrhythmia has caused, or is likely to cause, incapacity. If AV block documented, patients must not drive until 4 weeks after the cause has been identified and controlled.

Pacemaker

Patients must not drive for 1 week.

Syncope

Patients must not drive until the cause has been identified and controlled.

Heart failure, valvular heart disease and cardiomyopathy

Patients may continue to drive provided that there is no other disqualifying condition.

Group 2 entitlement (vocational driving)

Angina/MI/angioplasty/CABG

Patients must stop driving and inform the DVLA.

Relicensing is permitted once the patient is free of angina for 6 weeks with a satisfactory exercise test (see below).

Arrhythmia

Patients must not drive if the arrhythmia has caused, or is likely to cause, incapacity. Driving is permitted when the arrhythmia has been controlled for at least 3 months, provided that the LV ejection fraction is >0.4 and a satisfactory exercise test has been done.

Pacemaker

Patients must not drive for 6 weeks.

Syncope

Patients must not drive after single or recurrent episodes. Relicensing may be permitted after 3 months if specialist review and investigations are satisfactory.

Heart failure, valvular heart disease and cardiomyopathy

Patients must not drive if symptomatic. Relicensing possible if symptoms controlled and specialist review satisfactory.

Exercise test requirements

The patient must be off antianginal medication for 48 h.

The patient must complete the three stages of the Bruce protocol without any of the following:
- Angina
- Syncope
- Hypotension
- Sustained VT
- Horizontal or down-sloping ST segment shift >2 mm. Repeat every 3 years.

Angiography

This is not required for relicensing. If angiography has been undertaken, relicensing will not normally be permitted if the ejection fraction is ≤0.40 on ventriculography, or if there is significant proximal unrelieved coronary arterial stenosis (left main and proximal LAD ≥30% or proximal >50% elsewhere, unless subtending a completed infarction).

 http://www.dvla.gov.uk/at_a_glance/ch2_cardiovascular.htm.

Investigations and practical procedures

3.1 ECG

Principle

The ECG is a graphic representation of the electrical potentials of the heart. Each deflection represents electrical activity in the cardiac cycle:
• P wave: atrial depolarization. A further deflection that represents atrial repolarization is usually hidden within the QRS complex.
• PR interval: atrioventricular conduction time.
• QRS complex: ventricular depolarization. Q is the first negative deflection, R the first positive deflection and S the first negative deflection following a positive deflection.
• ST segment: from the end of the QRS to the start of the T wave.
• T wave: ventricular repolarization.
• U wave: after or in the end portion of the T wave. Cause unknown.

Adopting a systematic method of interpreting an ECG will enable you to approach the most complex of ECGs with confidence. If you approach all ECGs in this manner, certain patterns will become familiar, enabling rapid diagnosis of arrhythmias and possible structural cardiac abnormalities.

> **ECG interpretation scheme**
>
> After establishing the basic parameters, start at the P wave and progress through to the QRS and finally the T wave:
> • What is the rhythm? (regular/irregular)
> • What is the rate? [300/number of large squares between each QRS] (normal/bradycardia/tachycardia)
> • What is the QRS axis?
> • What is the P-wave axis?
> • Is the P-wave morphology normal?
> • Is the PR interval short/long?
> • Are there any δ waves?
> • Are there any Q waves?
> • Is the QRS morphology normal? (RBBB/LBBB)
> • Does the ST segment look normal in every lead?
> • Are any T waves inverted?
> • What is the QT interval?
> • Are there any additional features? (U waves)

QRS axis

To establish the QRS axis you need to do the following:

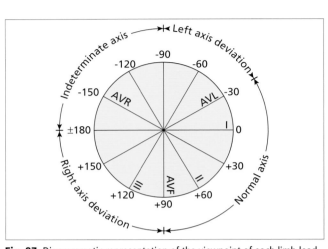

Fig. 87 Diagrammatic representation of the viewpoint of each limb lead.

• Identify the limb lead where the QRS is isoelectric—the axis will be 90° from this.
• Look at the limb lead whose axis is at 90° to the lead where the QRS is isoelectric (Fig. 87)—if deflection is positive, the axis is directed towards the positive pole of that lead (and if negative, away from it).

The normal axis is from −30° to +90°. Figure 88 demonstrates examples of the normal axis and right and left axis deviation.

Normal intervals

1 small square = 0.04 s

• PR interval (onset of P wave to first deflection of QRS) = 0.12 − 0.20 s
• QRS duration (<0.12 s)
• QT interval (onset of QRS complex to end of T wave) = 0.35 − 0.45 s
• QTc = QT adjusted for rate = $(QT/\sqrt{[R–R\ interval]})$ = 0.38 − 0.42 s.

Bradyarrhythmias/conduction disturbances

The key to identification of bradyarrhythmias is in establishing the relative relationship of the P wave and QRS complex. The following are the key features to identify:
• Rate
• Identify whether irregular/regular P waves/QRS complexes
• Plot all P waves and all QRS complexes
• No P wave before normal QRS suggests junctional rhythm
• No P wave before wide QRS suggests ventricular escape rhythm.

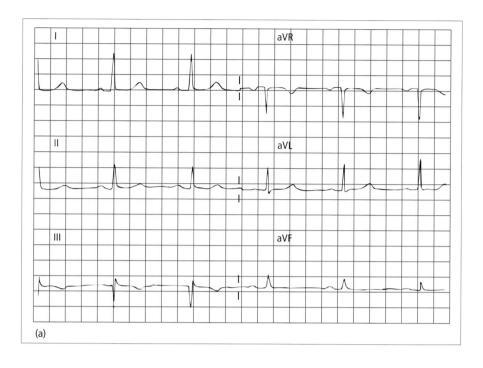

(a)

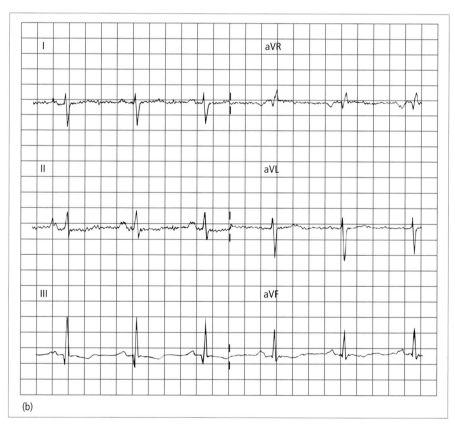

(b)

Fig. 88 Examples of (a) normal axis, (b) right and (c) left axis deviation.

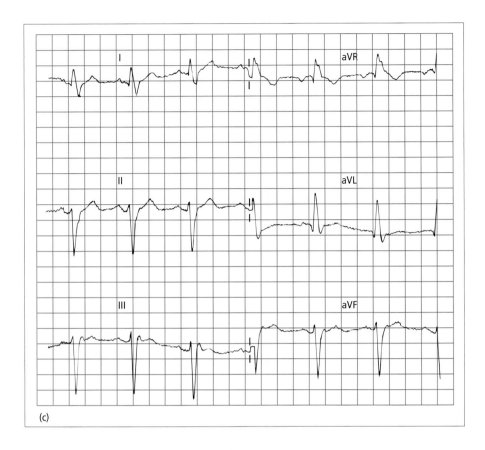

(c)

Fig. 88 *Continued*

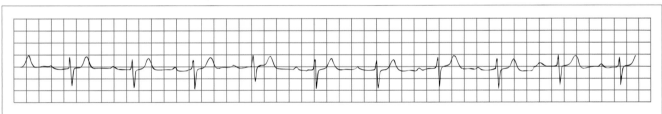

Fig. 89 Example of first-degree heart block. The PR interval is in excess of 0.20 s.

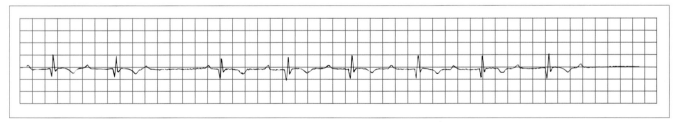

Fig. 90 Second-degree heart block (Wenckebach's or Mobitz, type I) with progressively increasing PR interval before failure of conduction with no QRS complex.

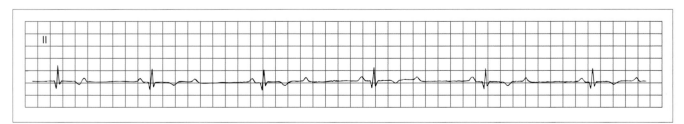

Fig. 91 Second-degree heart block (2 : 1): only alternate P waves are followed by a QRS complex. When there is failure of conduction without progressive increase in the PR interval, this is known as Mobitz, type II.

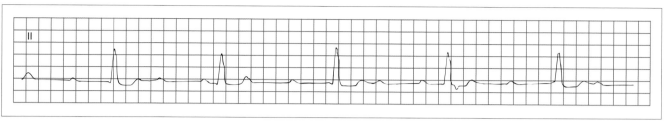

Fig. 92 Complete heart block: P waves and QRS complexes are not related. There is a slow ventricular escape rhythm (wider QRS complexes).

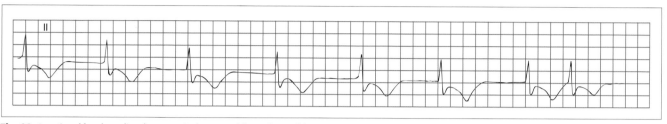

Fig. 93 Junctional bradycardia: slow ventricular rate with no discernible P waves.

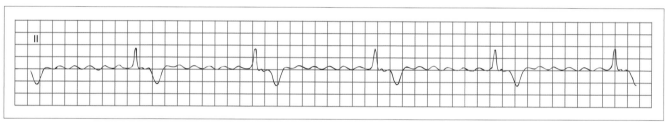

Fig. 94 Complete heart block in patient with atrial fibrillation as the underlying atrial rhythm.

Figures 89–94 illustrate varying degrees of atrioventricular block.

> Conduction abnormalities occur because of abnormalities of the normal depolarization from the AV node to the His bundle and bundle branches.
> • Abnormalities in AV node/His bundle conduction lead to degrees of heart block, e.g. coronary artery disease, myocarditis, digoxin toxicity, electrolyte abnormalities.
> • Abnormalities in conduction in the bundle branches leads to widened QRS complexes. Block of both bundles has the same effect as block of the His bundle, causing complete heart block (Table 31).

Table 31 Some key causes of bundle-branch block.

RBBB	LBBB
May be normal	Coronary artery disease
Coronary artery disease	Cardiomyopathy
Cardiomyopathy	Left ventricular hypertrophy
Atrial septal defect	(hypertension, aortic stenosis)
Ebstein's anomaly	Conduction system fibrosis
Massive pulmonary embolism	

LBBB, left bundle-branch block (wide [>0.12 s] notched, M- or plateau-shaped QRS complex in leads orientated to the left ventricle—V5, V6, AVL and I); RBBB, right bundle-branch block (M-shaped QRS complex in leads orientated to the right ventricle—V1 and V2).

Tachyarrhythmias

Find out whether there are any of the following:
• Narrow/broad complex?
• Identify whether irregular/regular.
• 'Saw-tooth' appearance of baseline suggests atrial flutter (ventricular rate may be irregular if variable block).
• Regular narrow complex tachycardia with no P waves seen suggests AVNRT (see Section 2.2.2).
• Consider differential diagnosis of SVT with aberration (Fig. 95) (Table 32).

Specific morphological changes in the ECG

Left ventricular hypertrophy

There are several criteria:
• Usually left axis deviation (>−30°)
• Amplitude of V1 or V2 + V5 or V6 >40 mm
• Note in young men with thin chest wall, criteria may be met without LVH.

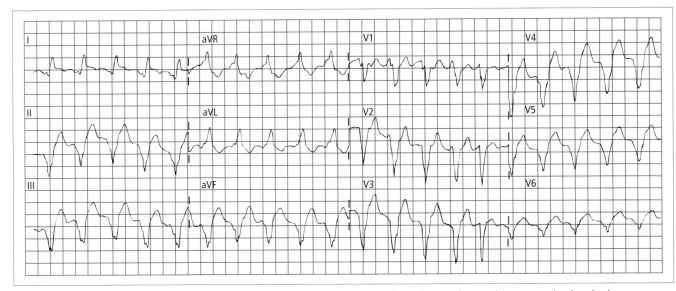

Fig. 95 Twelve-lead ECG of ventricular tachycardia with significant axis deviation, broad complexes and concordance across the chest leads.

Table 32 Differentiating ventricular tachycardia (VT) and supraventricular tachycardia (SVT).

Features supporting VT	Features supporting SVT
Very broad QRS complexes (>140 ms)	Termination with Valsalva manoeuvre/adenosine
Fusion beats	
Capture beats	Association of 'p' waves and QRS complexes
AV dissociation	
Significant axis deviation (right or left)	Onset following premature atrial beat
Concordance of the QRS deflexions in V1–6	
Onset following R on T	

Right ventricular hypertrophy

Criteria are the following:
- Right axis deviation (>90°)
- R V1 + S V6 >11 mm
- R V1 or S V6 >7 mm.

Metabolic abnormalities

- Hypercalcaemia: short QT, prominent U wave
- Hypocalcaemia: long QT
- Hyperkalaemia: flat/lost P waves, increased PR interval, wide QRS, tented T wave, arrhythmias
- Hypokalaemia: first-degree heart block, ST depression, U waves.

3.1.1 EXERCISE ECGs

Excercise ECGs are an extremely useful non-invasive investigation in appropriate clinical circumstances, but it is always important to remember that it can produce both false negatives and false positives. If significant diagnostic doubt remains in a patient who gives a good history of angina, further investigation should be considered (coronary angiography/myocardial perfusion imaging). Exercise testing in asymptomatic patients is of limited value.

Principle

The aim of the study is to document the electrophysiological and haemodynamic response to physical stress.

Indications

Exercise ECGs are indicated for the following:
- Establishing a diagnosis of angina in a patient with chest pain
- Obtaining a measure of exercise tolerance
- Evaluating a haemodynamic response to exercise
- Evaluation of exercise-induced arrhythmias.

Contraindications

There is a very low mortality if the test is used in appropriate patients: <1 : 20 000. The following are contraindications:
- Significant aortic stenosis
- Hypertrophic obstructive cardiomyopathy (for relative contraindications see Section 2.4.1)
- Acute pericarditis/myocarditis
- Acute MI/unstable angina
- Acute aortic dissection
- Systemic infection
- Physical impairment restricting patient from exercising.

Practical details

Before investigation

Omit antianginal medication if the test is for diagnostic reasons. Continue if a functional assessment on treatment is required. Note that β blockers and antihypertensives will mask the haemodynamic response.

The investigation

Close observation of the patient is required with full resuscitation facilities to hand. At least two qualified people should supervise the test.

After investigation

Continue to observe the patient closely. Dramatic haemodynamic changes can occur during the recovery period. Terminate the investigation only when all the parameters have returned to their normal level.

Results

Response to exercise

Normal ECG response to exercise:
• Ventricular rate increases
• P wave: increase in amplitude
• PR: shortens
• QRS: R-wave amplitude decreases
• ST: sharply up-sloping
• QT: shortens
• T wave: decrease in amplitude.
  Abnormal ECG response to exercise (Fig. 96):
• No increase in ventricular rate
• ST depression >1 mm (horizontal/down-sloping): myocardial ischaemia (the greater the degree and the longer it persists into recovery the greater the probability of coronary heart disease)
• ST elevation (horizontal/up-sloping): where previous MI suggests dyskinetic ventricle/aneurysm
• QRS: bundle-branch block may suggest ischaemia
• QT: prolongation of QTc may be a risk marker for *torsade de pointes*
• T wave: inversion suggests ischaemia
• Arrhythmias: ventricular arrhythmia suggests ischaemia.

Cleland JGF, Findlay IN, Gilligan D, Pennell DJ. *The Essentials of Exercise Electrocardiography.* London: Current Medical Literature Ltd, 1993.
Hampton JR. *The ECG Made Easy.* Edinburgh: Churchill Livingstone, 1997.
Xiao HB, Spicer M. How to do electrocardiography. *Br J Cardiol* 1996; 3: 148–150. (Seven part series).

3.2 Basic electrophysiology studies

Principle

Pace/sense electrodes are placed transvenously via the femoral vein and/or subclavian vein to various intracardiac locations. Electrograms are recorded during sinus rhythm. Arrhythmias are induced using pacing protocols with programmed extra stimuli.

Indications

Electrophysiology studies (EPS) may be helpful in the following circumstances:
• Narrow complex tachyarrhythmias: assessing for radio-frequency ablation
• Broad complex arrhythmias: assessing for radio-frequency ablation or implantation of an ICD
• Establishing a diagnosis in patients with palpitations/syncope
• Assessing bradyarrhythmias (limited value)
• Assessing effectiveness of antiarrhythmic to suppress arrhythmia.

Contraindications

EPS are not indicated for patients with the following:
• Reversible aetiology for arrhythmia
• Severe electrolyte abnormality.

Practical details

Before investigation

Antiarrhythmic medication is usually stopped 48 h before study.

The investigation

Intravenous sedative (often benzodiazepine) may be used before the procedure because some pacing protocols

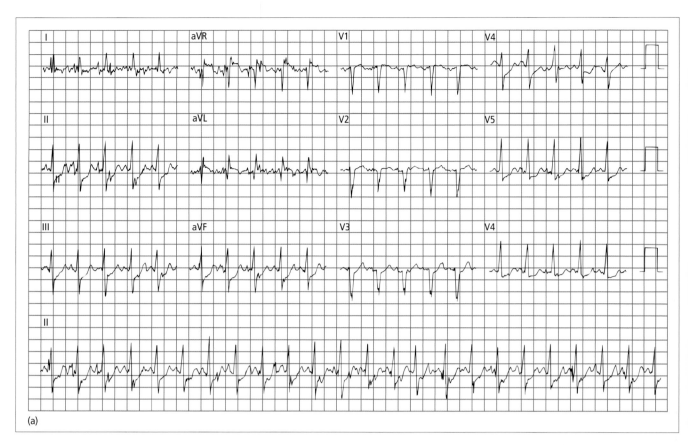

(a)

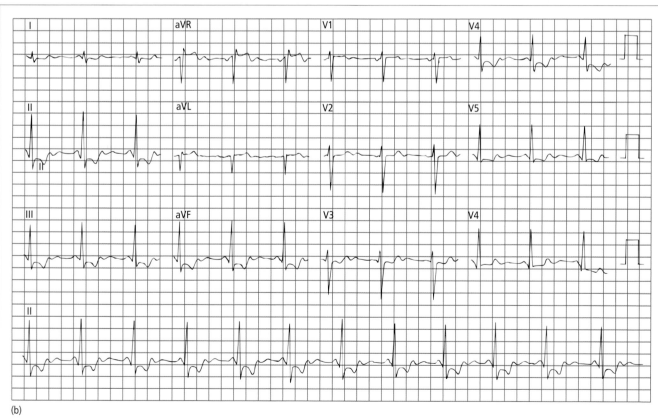

(b)

Fig. 96 Positive exercise ECG: note (a) the significant ST changes in the inferolateral leads which (b) become more marked in recovery.

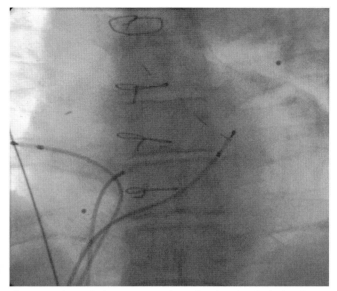

Fig. 97 Radiograph demonstrating electrodes placed in the high right atrium, right ventricular outflow tract and His bundle during an electrophysiological test. Sternal wires present from previous coronary bypass grafting.

produce extremely rapid heart rates. Bipolar electrodes are placed to obtain intracardiac electrograms (high right atrium, RV apex/outflow tract and His–Purkinje system) (Fig. 97). A multipolar electrode placed in the coronary sinus records electrograms from the left atrium. Arrhythmias are induced by delivering extra pacing beats after a train of paced beats in the atrium and ventricle. These extra stimuli are timed to occur during the refractory period in an attempt to establish a possible re-entry mechanism (Fig. 98). The timing of the individual electrograms will indicate whether there is a possible electrophysiological substrate for arrhythmias. Assessment of the function of the SA and AV nodes indicates whether permanent pacing might be required.

After investigation

Patients are observed for 24 h. Drug therapy may be changed as a result of the EPS.

Complications

- Femoral vein/subclavian vein (haematoma)
- Incessant arrhythmias requiring cardioversion, e.g. AF.

 Fogoros RN. *Electrophysiological Testing*, 2nd edn. Oxford: Blackwell Science, 1995.

3.3 Ambulatory monitoring

Principle

Documenting a single-channel electrocardiogram over 24 h can provide useful information in the investigation of patients with palpitations, arrhythmias and syncope. It is non-invasive and, with current analysis hardware/software, tapes can be analysed rapidly and accurately. It is always important when using Holter monitoring to appreciate that this provides only a brief snapshot of the patient's heart rhythm, and that a negative result does not mean that the patient's symptoms are not secondary to an arrhythmia.

Indications

Ambulatory monitoring is indicated for the following:
- Evaluation of patients with palpitations and syncope
- Monitoring the efficacy of antiarrhythmic therapy
- Evaluation of heart rate variability.

Practical details

There are a number of different methods by which heart rate and rhythm can be observed.

Twenty-four-hour Holter monitoring

This is used for patients with frequent symptoms. Even some patients who have infrequent symptoms may have asymptomatic arrhythmic episodes on a 24-h recording that may provide valuable information (Fig. 99).

Patient-activated devices

These are used for less frequent symptoms, e.g. Cardiomemo recorder. However, the efficacy of these devices relies on the patient activating the device, which is not always possible during or shortly after a symptomatic episode.

Implantable loop recorders

These are used for infrequent symptoms. They enable the patient to activate the device up to 40 min after the event and still record the heart rhythm (Figs 100 and 101).

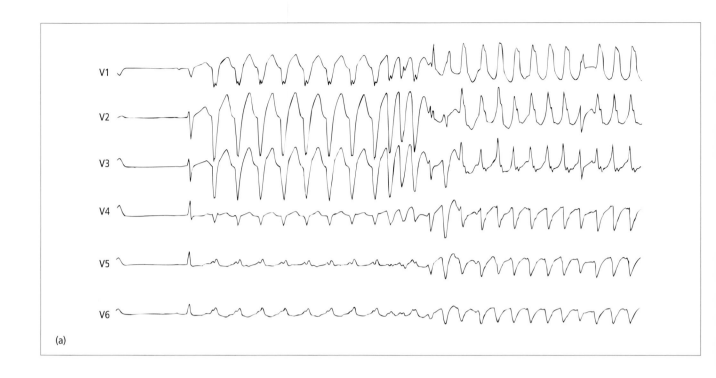

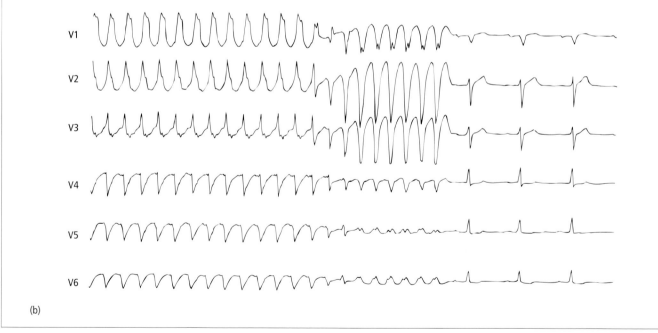

Fig. 98 Induction of ventricular tachycardia. (a) Note the train of paced beats followed by earlier extra stimuli and then onset of monomorphic ventricular tachycardia. (b) Ventricular tachycardia is then terminated with nine beats of overdrive pacing.

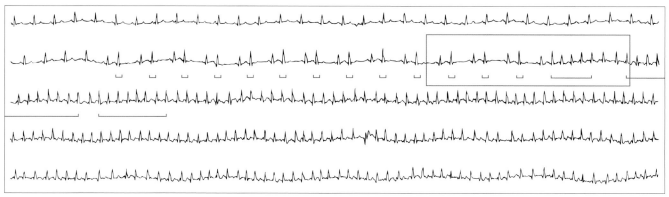

Fig. 99 Holter monitor recording demonstrating atrioventricular nodal re-entry tachycardia (AVNRT)/atrioventricular re-entry tachycardia (AVRT). Note the sudden onset after a short period of ventricular bigeminy.

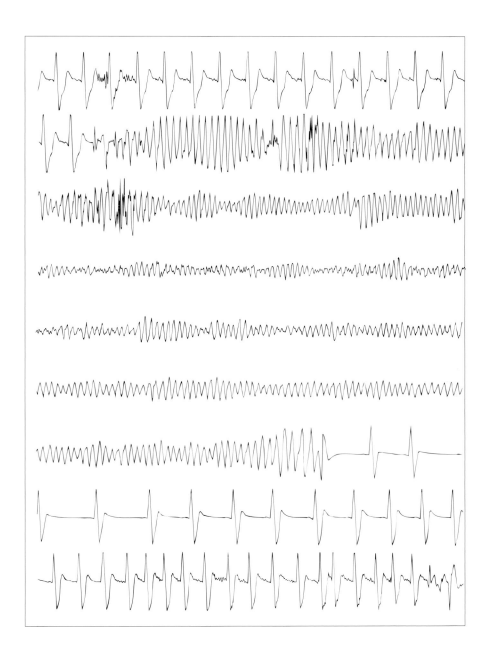

Fig. 100 Loop recording showing sinus tachycardia followed by *torsades de pointes* with spontaneous resolution.

129

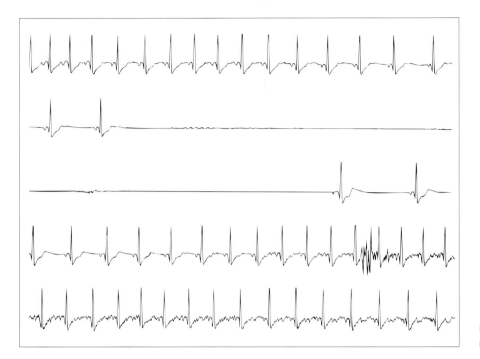

Fig. 101 Tracing from implantable loop recorder showing significant pause.

3.4 Radiofrequency ablation and implantable cardioverter defibrillators

3.4.1 RADIOFREQUENCY ABLATION

Principle

The basic idea is to place an electrode in a specific site in the heart and deliver damaging energy through the electrode to produce a discrete scar. As the scar is electrically inactive, the pathways necessary for tachyarrhythmias may be disrupted. Most tachyarrhythmias can be treated with radiofrequency (RF) ablation:

- AVNRT
- Wolff–Parkinson–White syndrome
- Concealed accessory pathways (AVRT)
- VT
- Focal atrial tachycardias
- AF (fast rates abolished by ablation of AV node and pacemaker implant)
- Most can be accessed via the right side of the heart from the femoral/subclavian veins; others (left-sided pathways/left-sided VT) have to be approached from either the femoral artery/aorta or via an atrial trans-septal approach.

Indications

Indications include those who have recurrent tachyarrhythmias despite antiarrhythmic therapy. Some patients (e.g. those with Wolff–Parkinson–White syndrome) who are at high risk should probably undergo RF ablation even with minimal symptoms.

Practical details

Before procedure

Antiarrhythmic drug therapy is usually stopped a few days before the procedure. Careful informed consent must be given.

The procedure

The treatment is usually performed under sedation.

After procedure

Most patients are discharged the following day.

Complications

The major complication of RF ablation procedures is the risk of unintentional damage to the AV node and the need for a permanent pacemaker. This occurs in <1%. A rare complication is cardiac perforation which may require pericardiocentesis or surgical repair.

Prognosis

- RF ablation is usually permanent
- <10% recurrence of the arrhythmia.

 1 Fogoros RN. *Electrophysiological Testing.* Oxford: Blackwell Science, 1995.

3.4.2 IMPLANTABLE CARDIOVERTER DEFIBRILLATOR

Principle

Patients who are at high risk of ventricular arrhythmias may benefit from implantable cardioverter defibrillators (ICDs). Once a ventricular arrhythmia is detected, an ICD can either deliver anti-tachycardia pacing (ATP) or shock therapy (electrodes in the right ventricle, superior vena cava and/or casing of the ICD) or a combination of both, depending on how the device is programmed.

Indications

In general, indications are becoming broader as larger prospective randomized trials are reported (e.g. AVID [1], MADIT [2], MUSTT [3]):
- Previous spontaneous VT/VF
- Syncope of undetermined aetiology with VT inducible during EPS. (See Section 3.2, p. 125.)

Contraindications

- Reversible cause for VT/VF
- Incessant VT/VF
- Surgical, medical or psychiatric contraindication.

Practical details

Before investigation

Patients are thoroughly investigated to exclude reversible cause of arrhythmia (echocardiography, cardiac catheterization, CT/MRI). Most will have an EPS to confirm the diagnosis and identify whether the arrhythmia can be pace terminated. (See Section 3.2, p. 125.)

The investigation

ICDs are implanted under sedation (e.g. midazolam) or general anaesthesia. The leads are placed transvenously via the subclavian/cephalic veins. The device is implanted either under the pectoralis major muscle or subcutane-

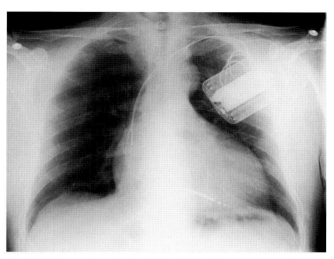

Fig. 102 Chest radiograph of patient with dual-chamber implantable cardioverter defibrillator. Note electrode in right ventricle with defibrillation coil at distal end. A pace/sense electrode is positioned in the right atrial appendage.

ously on the left side of the chest wall (Fig. 102). VF is produced to ensure that the device can successfully terminate it with shock therapy.

After investigation

After a few days, the device is checked to ensure correct function of the pacing systems: patients usually undergo a further VF induction under sedation.

Complications

Complications are similar to those associated with pacemaker implantation. (See Section 3.5, p. 132.)

Prognosis

Most patients with ICDs die as a result of cardiac pump failure or incessant ventricular arrhythmia. ICDs last between 5 and 10 years, depending on the number of shocks delivered.

 1 The Antiarrhythmic Versus Implantable Defibrillator (AVID) Investigation. A comparison of antiarrhythmic drug therapy with implantable defibrillators in patients resuscitated from near fatal ventricular arrhythmias. *N Engl J Med* 1997; 337: 1576–1583.
2 Moss A, Hall J, Cannon D *et al.* for the MADIT Investigation. Improved survival with an implanted defibrillator in patients with coronary disease at high risk of ventricular arrhythmias. *N Engl J Med* 1996; 335: 1933–1940.
3 Buxton A, Lee K, Fisher J *et al.* for the Multicenter Unsustained Tachycardia Trial (MUSTT) Investigation. A randomized study of the prevention of sudden death in patients with coronary artery disease. *N Engl J Med* 1999; 341: 1882–1990.

3.5 Pacemakers

Pacing of patients with non-reversible significant brady-arrhythmias can restore life expectancy to close to that of the normal population. Pacemakers have improved considerably over the last two decades. Devices have increased in longevity and been reduced in size. In addition, many technical innovations have resulted in pacemakers that are more physiological in their mode of action. The simplest of pacemakers consists of a single lead, with its tip in the right ventricular apex connected to the pulse generator in the subcutaneous tissue of the chest wall. Dual-chamber devices have a further lead with its tip positioned in the right atrial appendage (Fig. 103). Pacemakers have a designated terminology which describes the pacing and sensing functions of the device (Table 33).

Indications

Temporary pacemaker

Temporary pacing is useful in the following circumstances:
- As an interim measure before permanent pacemaker
- Inferior MI: second-/third-degree block and hypotension/heart failure
- Anterior MI: second-/third-degree block (usually large infarct to involve the AV node)
- Symptomatic/asymptomatic patients with trifascicular block undergoing general anaesthesia (should be assessed for permanent pacemaker)
- Drug overdose, e.g. digoxin, β blockers, verapamil.

Temporary pacing is not indicated for asymptomatic patients with bifascicular block who are undergoing general anaesthesia.

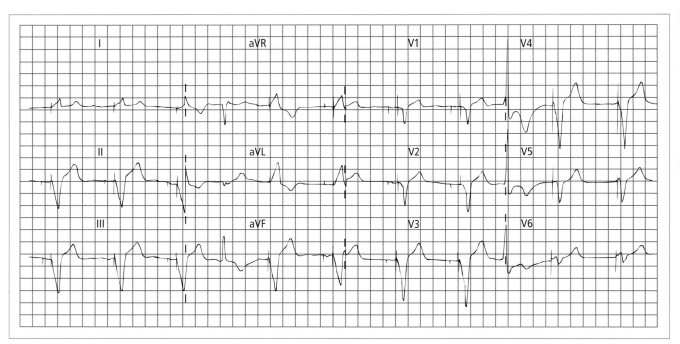

Fig. 103 ECG demonstrating dual-chamber pacing. Note the pacing 'spike' before most P waves and QRS complexes.

Paced chamber	Sensed chamber	Effect of sensing	Programming/rate responsiveness
0 = none	0 = none	0 = none	0 = none
A = atrium	A = atrium	T = triggered	P = simple
V = ventricle	V = ventricle	I = inhibited	M = multiprogrammable
D = dual (A + V)	D = dual (A + V)	D = dual (T + I)	C = communicating
			R = rate responsive

Table 33 Algorithm used to describe pacemaker function*.

*For example, a DDDR pacemaker both senses and paces in the atrium and ventricle, and triggers and inhibits, depending on what is or is not sensed. It also has a rate response which means that the heart rate will be paced faster if appropriate, e.g. during exercise.

Permanent pacemaker

The permanent pacemaker is useful for the following:
- Third-degree heart block
- Symptomatic, second-degree block
- Asymptomatic, type II, second-degree block
- AF with pauses >3.0 s
- Symptomatic documented sinus node dysfunction
- Recurrent syncope associated with >3.0 s pause with carotid sinus stimulation.

Practical details

Before procedure

Patients should give informed consent and be fasted.

The procedure

The procedure is usually performed under local anaesthesia. The pacemaker leads are placed transvenously via the cephalic/subclavian routes into the right ventricular apex and right atrial appendage under fluoroscopic guidance. The leads are checked to ensure correct pace/sense functions and the pulse generator is implanted subcutaneously.

After procedure

After a satisfactory pacemaker check the following day, most patients may be discharged from hospital, usually with 5 days of antibiotic therapy and after a lateral and posteroanterior chest radiograph (Fig. 104). For driving regulations, see Section 2.19, p. 118. Pacemakers can be programmed and interrogated by placing a 'wand' over the device; using electromagnetic induction, information can be received or transmitted to the pacemaker. Patients are usually seen every 6–12 months to monitor the pacemaker and re-program if necessary. The expected life of the battery is 8–12 years.

Complications of pacemakers

Although complications are rare, the following may occur.

Common

- Pneumothorax
- Pacemaker lead displacement (Fig. 105)
- Haematoma.

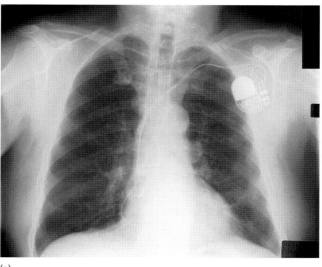

(a)

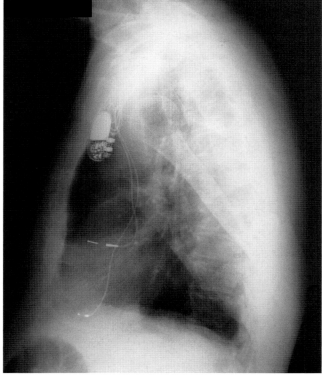

(b)

Fig. 104 Chest radiograph of dual-chamber pacemaker: (a) anteroposterior and (b) lateral.

Uncommon

- Local infection
- Pericardial effusion
- Thrombosis and thromboembolism
- Infective endocarditis
- Pacemaker syndrome: single-chamber pacing, leading to symptoms as a result of loss of AV synchrony.

133

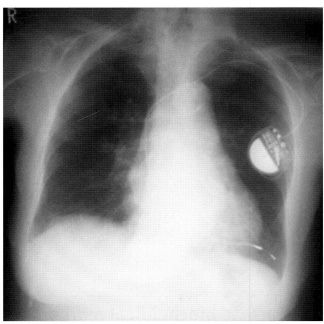

Fig. 105 Chest radiograph showing displacement of ventricular lead through ventricle to pericardial space.

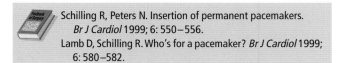

Fig. 106 Schematic diagram of cardiac silhouette on chest radiograph. AA, arch aorta; Asc A, ascending aorta; LA, left atrial appendage; LV, left ventricle; PA, pulmonary artery; RA, right atrium; SVC, superior vena cava.

Rare

- Twiddler's syndrome: patient consciously/subconsciously turns the pacemaker generator, leading to retraction and eventual displacement of the pacing lead
- Component failure: lead/pulse generator.

Schilling R, Peters N. Insertion of permanent pacemakers. *Br J Cardiol* 1999; 6: 550–556.

Lamb D, Schilling R. Who's for a pacemaker? *Br J Cardiol* 1999; 6: 580–582.

3.6 The chest radiograph in cardiac disease

Commonly encountered abnormalities

The normal cardiac silhouette is shown in Fig. 106. Below are the most commonly encountered abnormalities.

Cardiomegaly

Cardiothoracic ratio >0.5 on posteroanterior projection is a fairly specific indicator of cardiac disease, but may be falsely increased in pes excavatum and very thin patients. Echocardiography is much more sensitive.

Aortic enlargement

This is seen in hypertension, atherosclerosis or aortic regurgitation:

- Prominent aortic arch
- Ascending aorta protrudes further to the right side
- Tortuous descending aorta.

Mediastinal widening

This may indicate an aortic dissection.

Enlarged pulmonary artery

This is seen in the following:
- Pulmonary hypertension: COAD, primary pulmonary hypertension, Eisenmenger's syndrome
- Pulmonary stenosis: poststenotic dilatation as a result of turbulent blood flow
- Collagen disorders, e.g. Marfan's syndrome.

Left atrial enlargement

This is seen in mitral disease or replacement and LV impairment. It may be mimicked by mediastinal or pleural neoplasm. Occasionally, the left atrium may be so grossly enlarged that it forms the right heart border (i.e. lateral to the right atrium). In this situation, left atrial enlargement may be recognized by following the superior border of the left atrium, which will cross the midline. If the prominent right heart border is caused by right atrial

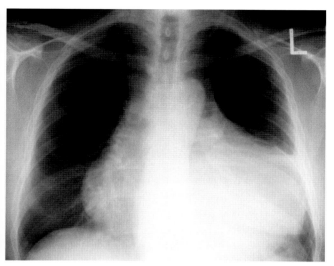

Fig. 107 Globular cardiomegaly caused by a large pericardial effusion. Note sternal wires from recent cardiac surgery.

enlargement, the contour is continuous with the superior vena cava.

Left ventricular enlargement

- Pressure overload: apex elevated and more rounded
- Volume overload: widening of cardiac shadow.

Right ventricle enlargement

The right ventricle does not normally form a cardiac border, but enlargement pushes the LV posteriorly and to the left, causing widening of the heart shadow.

Pericardial effusion

This may produce massive cardiomegaly, giving the cardiac contour a globular appearance, with clear lung fields (Fig. 107).

Common abnormalities of pulmonary vasculature

Increased pulmonary blood flow

- Enlarged pulmonary arteries
- Recruitment of upper lobe vessels.

Pulmonary hypertension

- Peripheral vasoconstriction (pruning)
- Further enlargement of pulmonary arteries
- Pulmonary artery calcification.

Pulmonary venous hypertension and oedema

In increasing order of severity:
- Upper lobe blood diversion
- Interlobular septal thickening (Kerley B lines): thin horizontal lines at lung bases
- Alveolar oedema, typically involving the inner two-thirds of the lung ('bat wing' hilar shadowing).

Pulmonary oedema is occasionally unilateral. After treatment, the radiographic appearances often lag behind clinical improvement. Prominent interstitial lines also occur in the following:
- Fibrosis
- Tumour infiltration
- Interstitial pneumonia.

3.7 Cardiac biochemical markers

Principle

Heart muscle damage, usually caused by acute ischaemia, causes release of proteins that can be detected in the blood stream.

CK-MB

This cardiospecific isoenzyme of creatine kinase (CK):
- is the most widely used marker of heart muscle damage
- has a reasonable specificity but only a moderate sensitivity
- an arbitrary cut-off point is used for retrospective diagnosis of MI
- is used in conjunction with the ECG to make the diagnosis of non-Q-wave (or subendocardial) infarction
- gives results that are often equivocal and may be uninterpretable in some circumstances, e.g. very high CK caused by coexisting skeletal muscle damage.

Troponin tests

These tests are now superseding CK-MB assays. Troponins are regulatory elements of the contractile apparatus in muscle; they exist in cardiac-specific isoforms and are highly sensitive. Rapid bedside assays for cardiac troponins T and I are available. They are normally very low/undetectable in the blood and appear 4–6 h after myocardial damage, peak at 24 h and persist for up to 14 days. In addition, they are raised in 30% of patients with unstable angina. A positive test is associated with a higher risk of death or MI—the higher level indicating a worse prognosis. They may be used to select high-risk unstable angina

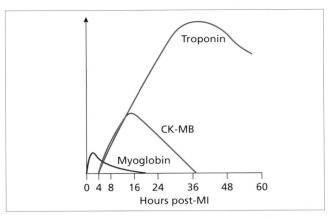

Fig. 108 Time course of cardiac markers after heart muscle damage. MI, myocardial infarction.

patients who would benefit from more aggressive treatment, e.g. low-molecular-weight heparin, glycoprotein IIb/IIIa receptor antagonists or early revascularization. A negative test may be used in conjunction with clinical and ECG criteria to identify low-risk patients who are suitable for early discharge without the need for overnight stay.

Myoglobin

Myoglobin is present in both skeletal and cardiac muscle, and released about 30 min after heart muscle damage. Elevated values may detect infarction much sooner after the onset of chest pain than CK-MB or troponins (Fig. 108). However, as a result of the poor specificity of myoglobin measurement, a positive test must be confirmed by troponin or CK-MB.

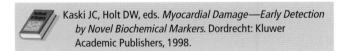
Kaski JC, Holt DW, eds. *Myocardial Damage—Early Detection by Novel Biochemical Markers*. Dordrecht: Kluwer Academic Publishers, 1998.

3.8 Cardiac catheterization, percutaneous transluminal coronary angioplasty and stenting

3.8.1 CARDIAC CATHETERIZATION

Principle

Catheters are introduced into the arterial or venous system and advanced to the left or right heart, respectively, allowing the following:
• Pressure measurements in the cardiac chambers and major vessels.

• Injection of radiographic contrast into cardiac chambers, major vessels or coronary arteries. Digital cineangiography provides a permanent versatile record of cardiac anatomy.
• Oxygen saturation measurements in blood sampled from the cardiac chambers and major vessels.

Indications

Left heart catheterization

• Angina (stable or unstable) not controlled by medical therapy, or with positive stress test at low/moderate workload. (See Section 2.1, p. 51.)
• Proposed heart valve surgery
• Suspected aortic dissection not clearly seen by other imaging methods. (See Section 2.11.1, p. 99.)

Right heart catheterization

This is indicated in suspected primary pulmonary hypertension and selected cases of pulmonary embolism.

Combined left and right heart catheterization

• Mitral stenosis and selected cases of mitral regurgitation before surgery
• Congenital heart disease: to confirm diagnosis and assess severity
• Pre-transplantation assessment.

Contraindications

Severely impaired coagulation. Pulmonary oedema and cardiogenic shock are relative contraindications because radiographic contrast may lead to haemodynamic deterioration, even death.

Practical details

Before investigation

• FBC, urea and electrolytes, INR if on warfarin
• ECG
• Informed consent
• Premedication with oral benzodiazepine.

The investigation

Lead aprons are worn to protect staff from radiation. Aseptic procedures are followed. Usually the right femoral artery and/or vein is punctured under local anaesthetic (but patients on warfarin with an INR of 1.5–3.0 may be safely catheterized from the arm). A 5–7 French gauge sheath (incorporating a haemostatic valve) is introduced

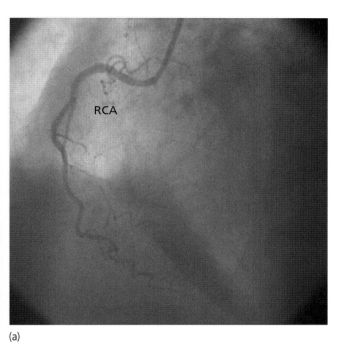

(a)

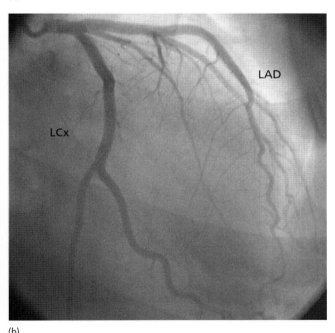

(b)

Fig. 109 Normal coronary angiogram: the right coronary artery is small (non-dominant) and shown in (a) with the left coronary demonstrated in (b). LAD, left anterior descending; LCx, left circumflex; RCA, right coronary artery.

Table 34 Normal intracardiac pressure values.

Pressure	Range (mmHg)
Right atrium mean	1–5
Right ventricle systolic	15–30
Right ventricle end-diastolic	1–8
Pulmonary artery systolic	15–30
Pulmonary artery diastolic	5–12
Pulmonary artery mean	9–16
Pulmonary capillary wedge mean	5–13
Left atrium mean	2–12
Left ventricle systolic	90–140
Left ventricle end-diastolic	5–12

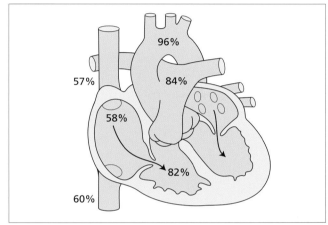

Fig. 110 Oxygen saturation measurements showing a 'step up' in the right ventricle, indicating a ventricular septal defect with left-to-right shunt.

The size of the shunt can be estimated from the ratio of pulmonary to systemic blood flow, using the following formula (derived from the Fick equation):

$$\frac{Qp}{Qs} = \frac{Ao - MV}{PV - PA}$$

where Qp = pulmonary flow; Qs = systemic flow; Ao = aortic saturation; MV = mixed venous saturation; PV = pulmonary venous saturation; PA = pulmonary arterial saturation. Pulmonary venous saturation is not usually measured directly, but is assumed to be 97%. From Fig. 110, the ratio of pulmonary to venous flow is calculated to be 2.9 : 1. A shunt >1.5 : 1 is regarded as significant.

After investigation

- Remove the sheath and press on the vessel to achieve haemostasis (arterial at least 10 min, venous 5 min). During this time, preliminary results may be given to the patient.
- Instruct patients on how to press on the vessel themselves.
- Arrange for return to the ward.
- Bedrest for 2–4 h after femoral artery puncture.
- Review and report catheter data.
- Review patient on the ward.
- Explain full results and plan.

using the Seldinger technique. Pre-shaped catheters are passed through the sheath (on a long J-tipped guidewire in the arterial system) and guided using continuous pressure monitoring and fluoroscopic imaging. A three-lead ECG is also monitored continuously.

Examples of images obtained from a left heart catheter are shown in Fig. 109. Normal values for pressure data are given in Table 34. Oxygen saturation measurement from a case of left-to-right shunting is illustrated in Fig. 110.

Complications

Minor

- Bruising in 50%
- Haematoma in 5%.

Major

- Femoral arterial damage requiring repair
- Stroke, MI or death.

Each of these complications has an incidence of about 1 per 1000.

> **Important information for patients**
>
> While obtaining consent, ensure that the patient understands why the procedure is being carried out, what is involved and what the risks are.
>
> Patients should not drive for 24 h afterwards, and must have someone staying with them if they are going home after a day-case procedure.

Miller GAH. *Handbook of Cardiac Catheterization*. Oxford: Blackwell Scientific Publications, 1990.

3.8.2 PERCUTANEOUS TRANSLUMINAL CORONARY ANGIOPLASTY AND STENTING

Principle

Angina is relieved by inflating a catheter-delivered balloon within a coronary artery at the site of stenosis.

Indications

- Patients with suitable stenoses in one or two coronary arteries who have angina (stable or unstable) that is not adequately controlled by medical therapy
- Recurrent angina after CABG (selected patients)
- Acute MI as primary treatment (primary angioplasty)
- Acute MI after unsuccessful thrombolysis (rescue angioplasty).

Contraindications

PTCA should not be undertaken in the following:
- Patients who would benefit prognostically from coronary bypass grafting. (See Section 2.1, p. 51.)
- Patients without angina (no evidence that life expectancy improved).

Practical details

Before procedure

This is as for cardiac catheterization (see Section 3.8.1, p. 136), but in addition insert an intravenous cannula.

The procedure

Usually a right femoral arterial approach is used. The coronary ostium is intubated with an angioplasty guide catheter. Heparin 10 000 units as an intravenous bolus is given at this stage. A guidewire is introduced through the guide catheter into the coronary artery lumen; it is advanced beyond the lesion using fluoroscopy and injections of radiographic contrast, given as necessary. A balloon catheter is passed over this guidewire, positioned at the site of narrowing and inflated for approximately 1 min. If a satisfactory result cannot be obtained using the balloon alone, a coronary stent may be deployed (Fig. 111). This is a latticework stainless steel tube mounted on a deflated balloon. After positioning at the site of narrowing, the balloon is inflated so that the stent is expanded and embedded in the coronary artery wall. When the balloon is deflated, the stent remains as a 'scaffold' to hold the artery open. If a stent is used, the activated clotting time (ACT) is checked and further heparin given if necessary to achieve an ACT of >350 s.

After procedure

The sheath is removed 4–6 h after the procedure, once the heparin has worn off. If a stent has been used, prescribe clopidogrel 300 mg stat dose, and 75 mg daily thereafter for 4 weeks, to reduce the risk of stent thrombosis. Patients may go home the day after an uncomplicated procedure.

Outcome

- The success rate is 95%
- The chance of re-stenosis in 6 months is 30% (slightly less if stented)
- If occlusion is chronic, there is a 50% chance of success and 50% chance of re-occlusion.

Complications

- Coronary dissection, acute vessel closure: usually controlled by stenting.
- Coronary thrombosis: most commonly seen in unstable angina. The glycoprotein IIb/IIIa receptor antagonists (e.g. abciximab) are intravenous antiplatelet agents which may be given to protect against this complication.

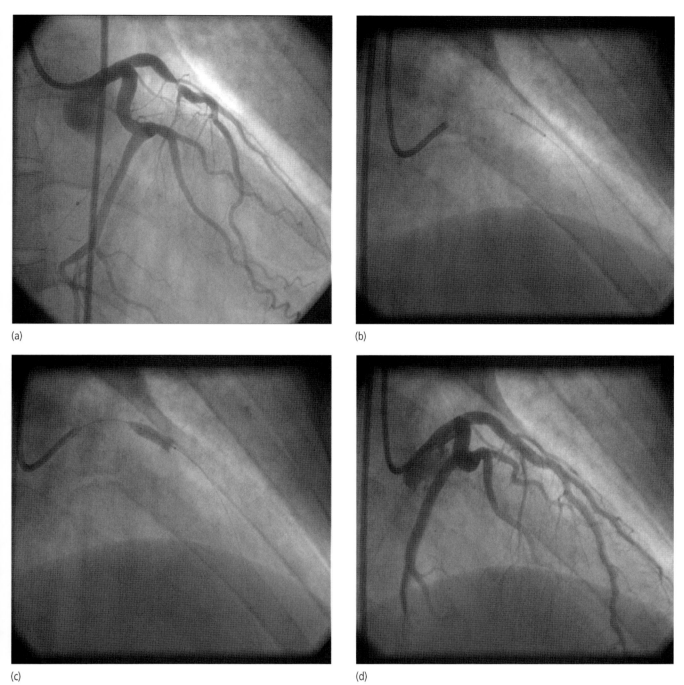

(a)

(b)

(c)

(d)

Fig. 111 Coronary artery stenting: (a) left coronary angiogram showing a tight stenosis in the left anterior descending coronary artery. (b) Positioning of a stent mounted on an angioplasty balloon. (c) Inflation of balloon to deploy stent. (d) Final result.

• Death, MI, emergency CABG, stroke about 1 per 200. (See also Section 3.8.1, p. 138.)

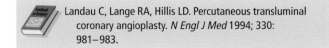 Landau C, Lange RA, Hillis LD. Percutaneous transluminal coronary angioplasty. *N Engl J Med* 1994; 330: 981–983.

 Important information for patients

• Expect transient angina during balloon inflations
• Get consent from all patients for angioplasty ± stent ± emergency CABG.

3.9 Computed tomography and magnetic resonance imaging

3.9.1 COMPUTED TOMOGRAPHY

Principle

Multiple radiography views are processed and a digital cross-sectional image produced, with different tissue densities displayed as different grey-scale values. In spiral CT the radiography tube rotates continuously around the slowly moving patient, scanning a large volume in a single breathhold and reducing artefacts. These images can be reconstructed in other (non-axial) planes.

Indications

- Pericardial disease: thickening, infiltration or effusion
- Spiral CT: contrast angiography of pulmonary vasculature down to the level of segmental branches ($\dot{V}/\dot{Q}$ or invasive pulmonary angiogram still better for smaller branches), aorta for aneurysms or dissection, renal or carotid stenoses.

Contraindications

- Contrast: known sensitivity or renal impairment (relative contraindication)
- Pregnancy: relative contraindication—large radiation dose but depends on risk/benefit balance and uterus can be shielded.

3.9.2 MAGNETIC RESONANCE IMAGING

Principle

The human body is about 60% hydrogen atoms. Inside a strong magnetic field, hydrogen nuclei (protons) align like small magnets. A further oscillating perpendicular magnetic field excites the protons and they move out of alignment. As they return to the equilibrium state they emit signals that are processed into images, reflecting different tissue characteristics.

Indications

Anatomy

- Aortic aneurysms, dissection or coarctation, and large arteries, e.g. carotid
- Congenital heart disease: very detailed three-dimensional anatomy

- Cardiomyopathies, ventricular mass and tumours
- Pericardial disease.

Function

- LV regional wall motion
- Myocardial perfusion.

Future clinical use—not currently

- Native coronaries and grafts.

Contraindications

- Embedded ferromagnetic objects: intracranial clips, foreign bodies, early Starr–Edwards valves
- Permanent pacemakers or implantable defibrillators (affects function)
- Later prosthetic valves and sternal wires safe, but cause an artefact.

Practical details

All ferromagnetic or magnetized objects (e.g. credit cards) must be removed. The ECG is used to 'gate' the image, i.e. it is only acquired during diastole when the heart is relatively still. ST-segment changes seen are artefactual. Irregular rhythms result in a poorer image quality. The magnet makes a knocking sound and a claustrophobic patient may find the experience unpleasant. A scan takes 30–60 min.

3.10 Ventilation–perfusion isotope scanning ($\dot{V}/\dot{Q}$)

Principle

The principle of this investigation is comparison of ventilation and perfusion in the lungs to detect areas of mismatch (i.e. ventilated but not perfused), which occur in acute pulmonary embolism. Many other conditions (e.g. tumour or consolidation) cause perfusion defects, but these are generally matched by ventilation defects and associated with chest radiograph abnormality.

Indication

A suspected pulmonary embolism, preferably with a normal chest radiograph. Ventilation–perfusion scan reports are useful if perfusion is normal and PE therefore excluded, or if definite unmatched defects are seen and the diagnosis confirmed; however, many scans do not produce clear-cut results and are reported as being of intermediate probability. The diagnostic yield is improved by correlation with clinical suspicion, but there are still many cases where other imaging modalities are required.

Contraindications

There are none. It is safe in pregnancy, although some centres modify the dose.

Practical details

- Inhalation of radioisotope (krypton-81m, xenon-133 or technetium-99m [^{99m}Tc]): patient needs to be able to inhale sufficiently
- Injection of ^{99m}Tc-labelled albumin macroaggregates or microspheres
- Scanning after each; some centres only perform a ventilation scan if the perfusion is abnormal
- Duration of about 40 min.

 PIOPED Investigators. Value of the ventilation/perfusion scan in acute pulmonary embolism. *JAMA* 1990; 263: 2753–2759.

3.11 Echocardiography

Principle

Ultrasonic waves are generated in pulses. As the ultrasonic wave travels through tissues, some of it is reflected back towards the transducer as an echo every time the sound crosses an interface—typically the junctions between blood and the heart valves or myocardium. Several modes of imaging are recognized.

M-mode

Ultrasonic pulses are directed along a single line and the interfaces displayed as a graph of depth against time. It allows detailed evaluation and measurement of particular structures (Fig. 112).

Two-dimensional echocardiography

The information is displayed as a fan-shaped image. Detailed information about cardiac structures and their movement can be observed. Standard transthoracic views

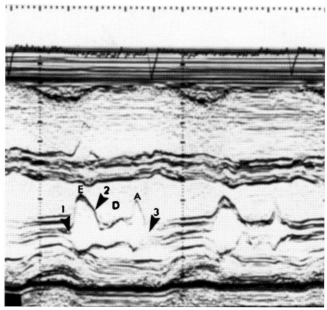

Fig. 112 Parasternal long axis M-mode at the level of the mitral valve leaflets. 1, at the end of systole the mitral valve begins to open; E, maximum excursion of anterior mitral leaflet; 2, initial diastolic closing wave; D, diastole; A, reopening of mitral valve caused by atrial systole; 3, mitral valve closes at onset of ventricular systole. (Courtesy of Dr J Chambers.)

include the parasternal short and long axes, and the apical long axis (Fig. 113).

Doppler echocardiography

Quantitative measurements of velocity can be made (continuous and pulsed-wave Doppler), allowing the estimation of pressure gradients, intracardiac pressures and valve areas, on which the determination of the severity of valve lesions depends. Qualitative information can be obtained by colour coding velocity information and displaying this superimposed on a two-dimensional image. Detection of abnormal flow patterns within the heart is made possible with this technique (see Fig. 53).

In some patients and indications, transthoracic images may not be of sufficient quality to allow diagnosis. TOE, where the ultrasonic transducer is positioned in the oesophagus, behind and close to the heart, allows much better image quality. This can be combined with exercise or dobutamine to assess reversible areas of hypokinesia, which suggest ischaemia if they occur on stress. The development of intravenous contrast agents, allowing echocardiographic imaging of perfusion, has enormous potential in this respect.

Dobutamine stress echocardiography can also be used to assess myocardial viability, and is finding an increasing role in the assessment of the functional significance of valve lesions.

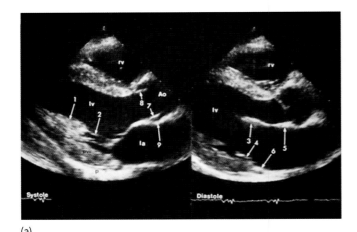

(a)

(b)

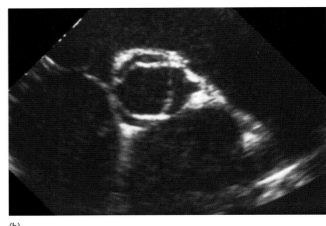

(c)

Fig. 113 Parasternal long (a) and short (b) axes (at the level of the aortic valve) and four-chamber views (c) of a normal heart. LA, left atrium; LV, left ventricle; RA, right atrium; RV, right ventricle; Ao, aorta. (Courtesy of Dr J Chambers.)

Indications

Echocardiography forms an essential part of the non-invasive assessment of valvular and structural heart disease, ventricular function and myocardial ischaemia viability.

Contraindications

- Unstable angina at the time of stress echocardiography.
- TOE: known pharyngeal pouch or severe oesophageal disease. If there is unexplained dysphagia, arrange barium swallow before considering TOE.

Practical details

Transoesophageal echocardiography

- Nil by mouth for at least 4 h; consider antibiotic prophylaxis if prosthetic valve
- Obtain written consent
- Insert intravenous cannula
- Check for loose teeth; remove false teeth
- Position patient
- Give sedation—e.g. midazolam 4 mg i.v. or diazepam 5–10 mg i.v.
- Monitor peripheral oxygen saturation continuously
- Insert mouth guard and perform test, ensuring that mouth secretions cleared using suction
- Monitor recovery; allow home with escort once free of sedation.

Stress echocardiography

Intravenous access is required for administration of dobutamine. Resting echocardiogram followed by stress with exercise or dobutamine, noting symptoms ± ECG changes. Monitor echocardiogram to assess development of wall motion abnormality (ischaemia) or recovery of function (viable myocardium). Monitor to ensure disappearance of symptoms and resolution of any ECG changes.

Complications

Transoesophageal echocardiography

- Oesophageal trauma ranging from inflammation to rupture
- Aspiration.

Important information for patients

Explain the following:
- The benefits and risks of the procedure
- The need for sedation, such that they may not remember the test
- That they will be drowsy afterwards, should not drive for the rest of the day and will need to be escorted home
- That they may have a sore throat for 1–2 days.

Stress echocardiography

- Supraventricular tachyarrhythmia
- VT/VF: 1 : 5000 treadmill tests
- Death as a result of resistant VF—1 : 10 000 treadmill tests
- Precipitation of acute coronary syndrome.

Important information for patients

Stress echocardiography
Stop β blockers for 48 h before test. Inform patients about the procedure and chosen stress modality. Make sure that they are aware that they may experience their angina pain during the test. Explain risk of arrhythmias.

Bach DS, Armstrong WF. Dobutamine stress echocardiography. *Am J Cardiol* 1992; 69: 90.
Chambers J. *Clinical Echocardiography*. London: BMJ Publishing Group, 1995.
Sanderson JE, Chan WW. Transoesophageal echocardiography. *Postgrad Med J* 1997; 73: 137–140.

3.12 Nuclear cardiology

3.12.1 MYOCARDIAL PERFUSION IMAGING

Thallium-201 is actively taken up by myocardial cells in a manner similar to potassium. Its concentration in the myocardium depends on both perfusion and integrity of the myocardial cell membrane. A graded colour representation of perfusion is obtained, allowing comparison between regions. Absolute values of blood flow are not obtained.

A scan after exercise or pharmacological stress with dipyridamole or adenosine is followed by a resting scan at 2–4 h. Defects seen during stress, which are not present at rest, represent ischaemia. Defects present in both scans ('fixed perfusion defect') usually indicate infarction (Fig. 114). The sensitivity for detection of significant coronary artery disease is 80–85% and specificity >90%.

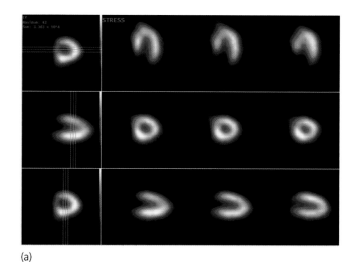

(a)

(b)

Fig. 114 (a) Normal and (b) abnormal stress thallium-201 perfusion scan, showing inferior ischaemia (b). (Courtesy of Dr Jan.)

Indications

Nuclear techniques are expensive. In most cases, myocardial perfusion imaging should be used when ECG morphology or patient morbidity precludes the interpretation or use of exercise ECG testing. Indications in common with exercise testing include the following:

• Prognostic stratification after MI
• Identification of ischaemia in symptomatic patients, especially atypical pain
• Risk stratification in patients with known or high risk of coronary artery disease before non-cardiac surgery.

3.12.2 POSITRON EMISSION TOMOGRAPHY

This technique uses positron-emitting radionuclides to produce tomographic images of coronary flow and metabolism. The technique also allows quantification of blood flow within specified regions of the heart. Rest and pharmacological stress scans are performed in a similar manner to thallium imaging. Myocardial viability is suggested by maintained glucose metabolism in an area with a fixed perfusion defect.

Dilsizian V, Bonow RO. Current diagnostic techniques of assessing myocardial viability in patients with hibernating and stunned myocardium. *Circulation* 1993; 87: 1–20.

Kotler TS, Diamond GA. Exercise thallium-201 scintigraphy in the diagnosis and prognosis of coronary artery disease. *Ann Intern Med* 1990; 113: 684–702.

Acknowledgements

The authors and editor would like to thank: Dr L.M. Shapiro, Dr R. Coulden, and the Pulmonary Vascular Diseases Unit, Papworth Hospital, Cambridge for their help in the preparation of this module.

4 Self-assessment

Answers are on pp. 257–260.

Question 1

A 67-year-old man presents with chest pain that came on suddenly while he was lying in bed. It radiated to the left shoulder, and he felt sweaty and nauseated. His past medical history was notable for duodenal ulceration, 20 years previously, and hypertension, for which he took bendrofluazide as his only regular medication. On examination he looked unwell, with pulse 110/min (regular), BP 120/60 mmHg in both arms, and jugular venous pressure elevated 5 cm. On auscultation of the heart he had a soft pericardial rub and a short early diastolic murmur. His chest radiograph is shown (Figure 115). What is the most likely diagnosis?

A myocardial infarction
B pericarditis
C aortic dissection
D pulmonary embolus
E perforated duodenal ulcer

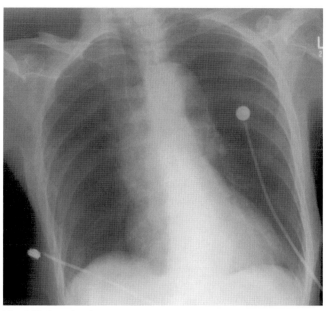

Fig. 115 Question 1.

Question 2

A 28-year-old woman becomes dizzy with a feeling of heaviness in the chest when jogging with a friend. She stops, sits down, and over a few minutes she improves so that she can walk home. The friend brings her to the Accident and Emergency department, where you are asked to assess her. Aside from dizziness and heaviness she was not aware of any other symptoms and she has not had the problem before. She has no significant past medical history and takes the oral contraceptive pill as her only regular medication. Physical examination is normal. Her ECG is shown (see Figure 116). What is the most likely diagnosis?

A acute myocardial infarction
B pulmonary embolism
C paroxysmal atrial fibrillation
D Wolff-Parkinson-White syndrome
E acute pericarditis

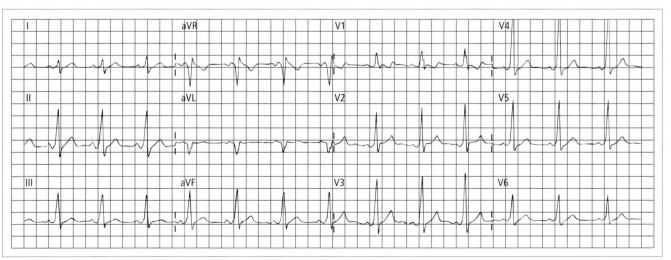

Fig. 116 Question 2.

145

Question 3

A 68-year-old man presents on the emergency medical take with breathlessness. His chest radiograph is shown (see Figure 117). Which is the best description of the radiograph?

A normal

B pulmonary oedema

C pulmonary oedema and cardiomegaly

D pulmonary oedema and cardiomegaly with enlarged right ventricle

E pulmonary oedema and cardiomegaly with enlarged left atrium

Question 4

A 58-year-old man presents with severe ischaemic chest pain. His ECG is shown (see Figure 118). Which is the best description of the ECG?

A acute anterior myocardial infarction

B acute anterolateral myocardial infarction

C acute anterolateral myocardial infarction with ventricular ectopics

D acute anterior myocardial infarction with ventricular ectopics

E acute anterolateral myocardial infarction with posterior extension

Question 5

A 70-year-old man, who is known to have ischaemic heart disease and has had short-lived episodes of atrial fibrillation in the past, presents with 48 hours of fatigue and breathlessness. He is not very ill, but his pulse is 150/min in atrial fibrillation. Which two drugs would be most appropriate to achieve 'chemical cardioversion'?

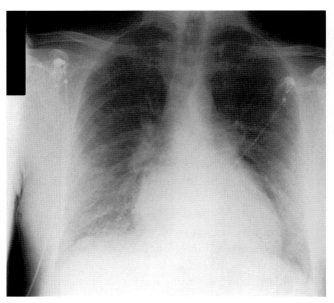

Fig. 117 Question 3.

A digoxin

B quinidine

C procainamide

D disopyramide

E sotalol

F atenolol

G propanolol

H verapamil

I amiodarone

J diltiazem

Question 6

A 45-year-old man is referred by his general practitioner

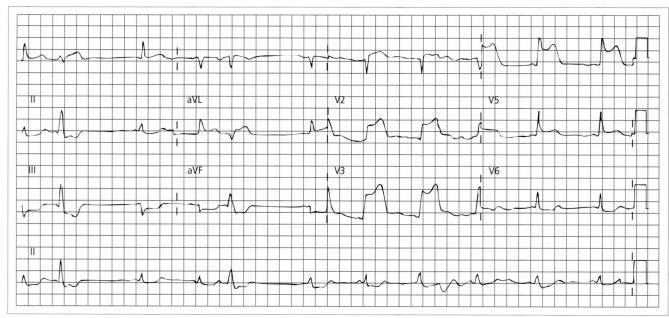

Fig. 118 Question 4.

with palpitations. He has no other associated symptoms and specifically he is not presyncopal. Holter monitoring has demonstrated short non-sustained runs of a monomorphic broad complex tachycardia. Which two of the following are the most likely arrhythmias?

A sinus tachycardia
B atrial fibrillation with intermittent rate associated bundle branch block
C right ventricular outflow tract tachycardia
D atrial flutter with one to one conduction
E tachycardia associated with Wolff-Parkinson-White syndrome
F ischaemic ventricular tachycardia
G atrioventricular nodal reentry tachycardia
H ventricular fibrillation
I torsades de pointes
J atrioventricular reentry tachycardia

Question 7

A 63-year-old man with Marfan's syndrome presents with chest pain and is found to have an acute aortic dissection. Which two of the following cardiac conditions are associated with Marfan's?

A atrial myxoma
B mitral stenosis
C pulmonary regurgitation
D ventricular tachycardia
E atrial septal defect
F ventricular septal defect
G cardiac amyloid
H sarcoidosis
I mitral valve prolapse
J aortic stenosis

Question 8

A 77-year-old man presents with 5 hours of chest pain at rest. He had undergone stenting to his left anterior descending artery 4 years previously. ECG shows inferior T-wave inversion, with ventricular ectopics. His troponin T is elevated at 0.4. He is already taking aspirin. Which two of the following would be considered appropriate initial therapeutic interventions?

A amiodarone
B change aspirin to clopidogrel
C coronary artery bypass grafting
D digoxin
E flecainide
F Glycoprotein IIb/IIa receptor blocker
G percutaneous coronary intervention
H dipyridamole (modified release)
I prophylactic dose of low molecular weight heparin
J thrombolysis

Question 9

A 48-year-old man is found to have a blood pressure of 176/112 mmHg when he attends his general practitioner for a 'new patient check-up'. He takes occasional anxiolytics for anxiety, but his past medical history is otherwise unremarkable. Physical examination is normal, excepting for obesity (BMI 32). A 'routine' biochemical screen is normal, excepting for potassium 3.3 mmol/l. The two most likely causes of his hypertension are:

A renal hypertension
B hypothyroidism
C renovascular hypertension
D Cushing's syndrome
E primary hyperaldosteronism (Conn's syndrome)
F acromegaly
G essential hypertension
H isolated clinic ('white coat') hypertension
I phaeochromocytoma
J coarctation of the aorta

Question 10

You find a middle aged man on a path in a park. He has no pulse and is not breathing. What is the appropriate next step:

A give two rescue breaths and initiate CPR at a ratio of 5 compressions to 2 breaths
B give two rescue breaths and initiate CPR at a ratio of 15 compressions to 2 breaths
C give a precordial thump
D give two rescue breaths and go for help
E go to call 999 (emergency services) immediately

Question 11

A 70-year-old man with a past history of anterior myocardial infarction presents with syncope and ventricular tachycardia (VT). Angiography reveals that the left anterior descending (LAD) artery is occluded and there is poor left ventricular function. Thallium (nuclear) imaging reveals a fixed anterior defect with no evidence of reversible ischaemia. What would be the optimal therapeutic strategy?

A amiodarone
B coronary artery bypass grafting and amiodarone
C implantable cardioverter defibrillator (ICD)
D implantable cardioverter defibrillator and beta-blocker
E percutaneous angioplasty to the LAD

Question 12

A 60-year-old woman presents with recurrent syncope; ECG reveals complete heart block. She is scheduled for a pacemaker. Which of the following pacemakers would be most appropriate?

A AOO
B DDD

C implantable cardioverter defibrillator (dual chamber)

D VVI

E VVIR

Question 13

A 70-year-old man is investigated for deteriorating anginal symptoms. Echo confirms a stenotic aortic valve with peak gradient 80 mmHg. Angiography demonstrates a discrete severe stenosis in his left anterior descending artery (LAD). Which would be the optimal treatment?

A aortic valve replacement

B aortic valve replacement and internal mammary artery graft to the LAD

C beta-blocker, aspirin, statin and review

D percutaneous coronary angioplasty to the LAD

E percutaneous aortic valvotomy and coronary angioplasty to the LAD

Question 14

A 50-year-old man presents 3 months after mitral valve replacement (metallic) with increasing shortness of breath, fever and weight loss. Clinically he is in pulmonary oedema. Transoesophageal echo (TOE) confirms severe paravalvular mitral regurgitation. The first blood culture is positive for *Staph epidermidis*. Which is the optimal therapeutic approach?

A intravenous antibiotics for 4 weeks and then repeat TOE

B oral antibiotics for 4 weeks and angiotensin-converting enzyme (ACE)—inhibitor

C start intravenous antibiotics and urgent re-do mitral valve replacement—bioprosthetic

D start intravenous antibiotics and urgent re-do mitral valve replacement—metallic

E withold antibiotics and repeat 3 sets of blood cultures

Question 15

A 32-year-old woman has been referred to you by her doctor, after complaining of syncope and breathlessness. Her sister died suddenly in her 20's. Clinically she has loud pulmonary second heart sound. What is the most likely diagnosis?

A aortic stenosis

B mitral stenosis

C tricuspid regurgitation

D primary pulmonary hypertension

E aortic regurgitation

Question 16

A 60-year-old man is being investigated for chest pain and undergoes exercise tolerance testing. Which of the following features is associated with a worse prognosis?

A increased heart rate with exercise

B ventricular tachycardia

C increase in blood pressure with exercise

D rapid resolution of heart rate in recovery

E absence of symptoms during exercise

Question 17

A 45-year-old man with dilated cardiomyopathy is being considered for cardiac transplantation. Which of the following is generally deemed to be a contraindication to cardiac transplantation?

A any previous cancer

B pulmonary artery wedge pressure <20 mmHg

C creatinine clearance <50 ml min^{-1}

D previous alcoholism

E hypertension

Question 18

A patient with documented systolic dysfunction has permanent atrial fibrillation. His resting heart rate is 100 and systolic blood pressure 120 mmHg; there is no evidence of fluid retention. Creatinine is normal and he is already receiving appropriate doses of furosemide and angiotensin-converting-enzyme (ACE) inhibitor. Which of the following would be the next therapy?

A amiodarone

B carvidolol

C DC cardioversion

D digoxin

E metoprolol

Question 19

A 78-year-old man with known ischaemic heart disease and congestive cardiac failure is admitted as an emergency with severe pulmonary oedema. He is sitting with his legs over the side of the casualty trolley and gasping. He has smoked 20 cigarettes per day for many years. What is the first treatment he should receive?

A furosemide 40 mg intravenously

B high flow oxygen via reservoir bag

C 35% oxygen

D diamorphine 2.5 mg intravenously, with anti-emetic

E isosorbide dinitrate by intravenous infusion at dose titrated against blood pressure

Question 20

A 60-year-old woman develops hypotension and a new systolic murmur 36 hours after being successfully thrombolysed for an anterior myocardial infarction. Which of the following statements is correct?

A acute mitral incompetence due to rupture of the posterior papillary muscle is the most likely diagnosis

B acute mitral incompetence due to rupture of the anterior papillary muscle is the most likely diagnosis

C a basal ventricular septal defect (VSD) is the most likely diagnosis

D an apical ventricular septal defect is the most likely diagnosis

E the systolic murmur is likely to be due to mitral valve prolapse

Question 21

A 70-year-old woman presents with 8 hours of chest pain. Her pulse rate is 40/minute and blood pressure 105/85. The ECG shows complete heart block, ST segment elevation and Q waves in leads II, III and AVF. Which of the following statements is correct?

A atropine should be given immediately

B an isoprenaline infusion should be set up immediately

C thrombolysis should be given immediately

D thrombolysis should be avoided because she has completed her myocardial infarction

E thrombolysis should be avoided because she may require a temporary pacing wire

Question 22

A 68-year-old man is admitted to the coronary care unit and thrombolysed for an inferior myocardial infarction. He makes an uneventful recovery. His total serum cholesterol on the admission blood test is 4.8 mmol/L. What action should be taken?

A he should be reassured that his cholesterol is normal

B he should have a repeat fasting serum cholesterol measured before discharge from hospital

C he should receive dietary advice and have his serum cholesterol measured in 3 month's time

D he should be started on an HMG Coenzyme A inhibitor.

E a full lipid profile should be obtained and lipid lowering drug treatment started if his LDL fraction is >3.5 mmol/L and his HDL is <1.0 mmol/L.

Question 23

A 20-year-old female student presents with central chest pain after four days of a 'flu-like illness. She has no significant past medical history and takes the oral contraceptive pill as her only regular medication. The most likely diagnosis is:

A acute viral pericarditis

B gastro-oesophageal reflux

C acute myocardial infarction

D systemic lupus erythematosus

E pulmonary embolism

Question 24

A 28-year-old woman presents with breathlessness and pleuritic chest pain. Which of the following test results is more than 90% specific for excluding pulmonary embolism (PE) in a patient presenting with a high clinical probability of the diagnosis?

A negative D-dimer

B normal lung perfusion on V/Q scan

C no evidence of PE on spiral CT

D normal chest radiograph and arterial blood gases

E no evidence of deep vein thrombosis (DVT) on lower limb venography

Question 25

A 59-year-old man with moderate chronic obstructive lung disease is admitted breathless following an episode of syncope while shopping. There is no previous history of syncope. Past history includes multiple stab ligations for bilateral varicose veins four weeks previously and open cholecystectomy 10 years before. On examination he is breathless at rest, apyrexial, pulse 104/min (regular), BP 110/60 mmHg. Heart sounds are normal. Chest examination reveals a few scattered wheezes. Neurological examination is normal. ECG shows sinus tachycardia with inverted T waves in leads V1-V3. Chest radiography normal. Oxygen saturation is 92% on 40% oxygen. PEFR is 290 L/min. What is the most likely diagnosis?

A acute pulmonary oedema

B acute exacerbation of chronic obstructive pulmonary disease

C pulmonary embolism

D acute myocardial infarction

E pneumocystis

Respiratory Medicine

AUTHORS:
P. Bhatia, M.I. Polkey and V.L.C. White

EDITOR:
M.I. Polkey

EDITOR-IN-CHIEF:
J.D. Firth

Clinical presentations

1.1 New breathlessness

Case history

A 52-year-old man presents with a 2-month history of increasing breathlessness.

Clinical approach

Breathlessness or dyspnoea is defined as difficult, laboured or uncomfortable awareness of breathing. It is a feature of many cardiac and respiratory conditions. The physician must seek to make a clinical diagnosis before attempting a definitive test. The main diagnostic categories are shown in Table 1. An important concern is to identify malignant disease as early as possible.

History of the presenting problem

 Listen to your patient. He is telling you the answer.
(René Laënnec)

When and how?

A careful description of the dyspnoea is required. Let patients tell their story in their own words, but clarify the following points if they do not emerge spontaneously.

Table 1 Causes of slow onset new breathlessness.

Common
Airways disease
Cardiac disease
Pleural effusion/disease
Lobar/lung collapse (from obstructing tumour)

Must consider
Thromboembolic disease
Anaemia

Other conditions
Pulmonary artery hypertension
Interstitial lung disease
Neuromuscular disease
Chest wall disease

- Is the dyspnoea really new or is this a progression of previous mild symptoms? Airways disease in particular often becomes a 'new' problem when the patient is unable to perform a particular task?
- When is it worse? Exertional dyspnoea is a nonspecific symptom, but the specific complaint of orthopnoea suggests heart failure (or rarely bilateral diaphragm paralysis).
- If the symptoms are worse lying on one side, this may suggest unilateral lung disease, e.g. a patient with right lung collapse may report a preference for sleeping on the right side.
- Nocturnal dyspnoea usually makes the clinician think of heart failure, but asthma is also worse at night.

Is the patient a smoker?

Is the patient a smoker—currently or previously? Does the patient have cancer? These points needs to be clarified early. In a smoker, lung cancer requires positive exclusion if there are ominous associated symptoms (particularly weight loss or haemoptysis). New breathlessness may also indicate a new perception of previously unrecognized airflow obstruction.

What is the patient's job?

The incidence of mesothelioma is set to peak in 2015. These symptoms could fit, especially if associated with unilateral pain and if the employment history indicates asbestos exposure. Some periods of such employment may have been temporary, hence—when relevant—it is necessary to reconstruct the patient's full work CV. (See Section 1.11, p. 178.)

Pets or unusual hobbies

Although the answer is usually 'no', this question is quick to ask.

Features to suggest infection

Infection would not be a common cause of dyspnoea of 2 months' duration. The exceptions to this are tuberculosis or lung abscess and you should therefore ask about fever, shivering attacks and sputum production. Is the patient at high risk of tuberculosis (for example an immigrant from an endemic area, or living on the streets).

Inhaled foreign body. Patients often have to be prompted to enable this diagnosis, which is suggested by lobar collapse or persistent cough.

Relevant past history

Previous pulmonary disease

A previous history of asthma, wheeziness or colds 'going to my chest' clearly raises the likelihood of airflow obstruction being the diagnosis. Remember that the patient may have had undiagnosed asthma at school (and therefore been unable to play sport or have disliked the playground in the winter) and grown out of it, only to have it relapse.

Examination

Always note the general appearance, followed by a full cardiac and respiratory examination.
- General appearance—breathless at rest; weight loss; pale (anaemic); jaundiced; can the patient lie supine?
- Give a cough—normal in character; productive
- Take big breath—stridor (a 'wheezing' found on inspiration)
- Hands—clubbing; muscle wasting
- Pulse rate—regular
- Eyes—anaemia; Horner's syndrome (if complaining of apical pain)
- Tongue—central cyanosis
- Lymph nodes—palpable; axillary examination not mandatory unless lymph nodes are palpable elsewhere or history of breast cancer
- Jugular venous pressure (JVP)—elevated?
- Apex—position
- Heart auscultation—added sounds and murmurs
- Tracheal position—centred
- Chest wall—scoliosis (may be surprisingly hidden by clothes); movement equal and adequate; paradoxical abdominal movement
- Tactile vocal fremitus—normal and equal
- Percussion—not forgetting the apices and lateral chest wall
- Auscultation—not forgetting the apices and lateral chest wall
- Ankles—swelling.

The measurement of peak expiratory flow (PEF), and ideally spirometry, should form part of the outpatient assessment unless a clear-cut diagnosis (e.g. large pleural effusion) is made on examination.

Approach to investigations and management

Investigations

Chest radiograph

The chest radiograph is almost an extension of physical examination. Most new patients attending the chest clinic have a chest radiograph before seeing the doctor. Frequently this will show an abnormality that initiates a standard diagnostic pathway, e.g. pleural effusion, a solitary lung mass or apical alveolar shadowing. It is important to check for cardiac enlargement.

If the chest radiograph appears to be normal, then carefully review the apices, the mediastinum and the bony structures.

A patient with dyspnoea and pain may have a pneumothorax. This is usually of sudden onset, but not always, and may be forgotten by the patient. A chest radiograph taken in expiration may demonstrate the condition, as shown in Fig. 1.

Blood tests

These are of limited value in the assessment of slow onset of new dyspnoea. The haemoglobin will exclude anaemia (and polycythaemia if there has been long-standing hypoxia). Blood tests may be diagnostic where the history and/or examination suggests a specific diagnosis, e.g. in avian extrinsic alveolitis, and clinical clues of malignancy should be pursued (e.g. measurement of liver function tests).

Sarcoid is notoriously variable in its presentation: measurement of serum angiotensin-converting enzyme (ACE) and calcium are indicated where this diagnosis is entertained.

Lung function

Lung function measurements are the next investigation for the breathless patient in whom the chest radiograph is non-contributory. Look for evidence of airflow obstruction or a restrictive lung defect. Lung volumes and gas transfer measurements are required where the diagnosis is genuinely uncertain.

Additional investigations

Further investigations are guided by the clinical features and results of the radiograph and lung function, but might include:
- high-resolution computed tomography (CT) of the thorax
- spiral protocol CT of the thorax
- ECG and echocardiogram (possibly with contrast)

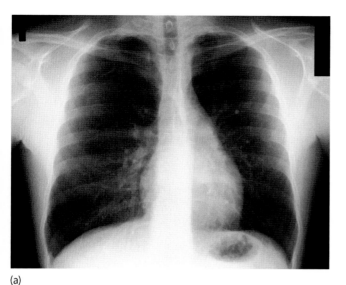

(a)

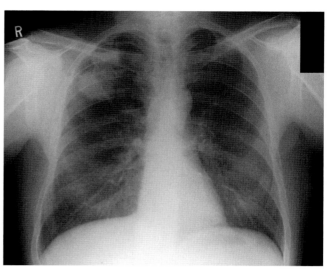

Fig. 2 Chest radiograph of patient showing right upper lobe nodule.

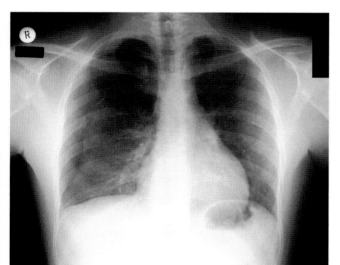

(b)

Fig. 1 A pair of radiographs taken in a patient with a right-sided pneumothorax. In the inspiratory film (a) the pneumothorax is around 20% which increases to around 60% in the expiratory film (b).

- bronchoscopy
- thoracoscopy
- lung biopsy
- respiratory muscle function tests.

 Consider respiratory muscle weakness if there is a restrictive defect with a normal or supernormal gas transfer in the presence of a normal chest radiograph [1]. A good screening test is to compare the erect and supine vital capacity, when a drop of >20% suggests bilateral diaphragm paralysis.

 1 Polkey MI, Green M & Moxham J. Measurement of respiratory muscle strength. *Thorax* 1995; 50: 1131–1135.

1.2 Solitary pulmonary nodule

Case history

A 48-year-old executive has a chest radiograph as part of his company's health screening programme. It shows a pulmonary nodule in the right upper lobe (Fig. 2).

Clinical approach

The most important differential is lung cancer. Other possibilities would be an old tuberculous (TB) nodule, a benign adenoma or a lung secondary (rarer possibilities are shown in Table 2).

History of the presenting problem

 Any old radiographs are extremely helpful: ask the patient—they may have had a chest radiograph performed previously, perhaps in another hospital, e.g. before elective surgery.

Table 2 Differential diagnosis of a solitary pulmonary nodule.

Common
Lung cancer
Lung secondary
Old tuberculous nodule

Uncommon
Infection, e.g. lung abscess
Benign tumour, e.g. adenoma, hamartoma, carcinoid
Arteriovenous malformation
Active granulomatous disease, e.g. tuberculosis, sarcoid, Wegener's granulomatosis, rheumatoid nodule

Is this lung cancer?

Find out the following.
- Smoking history—never, ex- or current smoker?
- Occupational history—the patient may not always have been an executive. (See Section 1.11, p. 178.)
- Is there any history of cough and/or haemoptysis?
- Any chest wall pain, brachial plexus symptoms or shortness of breath?
- Any recent weight loss or anorexia?
- Enquire about symptoms that might arise from systemic manifestations of cancer (e.g. bone pains from hypercalcaemia or metastases, weakness from Eaton–Lambert syndrome).

Could it be tuberculosis?

The lesion may be active TB or an old nodule. Check the following:
- ethnic origin, foreign travel or residence
- personal or family history of TB
- recent fevers or night sweats
- haemoptysis.

Other considerations

- Benign tumour—history of haemoptysis would make this less likely
- Lung secondary—any history of other tumours, weight loss or anorexia (Fig. 3).

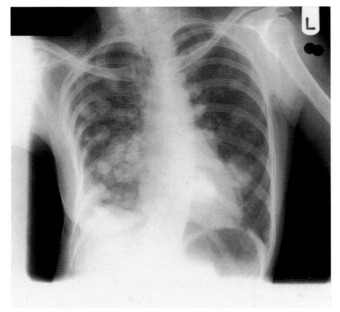

Fig. 3 Chest radiograph of a patient with a malignant salivary gland tumour showing multiple nodular pulmonary secondaries.

Relevant past history

Previous tuberculosis

Is there a history of prolonged hospital stays as a youngster? If treated for TB, were they given antibiotics, and if so, which ones and for how long (it may be impossible to find this information, but important to ask)?

Examination

General

Does the patient look unwell? Do they appear to have lost weight recently? Do they look pale? Is there ptosis or jaundice?

Respiratory

Look carefully for the following:
- cough—is this of normal character? Is it productive?
- stridor
- clubbing
- lymphadenopathy—both cervical, supraclavicular and axillary
- superior vena cava obstruction
- position of trachea
- chest expansion
- percussion
- breath sounds
- vocal and tactile fremitus
- dependant oedema
- hepatomegaly
- neurological signs
- telangectasia—may suggest arteriovenous malformations (AVMs).

A lung secondary

Feel for an abdominal mass and for groin lymphadenopathy. Examine the thyroid gland, and do not forget to examine the breasts in women and testes in men.

 Breast examination

- If a woman presents with a mass on her chest radiograph, explain why you need to examine her breasts: 'sometimes problems with the breasts can show up on a chest radiograph'.
- Do not forget to reassure if you find nothing abnormal: 'your breasts feel entirely normal, I don't think that they are the cause of the problem'.
- Ask for a chaperone if you think this appropriate.

Approach to investigations and management

Investigations of solitary pulmonary nodule
- Computed tomography scan of chest, liver and adrenals—preferably before bronchoscopy
- Bronchoscopy—ideally within a week: lateral chest radiograph is essential if computed tomography scan is not available beforehand
- Sputum for cytology, microbiology (including acid-fast bacilli (AFB))
- Blood tests for routine haematology, coagulation screen, electrolytes, calcium and liver function tests.

Investigations

Computed tomography scan of chest

This must include the liver and adrenals when lung cancer is in the differential. Normally both lung and soft tissue views are obtained; the former looking at the lung parenchyma, the latter for mediastinal lymphadenopathy (Fig. 4) (see *Haematology*, Sections 1.16 and 2.2).

Bronchoscopy

Seventy per cent of lung cancers are visible bronchoscopically. Endobronchial lesions should be biopsied if there are no contraindications and routine blood tests do not demonstrate coagulopathy. Most operators also brush the lesion and send washings for cytological analysis.

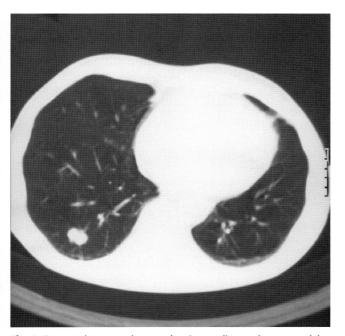

Fig. 4 Computed tomography scan showing a solitary pulmonary nodule in the posterior aspect of the right lower lobe, which was difficult to view on the plain chest radiograph. This patient was later diagnosed as having lymphoma.

- Bronchial biopsies should be sent for histology in formalin and for microscopy and culture in saline if TB is suspected.
- Bronchial washings and brushings should be sent for cytology and washings for microscopy and culture.
- Remember to request AFBs specifically when appropriate—they are not carried out automatically.

Cytological examination of sputum

This can yield a diagnosis in some patients but, because bronchoscopy is also required as a prelude to surgery, this approach is usually reserved for patients whose general health means that they will not receive active treatment for a tumour if one is found.

It is worth asking the physiotherapist to help obtain induced samples. Do not forget to send for microscopy and culture (specifically including AFB) as well as for cytology.

Blood tests

These should include a full blood count (FBC), erythrocyte sedimentation rate (ESR) (may be raised in active TB), clotting (before bronchoscopy or biopsy), blood biochemistry including electrolytes, calcium and liver function tests.

Do not miss hypercalcaemia associated with malignancy. (See *Endocrinology*, Section 1.2; *Emergency medicine*, Section 1.18.)

Computed tomography-guided biopsy

For peripheral lesions where bronchoscopic results are negative, percutaneous biopsy is the next procedure of choice. Lung function needs to be carefully assessed beforehand as there is a 10% chance of a pneumothorax: patients should be warned of this complication when they are consented.

Positron emission tomography

Fluorodeoxyglucose (FDG) positron emission tomography (PET) can be useful in the management of a solitary nodule. The principle is that metabolically active diseases will take up labelled glucose that can then be identified on images obtained by the PET scanner. The main indications are to provide reassurance if deciding against an open surgical biopsy or resection for undiagnosed nodules, or to look for otherwise covert metastases in patients being considered for a curative resection of a proven tumour.

Management

- Lung cancer: see Section 2.9.1, p. 220
- Chest infection/abscess
- Tuberculosis: see *Infectious diseases*, Section 2.6.1
- Sarcoidosis: see Section 2.8.2, p. 208
- Wegener's granulomatosis: see *Rheumatology and clinical immunology*, Section 2.5.2
- Benign tumour—resection is normally recommended to avoid the complications of bronchial obstruction, haemoptysis and possible mitotic transformation (2% of adenomas). However, the rate of growth of the tumour and general condition of the patient enter the risk–benefit equation and need to be taken into account.
- Pulmonary AVMs—only need to be treated if symptomatic. When part of an hereditary syndrome, bleeding elsewhere may cause greater problems. Pulmonary AVMs may be locally embolized using catheter techniques under radiological guidance. Occasionally lung resection may be necessary [1,2].

1 Temes RT, Paramsothy P, Endara, SA, Wernly JA. Resection of a solitary pulmonary arteriovenous malformation by video-assisted thoracic surgery. *J Thorac Cardiovasc Surg* 1998; 116: 878–879.
2 Puskas, JD, Allen MS, Moncure AC *et al.* Pulmonary arteriovenous malformations: therapeutic options. *Ann Thorac Surg* 1993; 56: 253–258.

1.3 Exertional dyspnoea with daily sputum

Case history

A 24-year-old man attends the chest clinic with a 7-month history of worsening exertional dyspnoea and coughing up a cupful of sputum daily. He remembers that as a child he was a frequent visitor to his general practitioner with cough. There is no history of wheeze. He also complains of intermittent abdominal pain for the last 12 months. He has smoked over 40 cigarettes daily since the age of 15 years.

Clinical approach

This young man has both pulmonary and abdominal symptoms. He is a very heavy smoker and coughing up excessive amounts of phlegm, which suggests an inflammatory process. Bronchiectasis, lung abscess and pneumonia can produce purulent sputum, which may be offensive

and blood tinged. Mucoid or mucopurulent sputum is characteristic of chronic bronchitis. In cystic fibrosis (CF), there may be copious purulent phlegm and frequent haemoptysis.

He is very young to be suffering from chronic bronchitis and emphysema, even if he has α_1-antitrypsin deficiency.

In any patient presenting with chronic exertional dyspnoea and sputum production, consider:
- chronic obstructive pulmonary disease (COPD) (history of smoking, wheeze, check spirometry)
- bronchiectasis (and any condition associated with bronchiectasis): see Section 2.4, p. 197
- bronchial asthma (history of wheeze, episodic)
- lung abscess, pneumonia (usually of acute onset, accompanied by fever)
- congestive cardiac failure.

History of the presenting problem

Extent of history

Was he perfectly well before this 7-month history of breathlessness? He remembers frequent visits to his general practitioner for treatment of cough. He could be suffering from asthma, but he denies wheeze. A 7-month history suggests a chronic disorder, but was respiratory function really normal prior to this? Could he play games at school? Could he keep up with his friends when he played football or went cycling?

Amount and character of sputum

He is coughing up a cupful (approximately 200 mL) of sputum in 24 h. Normally the mucous glands of the respiratory tract produce 100 mL of sputum daily and most of this is swallowed.

Abdominal pain related to pulmonary problem

Intermittent abdominal pain could be caused by a variety of problems (see *Gastroenterology and hepatology*, Sections 1.2 and 1.14), but might indicate underlying gallstone or a partial intestinal obstruction—meconium ileus equivalent in CF. Is he well built for his age? Malabsorption caused by CF may result in failure of linear growth in childhood and short stature in later life.

Nasal or sinus problems

This may suggest hypogammaglobulinaemia (see *Rheumatology and clinical immunology*, Sections 1.1 and 2.1.1).

Relevant past history

Childhood diseases

Did he suffer from measles, pneumonia or pertussis as a child? This may suggest underlying bronchiectasis.

Family history

This man is young to develop a chronic respiratory disorder. Is there a family history of such problems?
- Does he have any brothers or sisters, and do they (or could they) have CF—an autosomal recessive disorder with a carrier frequency of 1 in 22 in caucasians?
- Is there a family history of COPD? This might indicate α_1-antitrypsin deficiency—autosomal dominant and usually presenting at 20–40 years of age: smokers develop emphysema; 10–15% develop cirrhosis.

In a young patient with chronic exertional dyspnoea and sputum production, consider:
- bronchiectasis—may be caused by CF
- α_1-antitrypsin deficiency
- hypogammaglobulinemia—may be suggested by recurrent pneumonia or sinusitis.

Examination

Full general, respiratory and cardiac examinations are required (see Sections 1.1, p. 153 and 1.2, p. 155), but in this case pay particular attention to the following aspects.

General

- Look in the sputum pot: note quantity and character of sputum.
- Is the patient cachexic, of short stature, clubbed, cyanosed or oedematous (hypoproteinaemic/cor pulmonale) (CF)?

Respiratory

The auscultatory findings are only part of the picture, but concentrate on the following:
- Are the breath sounds vesicular or bronchial (underlying consolidation)?
- Is expiration prolonged (COPD)?
- Are crackles persistently heard over the same area (bronchiectasis)?
- Are breath sounds impaired over a specific area (lung abscess)?

Abdominal

As this patient could be suffering from CF, it is essential to examine the abdomen carefully. A mobile right lower quadrant mass may be palpable. Intermittent abdominal pain in CF can be caused by intermittent partial obstruction, low-grade appendicitis, duodenal irritation as a result of failure to buffer gastric acid, or cholelithiasis.

Look for signs of cirrhosis, which can occur in both CF and α_1-antitrypsin deficiency (see *Gastroenterology and hepatology*, Sections 1.4, 1.6 and 2.10).

Approach to investigations and management

Investigations

Blood tests

A raised white cell count with neutrophilia suggests underlying bacterial infection. Secondary polycythaemia suggests chronic hypoxia. Serum α_1-antitrypsin level may be low suggesting its deficiency and underlying emphysema. Liver function tests can exclude hepatic involvement in both CF and α_1-antitrypsin deficiency.

Chest radiograph

A chest radiograph is helpful to exclude an acute infection. It may also reveal features of COPD, bronchiectasis, lung abscess or cardiomegaly in congestive cardiac failure. Dextrocardia may be present.

Sputum examination

Send for microscopy, culture and sensitivity, including AFB.

Lung function tests

These will determine if there is airway obstruction, and in cases of COPD will help evaluate treatment. It is important to request full lung function tests comprising static lung volumes, spirometry and transfer factor.

Other investigations

- Arterial blood gases—indicated if fingertip SaO_2 <94% to check whether there is any respiratory failure (type I or II)
- Electrocardiogram—is there cor pulmonale?
- Sweat sodium concentration—in CF the sweat sodium concentration is usually high (>60 mmol)
- High-resolution CT scan of the lungs—can diagnose bronchiectasis, emphysema or presence of bullae
- Ultrasound examination of the hepatobiliary system—looking for cirrhosis and/or gall stones.

Management

- Cystic fibrosis: see Section 2.5, p. 199
- Bronchiectasis: see Section 2.4, p. 197
- COPD: see Section 2.3, p. 194
- Pulmonary infections (lung abscess/pneumonia): see *Infectious diseases*, Sections 1.5 and 2.5
- Hypogammaglobulinaemia: see *Rheumatology and clinical immunology*, Section 2.1.1.

MacNee W. Chronic obstructive pulmonary disease: causes and pathology. *Medicine* 1999; 27(9): 68–72.
Calverley, PMA. Management of chronic obstructive pulmonary disease. *Medicine* 1999; 27(9): 73–78.
Peckham DG, Conway S. Cystic fibrosis. *Medicine* 1999; 27(9): 82–87.

1.4 Dyspnoea and fine inspiratory crackles

Case history

A 53-year-old retired car salesman presents with a history of breathing difficulty. He has long-standing atrial fibrillation and is on amiodarone 200 mg once daily and warfarin. On examination he is dyspnoeic on transferring to the couch and has fine bibasal crackles.

Clinical approach

Breathlessness is a cardinal symptom of both cardiac and pulmonary disease. In this case it is obviously critical to determine whether the main cause is cardiac or pulmonary. Note that myocardial ischaemia may be silent and hence this cause of impaired left ventricular function and breathlessness may not be obvious.

History of the presenting problem

History of sputum production

Dyspnoea along with bibasal crackles may be a feature of bronchiectasis, which is typically accompanied by copious sputum. Chronic bronchitis and emphysema are also characterized by dyspnoea and bibasal crackles may represent superadded infection. Diffuse interstitial lung diseases may be accompanied by a dry cough.

Swelling of the ankles

Congestive cardiac failure or cor pulmonale may be accompanied by pedal and sacral oedema.

History of wheeze

Obstructive airways disease is accompanied by wheeze, but wheeze can also be a feature of cardiac failure.

Is breathlessness cardiac?

Can the patient sleep lying flat? Does the patient wake up with breathing difficulty at night? Orthopnoea and paroxysmal nocturnal dyspnoea suggest cardiac failure. When the patient gets breathless, is there any tightness in the chest? Breathlessness of many sorts can be associated with chest discomfort, but this might indicate angina and ischaemic left ventricular failure as the cause of breathing difficulty in this case. (See *Cardiology*, Sections 1.6, 2.3 and 2.4.)

Exercise tolerance limited by dyspnoea?

What activities are limited by breathlessness? This is not helpful in arriving at a differential diagnosis, but provides an estimate of disability and is essential in monitoring the response of disease to treatment.

Relevant past history

- This man has long-standing atrial fibrillation. This may be 'lone' (when by definition there is no other evidence of cardiac disease), but any history of cardiac disease (the most common form of which is ischaemic heart disease) makes breathlessness resulting from cardiac failure more likely than otherwise.
- Childhood pneumonia, measles, mumps or pertussis could cause bronchiectasis.
- A history of painful nodules on the shins (erythema nodosum) may point to sarcoidosis.
- Associated rheumalogical disease suggests pulmonary fibrosis.

Occupational and drug history

A detailed occupational and drug history is important to determine whether the patient has been in contact with any agent associated with diffuse interstitial lung disease (Table 3). Amiodarone is an obvious worry in this case.

Recreational history

Does the patient breed pigeons or keep a budgerigar? (Bird fancier's lung).

Family history

A family history of dyspnoea in young adults might

Table 3 Classification of interstitial lung disease.

Classification	Examples
Connective tissue disorder	Rheumatoid arthritis, scleroderma, systemic lupus erythematosus, ankylosing spondylitis, mixed connective tissue disorder, Sjögren's syndrome, polymyositis–dermatomyositis
Occupational/environmental	Silicosis, asbestosis, berylliosis, coal worker's pneumoconiosis, siderosis, stanosis, aluminium oxide fibrosis, bird fancier's lung, farmer's lung, malt worker's lung, mushroom worker's lung, humidifier lung, bagassosis
Autoimmune	Inflammatory bowel disease, primary biliary cirrhosis, Wegener's granulomatosis
Idiopathic	Cryptogenic fibrosing alveolitis, bronchiolitis obliterans organizing pneumonia, sarcoidosis
Drug induced	Antibiotics (sulfasalazine, furantoin), antiarrythmics (amiodarone, propranolol), anti-inflammatory (gold, penicillamine), anticonvulsants (phenytoin), chemotherapeutic agents (busulfan, bleomycin, cyclophosphamide), paraquat, crack cocaine inhalation
Rarities	Irradiation, amyloidosis, postinfectious, lymphangioleiomyomatosis, neurofibromatosis, Gaucher's disease, lipoid pneumonia, tuberous sclerosis, acquired immune deficiency syndrome, eosinophilic pneumonia, adult respiratory distress syndrome

suggest α_1-antitrypsin deficiency. Cryptogenic fibrosing alveolitis may be familial.

Examination

Full general, respiratory and cardiac examinations are required (see Sections 1.1, p. 153 and 1.2, p. 155), but in this case pay particular attention to the following aspects.

General

- Finger clubbing (cryptogenic fibrosing alveolitis, bronchiectasis, CF)
- Erythema nodosum (sarcoid—rare)
- Side effects of amiodarone (slate grey discoloration of the skin, signs of hypo/hyperthyroidism).

Cardiovascular

Does the patient have cardiac failure? If yes: is it right ventricular (cor pulmonale or disease of heart alone), left ventricular or biventricular (both suggesting heart disease other than cor pulmonale)?

Note the following:
- Pulse rate, rhythm and character (does the patient still need to be on amiodarone?)
- JVP—is this elevated?
- Cardiac apex—is this displaced? (Suggests cardiac disease other than cor pulmonale)
- Left or right ventricular heaves—are these present?

(Left ventricular heave suggests cardiac disease other than cor pulmonale)
- Cardiac murmurs or added sounds—are these present? (Murmurs or added sounds loudest at the apex suggest cardiac disease other than cor pulmonale)
- Palpate for the liver—is this enlarged? Is it pulsatile?
- Peripheral oedema.

Respiratory

Take special care to note the following.

Palpation

The movement of the thoracic cage is symmetrically diminished in diffuse fibrosis. The trachea may be pulled to the affected side if fibrosis is unilateral or asymmetrical.

Percussion

The percussion note at the bases is dull with pleural effusions (perhaps caused by cardiac failure in this case), but is normal in fibrosis.

Auscultation

Bilateral fine end-inspiratory crackles are characteristic of cryptogenic fibrosing alveolitis. Ask the patient to cough. The crackles of alveolitis are not influenced by cough, whereas they often lessen in pulmonary oedema.

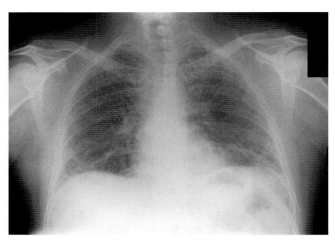

Fig. 5 Plain chest radiograph of a woman with fibrosing alveolitis; there is bilateral alveolar shadowing.

Approach to investigations and management

Investigations

Chest radiograph

Look for honeycomb appearance of diffuse lung fibrosis (Fig. 5), bilateral hilar lymphadenopathy in sarcoidosis, pleural plaques in asbestos exposure and asbestosis. Look for an enlarged heart and Kerley B lines, which would suggest cardiac failure.

Spirometry

In fibrosis both forced expiratory volume in 1 s (FEV_1) and forced vital capacity (FVC) are reduced and hence their ratio remains constant. The total lung capacity (TLC) and the transfer factor are both reduced.

High-resolution computed tomography scanning

High-resolution CT (2–3 mm slices) is superior to conventional CT scanning (Fig. 6). It helps to diagnose the presence of lung fibrosis and may also determine the aetiology in some cases, avoiding lung biopsy.

Echocardiography

The finding, by echocardiography or other means, of good left ventricular function can be helpful in excluding heart failure as a cause of dyspnoea and crackles.

Blood tests

Check full blood count for anaemia, or for polycythaemia caused by hypoxia. It is appropriate to test for inflammatory markers (C-reactive protein (CRP), ESR), rheumatoid factor, antinuclear antibodies, serum ACE and calcium level (sarcoidosis), antineutrophil cytoplasmic antibodies (Wegener's granulomatosis) and relevant precipitins (extrinsic allergic alveolitis).

Arterial blood gases

If SaO_2 <94% when breathing air, measure arterial blood gases to assess severity.

Electrocardiogram

Look for features of pulmonary hypertension—right axis deviation, P pulmonale in lead II (in patient who is not in atrial fibrillation), dominant R in V1.

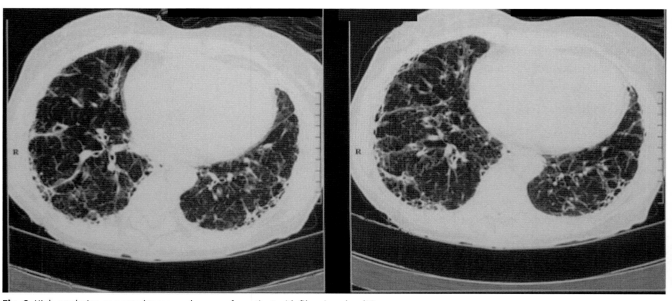

Fig. 6 High-resolution computed tomography scan of a patient with fibrosing alveolitis.

Lung biopsy

This may have to be performed to determine the aetiology if all other tests are unhelpful. Transbronchial biopsy is helpful if sarcoidosis is suspected, but as the sample size is small it may not be of use in other causes of lung fibrosis. Open lung biopsy or video-assisted thoracoscopic biopsy may be required.

Management

Whether or not amiodarone is the culprit, the strength of the indication should be reviewed and the drug stopped if possible.
- If the diagnosis is amiodarone pneumonitis, high-dose oral prednisolone is indicated.
- If the diagnosis is left ventricular failure, the management is of this condition. (See *Cardiology*, Sections 1.6, 2.3 and 2.4.)

Otherwise management depends on the final diagnosis reached.

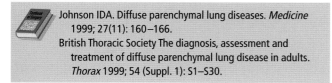

Johnson IDA. Diffuse parenchymal lung diseases. *Medicine* 1999; 27(11): 160–166.
British Thoracic Society The diagnosis, assessment and treatment of diffuse parenchymal lung disease in adults. *Thorax* 1999; 54 (Suppl. 1): S1–S30.

1.5 Pleuritic chest pain

Case history

A 54-year-old previously fit woman is admitted with left-sided pleuritic chest pain that began suddenly 8 h ago. On examination she is tachypnoeic at rest, with a respiratory rate of 28/min. She also gives a history of recent constipation and digital examination reveals a hard mass in the rectum.

Clinical approach

The visceral and parietal pleurae consist of single layers of cells separated by the pleural space. Pleuritic pain is characteristically triggered by deep inhalation, cough or movement of the thorax. It is usually unilateral, sharp, and can be referred to the shoulder, neck or abdominal wall. The following diagnoses should be considered:
- pulmonary embolism with pulmonary infarction (sudden onset, risk factors for thromboembolism)
- pneumothorax (sudden onset)
- pneumonia with infective pleurisy (recent history of purulent phlegm, fever)
- musculoskeletal causes (history of trauma or osteoporosis)
- malignant disease (often a duller and steady pain of some duration)
- non-infective pleurisy (systemic lupus erythematosus (SLE), rheumatoid arthritis).

In most cases, including this, the first priority is to exclude pulmonary embolism.

History of the presenting problem

Pain

Is the pain really pleuritic? Did it develop suddenly? Sudden pleuritic chest pain is most likely to be due to a pulmonary embolus with pulmonary infarction or a pneumothorax. Sudden onset of unilateral chest pain/discomfort and breathlessness should make you think immediately of pneumothorax, particularly in a tall, thin 'Marfanoid' man.

What was the patient doing in the hours before and at the moment when the pain came on? Unaccustomed or vigorous activity, e.g. painting the ceiling, is likely to precipitate musculoskeletal pain.

Breathlessness

Was the breathlessness sudden? Sudden onset of breathlessness with tachycardia and light-headedness caused by hypotension are suggestive of substantial pneumothorax or major pulmonary artery embolism.

Was there any haemoptysis? Haemoptysis occurs because of pulmonary infarction and strongly supports the diagnosis of pulmonary embolism.

Thromboembolic risk factors

Are there any risk factors for thromboembolism? In this case clearly the findings on rectal examination suggest the possibility of a rectal tumour. Cancer is a risk factor for thromboembolic disease. Other risk factors are:
- previous thromboembolism
- recent surgery: particularly major abdominal, pelvic, hip or knee surgery
- immobility, e.g. long haul aeroplane flights
- pregnancy/puerperium
- thrombophilia: protein C, protein S or antithrombin III deficiency; factor V Leiden mutation; family history of thromboembolism
- obstruction to venous flow (may be present if there is local spread of a tumour)
- smoking
- obesity
- age over 40 years.

Fever

Has there been fever? It is probable that this woman has had a pulmonary embolus, but ask about fevers, sweats or rigors. Most patients with pulmonary embolism are feverish, but high fever ($T > 38.5°C$), sweats or rigors make the diagnosis of pneumonia more likely.

Contraindications to anticoagulation

It is unlikely that this woman will have any contraindications to anticoagulation, but ask about these, the most common being a history of gastrointestinal bleeding. It is probable that you would decide to anticoagulate someone proven to have pulmonary embolism, but in the presence of a relative contraindication you would advise particularly close monitoring and counsel the patient to report problems immediately, e.g. change in colour of bowel motions, feeling of dizziness.

Examination

Full general, respiratory and cardiac examinations are required (see Section 1.1, p. 153 and 1.2, p. 155), but in this case pay particular attention to the following aspects.

General

Is the patient seriously ill? Does the patient need resuscitation of airway, breathing and circulation? If yes, resuscitate and seek immediate help from intensive care (see *Emergency medicine*, Sections 1.2 and 1.8).

If the patient is not gravely ill, note respiratory rate (tachypnoea is defined as a respiratory rate >20/min) and look for central cyanosis. Is there any evidence of deep venous thrombosis? Is there any evidence of metastatic spread (nodes)?

Cardiovascular

There should be particular emphasis on signs of acute pulmonary artery obstruction and/or pulmonary hypertension, which would be likely to be caused by subacute or chronic pulmonary embolism in this case:
- tachycardia
- hypotension
- elevated JVP
- right ventricular heave (along the left sternal border)*
- loud P2 and right ventricular S3.*

(*Features more typical of pulmonary hypertension.)

Respiratory

Respiration may be entirely normal, but listen carefully for a pleural rub. This can be very localized: ask the patient to put a finger on the spot that hurts most and listen carefully at and around that point. Consolidation typically gives bronchial breathing and dullness to percussion.

Musculoskeletal

Can the pain be reproduced by any movement or by localized pressure? If it can, then this supports a musculoskeletal cause of pleuritic pain. However, remember that pleurisy is exacerbated by anything that causes pleural movement. If in doubt, assume pulmonary embolism: be safe and not sorry.

Pulmonary embolism
- Sudden unexplained dyspnoea is the most common and often the only symptom.
- The combination of dyspnoea plus tachypnoea is present in 90% of patients.
- Only 3% of patients do not have one of the following: dyspnoea, tachypnoea or pleuritic chest pain.
- Examination may be normal.
- Tachycardia is a consistent but non-specific finding.
- Carefully search for risk factors for thromboembolism.

Approach to investigations and management

Investigations

Chest radiograph

This may be normal, but common findings in pulmonary embolism are linear infiltrates, segmental collapse, raised hemidiaphragm and pleural effusion. Look for other causes of pleuritic chest pain, in particular pneumothorax, but also for pneumonic consolidation. Remember that a normal chest radiograph in an acutely breathless hypoxic patient increases the likelihood of pulmonary embolism.

Electrocardiogram

The most common abnormalities are tachycardia and non-specific ST/T wave changes. Look for acute right heart strain with tall P waves, right axis deviation and ST/T wave changes in right ventricular leads (V1 and V2), and remember that the 'classical' S1Q3T3 pattern is seen in fewer than 10% of cases of proven pulmonary embolism.

Arterial blood gases

Occlusion of a pulmonary artery or its branches results in an area of lung that is ventilated but not perfused. This part of the lung does not then participate in gas exchange and hence results in wasted ventilation. Because of this ventilation–perfusion mismatching and hyperventilation the arterial blood gases in pulmonary embolism frequently show arterial hypoxaemia, hypocapnia and respiratory alkalosis. However, do not forget that a normal PaO_2 does not exclude pulmonary embolism.

Plasma D-dimer

D-dimer is a breakdown product of cross-linked fibrin and is elevated in active venous thromboembolism. A normal value can be used to exclude thromboembolism. The enzyme-linked immunosorbent assay (ELISA) is more accurate than the rapid latex test.

Echocardiography

In pulmonary embolism this is only helpful if a large embolus is suspected, when there may be right ventricular dilatation and hypokinesis, pulmonary artery enlargement, tricuspid regurgitation, abnormal septal movement, and failure of the inferior vena cava to collapse during inspiration.

Specific tests for pulmonary embolism

VENTILATION–PERFUSION ISOTOPE SCANNING

Ventilation scans are obtained using krypton-81m, technegas or xenon-133 and perfusion scans with intravenous ^{99m}Tc-labelled macroaggregates of albumin (Fig. 7). Scanning should ideally be performed within 24 h of clinical suspicion as appearances can revert to normal within a few days, and 50% do so within a week. The scans are interpreted as being normal, or of low, intermediate or high probability: reports need to be interpreted in the clinical context.

PULMONARY ANGIOGRAPHY

This is not routinely available in most hospitals in the UK. It is regarded by some as the 'gold standard' for diagnosing pulmonary embolism, but is invasive—with major or fatal complications in 0.5–1.3% of investigations, and minor complications in 2%—and interpretation is not always straightforward, particularly for those who do not perform the test regularly. The most common finding is a filling defect in the pulmonary artery as the radio-opaque dye flows around the embolus (Fig. 8).

SPIRAL COMPUTED TOMOGRAPHY

This can detect intravascular clot from the pulmonary trunk down to the segmental arteries, but unlike pulmonary angiography it cannot visualize emboli in the subsegmental arteries. In many centres this has become the investigation of choice, particularly for patients with pre-existing lung disease, which renders the interpretation of ventilation–perfusion scans difficult or impossible.

Investigations relevant to the rectal mass

Most cases of pulmonary embolism will not have a rectal mass, but in this case appropriate investigation would include sigmoidoscopy and biopsy. (See *Gastroenterology and hepatology*, Sections 1.5, 1.11 and 2.7.2.)

Management

If the patient is in shock administer high-flow oxygen and intravenous fluids, and immediately seek intensive care help.

Anticoagulation reduces the incidence of fatal recurrent embolism, and heparin should be started immediately pending the results of investigations when there is high or intermediate clinical suspicion.

Low-molecular-weight heparin is as effective as standard unfractionated heparin in non-life-threatening pulmonary embolism and has the advantages of rapid anticoagulation, simple once-daily administration and no need for laboratory monitoring.

Warfarin should be started once the diagnosis is confirmed.

 In patients without a contraindication to warfarin it is reasonable to start this at the same time as heparin, even in patients in whom the diagnosis is unsure. It can be stopped if the diagnosis of pulmonary embolism is subsequently excluded. If pulmonary embolism is confirmed, then the patient may be able to return home earlier.

Thrombolytic treatment is recommended for patients who are haemodynamically unstable. This is given peripherally, the doses used often being different from those used in myocardial infarction [1].

Pulmonary embolectomy is now reserved for patients who do not respond to thrombolysis or who have a contraindication to thrombolysis. Active bleeding from a rectal tumour would be a contraindication in this case.

Inferior vena caval filters should be considered in patients at high risk of emboli in whom anticoagulation is contraindicated and in those with recurrent embolism despite adequate anticoagulation.

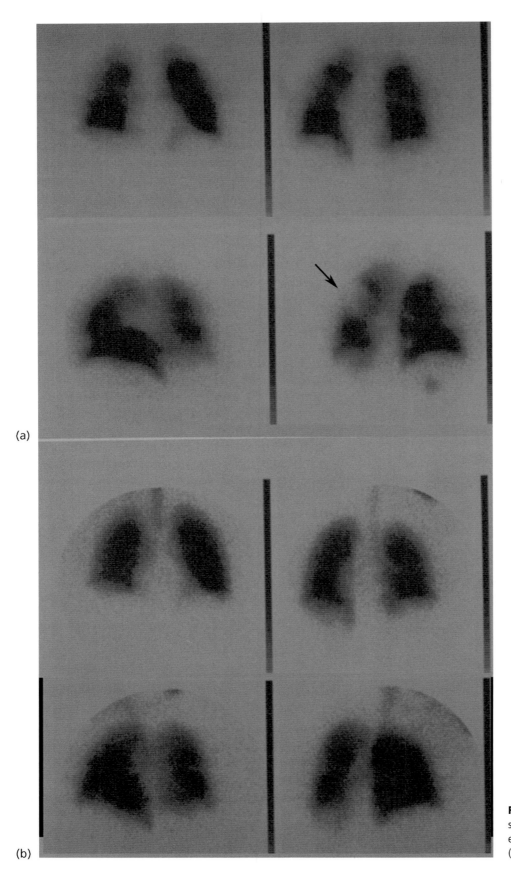

(a)

(b)

Fig. 7 Ventilation–perfusion scan showing right mid zone pulmonary embolism (arrowed): (a) perfusion; (b) ventilation images.

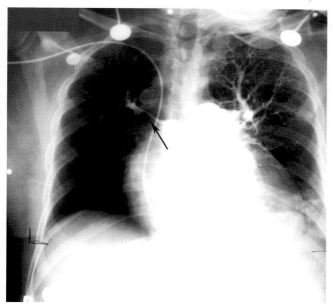

Fig. 8 Pulmonary angiogram showing large right pulmonary embolus (arrow). There are also clear abnormalities of perfusion in the left middle and lower zones.

See *Emergency medicine*, Sections 1.2 and 1.8
See *Haematology and oncology*, Section 3.6
See *Cardiology*, Sections 1.9, 2.18 and 3.10
British Thoracic Society. Suspected acute pulmonary embolism: a practical approach. *Thorax* 1997; 52: Supplement 4.
Arcasoy SM, Kreit JW. Thrombolytic therapy of pulmonary embolism: a comprehensive review of current evidence. *Chest* 1999; 115(6): 1695–1707.
1 The PIOPED investigators. Value of the ventilation/perfusion scan in acute pulmonary embolism. *JAMA* 1990; 263: 2753–9.

1.6 Unexplained hypoxia

Case history

A 44-year-old man has been admitted with a 2-week history of non-specific symptoms of tiredness and being

Table 4 Pathophysiologic processes leading to hypoxia.

Process	Example
Insufficient inspired oxygen	Altitude, anaesthetic mishaps
Right-to-left shunt	Anatomical shunts (cardiac, AVM), physiological shunts (e.g. resulting from atelectasis)
V/Q imbalance	Many causes, e.g. asthma, pneumonia, fibrosis, thromboembolic disease
Alveolar hypoventilation	Severe obstructive sleep apnoea, neurological/neuromuscular disease
Impaired diffusion	Fibrosis

AVM, arteriovenous malformation.

unwell. His chest radiograph is reported as normal but he is found to be hypoxic with a PaO_2 of 8.4 kPa.

Clinical approach

It is reasonable to assume that the patient has new-onset hypoxia, given that he is experiencing new symptoms. There are five physiological processes that can give rise to hypoxia (Table 4). In this case the finding of a normal chest radiograph makes some of these causes less probable.

History of the presenting problem

In practical terms the main issue is to distinguish between a genuinely new condition and the recent identification of something that is gradually progressive. With the chest radiograph reported as normal the main differential diagnoses in this case are shown in Table 5 and the history should pursue these possibilities.

Is the problem really acute?

Try to identify whether—with hindsight—the patient has had respiratory symptoms previously, perhaps on exercise. Has the patient had to stop doing anything or slow down recently?

If the problem seems to be long standing:

• Are there any respiratory or cardiac clues to the diagnosis?

Table 5 Differential diagnosis of hypoxia with a 'normal' chest radiograph.

	Long-standing problem	New condition
Likely diagnoses	Airways disease Interstitial lung disease Obstructive sleep apnoea	Pulmonary embolus Pneumonic process without chest radiograph changes, e.g. atypical pneumonia, miliary tuberculosis, *Pneumocystic carinii* pneumonia
Rare	Restrictive lung disease Upper airway obstruction Neuromuscular disease Cardiac shunts Pulmonary arteriovenous malformation Hepatopulmonary syndrome	Extrinsic alveolitis

- Are there features of untreated asthma, e.g. nocturnal cough, diurnal variation or atopy?
- Are there features of sleep disordered breathing? If this is severe enough to cause daytime hypoxia, then it should be associated with excessive daytime somnolence
- Is there anything to suggest a cardiac problem, e.g. report of a heart murmur?
- Is the patient at risk of interstitial lung disease? (See Section 1.4, p. 160.)

Always remember thromboembolic disease, which may not be associated with chest pain when chronic.

Consider other risks

What acute conditions is the patient at risk of?
- Pulmonary embolism may be suggested by recognized risk factors for thromboembolic disease. (See Section 1.5, p. 163.)
- The risk of atypical pneumonia is increased by exposure to air-conditioning systems (*Legionella*) or birds (*Chlamydia*).
- Miliary TB should be carefully considered in those at high risk, e.g. patients from particular ethnic groups.
- *Pneumocystis carinii* pneumonia (PCP) may present with isolated hypoxia and questioning about risk factors for human immunodeficiency virus (HIV) may be required. This needs tact and discretion and should be left to the end of the history and examination (see *General clinical issues*, Section 2).

Examination

Full general, respiratory and cardiac examinations are required (see Sections 1.1, p. 153 and 1.2, p. 155), but in this case pay particular attention to the following aspects.

General

- Does the patient have a fever or look toxic? These would favour an acute pneumonic process.
- Does the patient look as though he or she has lost weight? In this case weight loss might suggest miliary TB, or *Pneumocystis* as a complication of acquired immune deficiency syndrome (AIDS).
- Are there any other features to suggest AIDS, e.g. oral candidiasis?
- Is the patient likely to have obstructive sleep apnoea (OSA), e.g. obese, thick neck?
- Is the patient clubbed, which might suggest interstitial lung disease or a congenital cardiac shunt in this context?

Respiratory and cardiac

- Are there features of airways disease? Are there crackles in the chest, which might suggest interstitial lung disease in this context?
- Are there cardiac features to suggest pulmonary embolism (see Section 1.5, p. 163)? Are there any cardiac murmurs?

The measurement of PEF, and ideally spirometry, should form part of the clinical assessment—airways disease is common and should not be overlooked.

Neuromuscular

Is there evidence of neuropathy or myopathy? In particular, does the diaphragm move normally?

Approach to investigations and management

Investigations

Chest radiograph

Review the chest radiograph carefully. Take it back to the radiologist for further scrutiny with additional clinical information.
- Is the cardiac silhouette really normal?
- Is there subtle evidence of airspace shadowing (Fig. 9)? This would suggest interstitial lung disease or a pneumonic process.
- Are both hemidiaphragms clearly visible? Check that you are not missing left lower lobe consolidation, which is easy to neglect.
- Are both costophrenic angles clearly visible? A small pleural effusion might be caused by a pneumonic process or to thromboembolism. Sampling of pleural fluid could be diagnostic. (See Section 1.10, p. 176.)

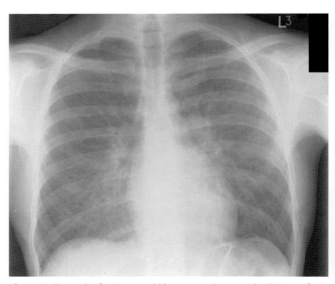

Fig. 9 Radiograph of a 29-year-old homosexual man with a history of dyspnoea and weight loss. Diagnostic possibilities include *Pneumocystis carinii* pneumonia.

Arterial blood gases

An increased $PaCO_2$ (or the demonstration, by calculation, of a normal arterial–alveolar (a–A) oxygen gradient) would suggest true alveolar hypoventilation. Comparison of arterial blood gases measured on room air and 100% oxygen allows calculation of the anatomical shunt, which in normal subjects is less than 5%.

Peak flow, spirometry and lung function

These measurements should be abnormal if there is occult airways disease of sufficient severity to cause hypoxia. In interstitial lung disease there will be a restrictive defect. Upper airway obstruction is an unlikely diagnosis in this case, but would be revealed by the flow–volume loop. (See Section 1.14, p. 184.)

Blood tests

Routine full blood count, biochemistry and inflammatory markers are indicated because of the non-specific nature of symptoms in this case. Serum ACE and calcium are indicated if sarcoid is possible. Atypical pneumonia titres or avian precipitins would be indicated if the history is appropriate.

It may be appropriate, after discussion, to test this patient for HIV (see *General clinical issues*, Section 2 and *Infectious diseases*, Section 1.24).

Computed tomography scan of thorax

This is likely to be a very helpful investigation, but the way in which the study is performed will depend on what is considered to be the most likely diagnosis. Discussion with the radiologist is required: not just an order form stating 'hypoxia—cause?'.
- For suspected thromboembolic disease a spiral protocol is used.
- For suspected interstitial lung disease a high-resolution scan gives the best images and is preferred. Significant pulmonary fibrosis may be invisible on a plain radiograph but seen on CT.

Further investigation for thromboembolism

If the clinical suspicion of thromboembolism is high, then specific tests as discussed in Section 1.5, p. 163, would be appropriate.

BRONCHOSCOPY

Analysis of bronchial lavage fluid is indicated to diagnose PCP and miliary TB. If there is CT evidence of interstitial lung disease transbronchial biopsy is likely to be required; open lung biopsy may be preferred in selected patients.

ECHOCARDIOGRAPHY

A contrast echo is the first choice investigation if an anatomic shunt is identified (estimation of pulmonary artery pressure is a useful piece of extra data from this study). If there is no cardiac shunt then a CT scan will usually identify a pulmonary AVM.

 The most useful investigation in respiratory medicine is the old radiograph. This adage normally applies when trying to decide the nature of a solitary pulmonary nodule. However, the principle can be applied prospectively; for patients who you feel uneasy about but are unable to diagnose, it can be helpful to recall them to clinic and repeat their radiograph.

Management

Clearly the management in this case is of the underlying condition. If the underlying condition is untreatable, oxygen should be considered for palliation of symptoms.

 Lennox AF, Nicolaides AN. Rapid D-dimer testing as an adjunct to clinical findings in excluding pulmonary embolism. *Thorax* 1999; 54(S2): S33–S36.
The PIOPED investigators. Value of the ventilation–perfusion scan in acute pulmonary embolism. Results of the prospective investigation of pulmonary embolism diagnosis (PIOPED). *JAMA* 1990; 263: 2753–2759.

1.7 Nocturnal cough

Case history

A 45-year-old woman, who has been a life-long non-smoker, is referred with a 6-month history of an annoying dry nocturnal cough. She has no previous history of respiratory problems.

Clinical approach

A chronic persistent cough can be defined as a cough that lasts more than 3 weeks. Causes can be divided according to whether the cough is productive or non-productive (Table 6).

Overall the most common cause of cough is smoking, and the most likely pathology is asthma, COPD or hyperreactive airways, possibly precipitated some time before by an upper respiratory tract infection. In smokers it is always crucial to rule out an underlying malignancy

Table 6 Differential diagnosis of a chronic cough.

Type of cough		Example
Productive	Common	Smoking, COPD/chronic bronchitis, asthma, bronchiectasis
	Consider	Tumour, tuberculosis, pulmonary emboli, congestive heart failure
	Other	Inhaled foreign body
Non-productive	Common	Smoking, asthma, postnasal drip, oesophageal reflux, ACE inhibitors
	Consider	Inflammatory lung disease, e.g. sarcoidosis, connective tissue disease, congestive heart failure, tumour
	Other	Middle ear disease, psychogenic

ACE, angiotensin-converting enzyme; COPD, chronic obstructive pulmonary disease.

such as a lung or throat neoplasm. However, this patient is a non-smoker and there are a number of important causes of chronic cough that are often overlooked:
• postnasal drip
• gastro-oesophageal reflux
• ear and throat problems.

History of the presenting problem

After the patient has told her story, address the following issues with direct questions if they have not already been covered.

Asthma

• When did the problem start? Was it related to a viral illness?
• Have you ever been wheezy, particularly during coughs and colds?
• Do you ever wake up feeling breathless or wheezy in the middle of the night?
• Is there a family history of atopy, i.e. asthma, hayfever, eczema?
• What is your job?

Postnasal drip

There may be a history of hayfever or simply a very runny nose. If asked, some patients can describe a dripping sensation at the back of their throat or swallowing lots of catarrh.

Oesophageal reflux

Many patients with oesophageal reflux will have no symptoms, but check for history of peptic ulceration, indigestion or heart burn.

Cardiac disease

Patients may cough with cardiac failure, or secondary to their medication, especially ACE inhibitors. Are there any risk factors or symptoms of thromoembolic disease? (See Section 1.5, p. 163.)

Inflammatory lung disease

Sarcoidosis or lung manifestations of autoimmune rheumatic disease can simply present with a chronic cough. Look for other manifestations such as joint problems.

Ear and throat disease

Middle ear disease can lead to a cough. Ask about alternations in voice, as underlying vocal cord polyp or malignancy are possible (see *Oncology*, Section 2.6). Ask about sinusitis.

Relevant past history

Asthma

Is there any personal or family history that helps support the diagnosis? For example 'I was always chesty as a child.' 'All my cousins have asthma and my nephew's just been given an inhaler.'

Are there underlying or precipitating factors? For example, allergies—food, pets, eczema and hayfever. Has the patient ever smoked? Do the symptoms get worse in pubs or clubs, or other smoky atmospheres?

Bronchiectasis

If the cough is productive, ask about childhood illness such as pneumonia, TB and diphtheria that would predispose to bronchiectasis.

Examination

Full general, respiratory and cardiac examinations are required (see Sections 1.1, p. 153 and 1.2, p. 155), but examination is unremarkable in many cases presenting with cough as the only symptom. Even so, it is important to look carefully for clues, particularly of the more unusual causes, e.g. autoimmune rheumatic disease, where something such as evidence of small joint disease could be crucial in making the diagnosis.

Respiratory and cardiac

Examine particularly for wheeze and stridor, and for problems in the nose and throat. Use a torch to look for nasal polyps and catarrh dripping down the pharynx. Listen for crackles on inspiration that do not clear on coughing, indicative of inflammatory lung disease. Examine for signs of congestive heart failure.

Approach to investigations and management

> **Investigations of chronic cough**
>
> - Chest radiograph—mandatory in all patients
> - Lung function tests—pre- and postbronchodilator
> - Sputum examination
> - ENT referral and examination.
>
> Other investigations if no diagnosis made:
> - bronchoscopy
> - upper gastrointestinal endoscopy
> - high-resolution computed tomography scan of chest.

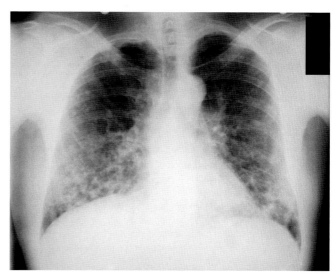

Fig. 10 Chest radiograph of 55-year-old non-smoker who presented to his general practitioner with a mild, but persistent, cough; he was later diagnosed as having diffuse alveolo-adenocarcinoma of the lung.

Investigations

Chest radiograph

This is crucial to rule out an obvious mass, tumour or cavity (Fig. 10). It may also reveal evidence of infection, cardiac failure or interstitial changes. If any of these are present, further investigation should follow as appropriate.

Lung function tests

It is important to request pre- and postbronchodilator values as these may not be performed automatically (Table 7). Lung volumes, flow–volume loops and gas transfer results may also help in establishing a diagnosis. The patient can be asked to undertake peak flow monitoring—at work as well as at home if appropriate.

Sputum examination

Send for microscopy, culture and sensitivity (MCS), including AFB, and cytology. Patients with other chronic diseases such as connective tissue disorders or diabetes may harbour chronic bacterial infections that can be cleared with an extended cause of antibiotics.

ENT referral and examination

It is important to arrange this early on if lung tumour, asthma, COPD and infection have been ruled out. Sinus radiographs are helpful in excluding potential sites of chronic infection.

Table 7 Lung function tests of a man who complained of a persistent cough that kept him awake at night; note the modest, but significant reversibility after bronchodilatator. Because the forced expiratory volume after 1 s (FEV_1) increase is >200 mL and >10% this patient just achieves the threshold to be a responder in terms of obstructive lung disease.

Spirometry (BTPS)	Predicted mean	Observed		Observed		
		pre	% pred	post	% pred	Percentage change
SVC (L)	3.80	2.33	61			
FVC (L)	3.67	2.15	59	2.33	63	+8
FEV_1 (L)	2.88	1.74	61	1.96	68	+13
FEV_1/FVC (%)	76	81		84		+4
MMEF (L/min)	192	1.67	52	2.60	81	+56
PEF (L/min)	463	322.0	72	322.6	72	+0
FIVC (L)	3.80	2.16	57	0.79	21	−64
PIF (L/min)	393.6	179.1	45	164.0	42	−8

FIVC, forced inspiratory vital capacity; FVC, forced vital capacity; MMEF, maximal mid-expiratory flow; PEF, peak expiratory flow; PIF, peak inspiratory flow; SVC, slow vital capacity.

Management

- Asthma (see Section 2.2.2, p. 191)
- Postnasal drip—often relieved by beclamethasone nasal spray
- Gastro-oesophageal reflux (see *Gastroenterology and hepatology*, Sections 1.2 and 2.2.2)
- Chest infection
- Inflammatory lung disease (see Section 2.7, p. 204)
- ENT problems: surgical therapy if appropriate.

 In younger patients (<40 years) it can be worth treating postulated gastrointestinal reflux 'blind' as a diagnostic trial using a proton pump inhibitor. If the trial is successful you will need to consider, on a balance of risks, whether formal investigation of the GI tract is worthwhile.

 Chung KF, Lalloo UG. Diagnosis and management of chronic persistent dry cough. *Postgrad Med J* 1996; 2: 594–598. McGarvey LPA, Heaney LG, Lawson JT *et al.* Evaluation and outcome of patients with chronic non-productive cough using a comprehensive diagnostic protocol. *Thorax* 1998; 98: 738–743.

1.8 Daytime sleepiness and morning headache

Case history

A 38-year-old woman, who weighs 85 kg, is found to be polycythaemic. Direct questioning reveals a 6-month history of morning headache and daytime somnolence.

Clinical approach

Polycythaemia could be caused by a primary haematological problem (see *Haematology*, Sections 1.14, 2.2.7 and 2.6), but the history of headache and somnolence suggests it is likely that the patient has nocturnal hypoxia as the cause, with carbon dioxide retention. For treatment purposes it is useful to distinguish between obstructive sleep aphoea (OSA) and chronic type II ventilatory failure.

History of the presenting problem

Determine the following:
- Does the patient snore? Snoring is a marker of OSA. The patient may not be the best witness: has her partner, or anyone else, ever complained about her snoring? Has anyone ever said that she made odd sounds or had funny breathing at night?

Table 8 Causes of chronic respiratory failure.

Classification	Examples
Increased load	Chronic lung disease (esp. COPD), skeletal chest wall disease, e.g. post-tuberculous sequelae, kyphoscoliosis, morbid obesity
Reduced respiratory muscle pump function	Reduced drive (e.g. sedative drugs), respiratory muscle weakness (e.g. motor neuron disease)

COPD, chronic obstructive pulmonary disease.

- Are there other features of OSA: enuresis, witnessed apnoeas, daytime sleepiness (as opposed to tiredness). Has she ever fallen asleep when she was not intending to, e.g. when driving?
- If there is hypersomnolence, are there features to suggest other causes? Cataplexy, hypnogogic/hypnopompic hallucinations (occurring on falling asleep or on waking) and automatic behaviours suggest narcolepsy. Reports of limb twitching suggest periodic limb movement syndrome.
- Are sleep opportunity and sleep hygiene satisfactory? Does the woman have young children who keep her awake all night? Is the patient working a shift pattern that makes it difficult or impossible to get into a sensible routine of sleeping and waking? Does the patient take 'cat naps' during the day?
- Does the patient have a recognized cause of chronic ventilatory failure (Table 8)?

Examination

Full general, respiratory and cardiac examinations are required (see Sections 1.1, p. 153 and 1.2, p. 155), but in this case pay particular attention to the following aspects:
- Is the patient hypertensive?—a common feature of OSA
- Is there evidence of cor pulmonale?—a feature of severe chronic lung disease and OSA
- Is there evidence of chronic lung disease?—clubbing, hyperinflation, chest signs, chest wall deformity (Fig. 11)
- Is there evidence of neurological disease?—wasting of the muscles, fasciculation
- Are there upper airway problems?—look for tonsillar enlargement, nasal polyps (Fig. 12).

Approach to investigations and management

Investigations

Routine

The aim of routine investigations is to detect common pathologies and to quantify end-organ complications.

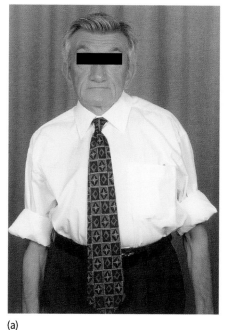 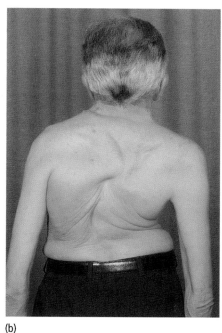

Fig. 11 The same patient shown (a) from the front, dressed, and (b) closer up, from behind and undressed. Kyphoscoliosis can be missed on superficial examination.

(a)   (b)

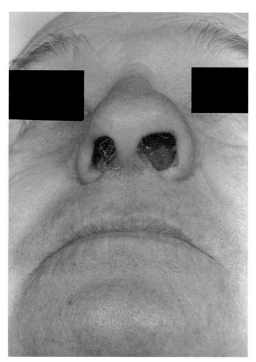

Fig. 12 This patient has snoring and obstructive sleep apnoea. Simple examination shows a polyp which, if treated may improve symptoms.

- Daytime arterial blood gases—the demonstration of daytime hypercapnia will influence the urgency and, possibly, mode of treatment
- Repeat full blood count—to confirm polycythaemia
- Thyroid function tests—hypothyroidism can precipitate weight gain and (rarely) OSA
- Chest radiograph—to exclude lung disease; look also for cardiomegaly

- ECG—may reveal left ventricular hypertrophy or right heart strain
- Spirometry, lung volumes, lying and standing vital capacity or mouth pressures
- Formal ENT evaluation.

Sleep orientated

Overnight oximetry is a useful screening investigation that may be done at home. The diagnosis of polycythaemia secondary to nocturnal hypoxia must be reviewed if the patient reports that she sleeps and there is no desaturation. The absence of nocturnal desaturation would require the assumption of an alternative cause of hypersomnolence (e.g. narcolepsy) occurring with an alternative cause of polycythaemia. However, note that a normal overnight SaO_2 does not exclude the diagnosis of OSA in patients with appropriate symptoms but without polycythaemia.

If the patient has an overnight SaO_2 trace suggestive of OSA, and examination or investigation does not reveal chronic respiratory failure (CRF; or risk factors for CRF), then it is reasonable to manage the patient as having OSA.

If the patient has nocturnal desaturation and risk factors for CRF (e.g. obesity and tobacco-related lung disease) then a more accurate assessment is required. This may involve a limited respiratory sleep study with transcutaneous carbon dioxide monitoring. Full polysomnography with carbon dioxide monitoring is used in some centres. These tests are required because the mode of ventilatory support is determined by the precise diagnosis.

173

After the institution of mechanical ventilatory support a repeat study is useful to confirm the adequacy of treatment.

> If a patient has daytime sleepiness secondary to OSA that is sufficiently severe to require nasal continuous positive airway pressure (CPAP) ventilatory assistance, they must inform both the DVLA and their motor insurer of the diagnosis.

Management

See Section 2.12, p. 231.

> Chesson AL, Ferber RA, Fry JM *et al.* The indications for polysomnography and related procedures. *Sleep* 1997; 20: 423–487.
> Gugger M. Comparison of ResMed Autoset (version 3.03) with polysomnography in the diagnosis of the sleep apnoea/ hypopoea syndrome. *Eur Resp J* 1997; 10: 587–591.

1.9 Haemoptysis and weight loss

Case history

A 35-year-old man, who came as a political refugee to the UK 5 years ago, presents with haemoptysis and weight loss. He has been previously fit and well. His chest radiograph is shown in Fig. 13.

Clinical approach

The presentation is vague about the patient's ethnic background and says nothing of his travel history, details of which are critical in this case. Apart from TB, much the most likely diagnosis, other causes of haemoptysis in a young patient are shown in Table 9.

History of the presenting problem

Communication may be difficult: unless the man has good command of English it is unlikely that you will be able to obtain a thorough history without the benefit of an interpreter.

The first thing to do is to establish if haemoptysis is the problem. How long has the patient been coughing up blood? Is the patient sure that the blood is in the phlegm and not in vomit or coming from the throat?

Haemoptysis caused by tuberculosis

A detailed personal, social, family and travel history is required, with particular emphasis on the following:

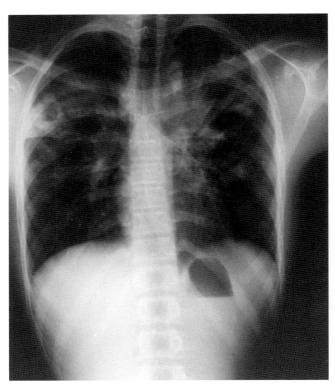

Fig. 13 Chest radiograph of this patient; note the bilateral apical changes, consistent with *Mycobacterium tuberculosis* infection, as well as the cavity on the periphery of the right upper lobe.

Table 9 Causes of haemoptysis in a young person.

Classification	Examples
Common	Infection, e.g. pyogenic bacteria or MTB
Consider	Bronchiectasis, pulmonary emboli
Rare	Tumour (benign or malignant), Goodpasture's or other vasculitis

MTB, *Mycobacterium tuberculosis*.

• Has the patient been treated for TB in the past? If so, was the patient given antituberculous medication, and how many drugs? Few people remember the names of the tablets: ask for descriptions of them—combination preparations that have distinctive colours and shapes are often used, e.g. Rifater, Rifinah.
• Have family members or close household contacts ever been treated for TB? Many patients deny this, particularly before a diagnosis has been made, because of the stigmas surrounding the disease.
• Where was the patient born? In which countries has the patient lived before coming to the UK? What sort of places has the patient lived in—refugee camps, hostels? The incidence of single-drug- and multidrug-resistant TB varies from region to region and this should be taken into consideration in any subsequent treatment. Remember also that some areas of Western Africa have much higher rates of HIV infection than, say, Bangladesh.

• Where is the patient living now? How many people are living in the patient's home? Many immigrants live in overcrowded housing: from the point of view of contact tracing and subsequent screening it is important to know who the patient's close contacts are.
• Has the patient lost any weight? How is the patient's appetite? Has the patient had any fevers or drenching night sweats? Has the patient needed to change the bedclothes? Weight loss, anorexia, fevers and sweats would all be expected in TB, and their absence would cast doubt on the diagnosis.

Other

• Bronchiectasis—is the patient producing any sputum? How much? Teaspoonfuls or cupfuls? Ask about childhood respiratory infections, including TB and whooping cough, which would predispose to this condition. (See Section 1.3, p. 158)
• Pulmonary emboli—is the patient at risk? (See Section 1.5, p. 163)
• Goodpasture's—exceedingly unlikely in this case, but is there a history of occupational exposure to solvents, paints or petrol?

Examination

Full general, respiratory and cardiac examinations are needed (see Sections 1.1, p. 153 and 1.2, p. 155), but particular attention to the following is required:
• Does the patient look unwell and cachetic? Does the patient appear hot and feverish?
• Is there lymphadenopathy, which would support the diagnosis of TB?
• Is there clubbing and inspiratory crackles that do not clear on coughing, which would support the diagnosis of bronchiectasis?
• What are the signs in the chest? In particular, are there pleural effusions that could be tapped and the pleura biopsied?
• Are there cardiac or pulmonary signs to suggest pulmonary emboli? (See Section 1.5, p. 163.)

Approach to investigations and management

Investigations of haemoptysis
• Chest radiograph—immediate
• Sputum examination for AFB
• Bronchoscopy—within a week if diagnosis not made.

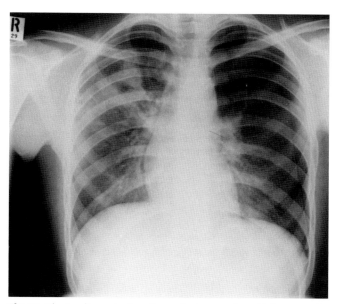

Fig. 14 Chest radiograph of another patient presenting with haemoptysis and later found to have tuberculosis; he had coughed so much that he had a left-sided pneumothorax, which had led to right mediastinal shift. This resolved spontaneously with conservative treatment. His tuberculosis was treated with quadruple therapy.

Investigations

Chest radiograph

This may help narrow down the diagnostic possibilities, but do not forget that TB can mimic many other pathologies, such as lung cancer, other bacterial infections and pneumonitis. Do not forget to look for pleural thickening and evidence of calcification, also for the unexpected (Fig. 14).

Sputum examination

Urgent (same day) examination for MCS and AFB. Send for cytology as well.

Bronchoscopy

Bronchial biopsies, if taken, must be sent both for histology (in formalin) and microbiology (in normal saline). It is good practice for bronchial lavage to be performed and sent for cytology (for malignant cells) and microbiology and virology. Silver staining is not indicated unless there are other reasons to suggest PCP.

Management

Will be according to diagnosis:
• TB: see *Infectious diseases*, Section 2.6
• Bronchiectasis: see Section 2.4, p. 197
• Pulmonary emboli: see *Cardiology*, Section 2.18 and *Haematology and oncology*, Section 3.6.

1.10 Pleural effusion and fever

Case history

A 43-year-old woman is admitted to the hospital with fever for the last 7–8 days. Her chest radiograph shows a pleural effusion on the right side (Fig. 15).

Clinical approach

Here the main symptom is fever, suggesting an underlying inflammatory or infective process. The history is short, indicating an acute problem. A pleural effusion on chest radiograph suggests the lungs as the primary site of pathology, but there are other causes of effusion, e.g. cardiac failure, but they are unlikely in this case.

Fever and pleural effusion

Pneumonia with an effusion and empyema are the likeliest diagnoses, but consider:
• TB
• Connective tissue disorder (rheumatoid arthritis/SLE)
• Malignancy (primary bronchial/secondary)
• Mesothelioma
• Pulmonary emboli
• Familial Mediterranean fever (seen in Jewish and Arabic people; recurrent attacks of fever, arthritis, and pleurisy. Prevented by colchicine).

History of the presenting problem

It is important to determine whether the problem really is new or, with hindsight, whether other features were present beforehand. Fever and pleural effusion developing acutely in a previously healthy person are most likely to be caused by an infective pathology. Has there been recent cough and purulent phlegm? Ask about the following if they do not emerge spontaneously in the history:
• Is there any pleuritic chest pain? (bacterial pneumonia/pulmonary embolism).
• Has the patient coughed up blood? (bacterial pneumonia/TB/malignancy).
• Has the patient lost any weight? (tuberculosis/malignancy).
• Has the patient travelled abroad recently? (infection/pulmonary embolism).
• Is the patient a smoker? (bronchial carcinoma).
• Is there any history of night sweats and evening rise of temperature? (TB).
• Has the patient been in contact with anyone with TB?
• Has there been a rash? (may suggest mycoplasma).
• Does the patient suffer from any joint pains in the hands? (rheumatoid arthritis/SLE).

Relevant past history

• Any history of joint pains? (rheumatoid arthritis/SLE).
• Any history of malignancy? (breast, ovarian, lymphoma).

Social and occupational history

• Does the patient smoke?
• Any exposure to asbestos? (benign effusions/mesothelioma).
• A nurse/doctor or other health worker may unwittingly have been in contact with TB.

Examination

Full general, respiratory and cardiac examinations are needed (see Sections 1.1, p. 153 and 1.2, p. 155), but particular attention to the following is required.

General

Look for cachexia, lymphadenopathy (malignancy, TB), jaundice (hepatic metastasis), sputum pot, rash of SLE, rheumatoid hands and nodules. Examine the breasts for any mass (with chaperone if appropriate).

Respiratory

The signs of a pleural effusion (reduced expansion, reduced breath/absent breath sounds and stony dullness) will be present if the effusion is big enough, but these do not help the differential diagnosis.

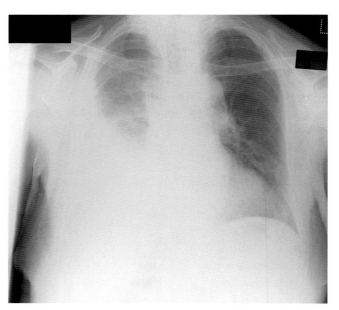

Fig. 15 Posteroanterior chest radiograph showing a right pleural effusion.

Approach to investigations and management

Investigations

Blood tests

Check full blood count, ESR, CRP, rheumatoid factor, antinuclear antibodies, calcium level and liver function tests.

Sputum

For microscopy and culture (specifically including for TB), and for cytology.

Pleural fluid

Examining the pleural fluid is critical.
- If there is associated pneumonia: is the fluid parapneumonic or is it an empyema? If it is opaque/turbid and with a foul smell, then it is clearly an empyema. In cases that are less clear-cut the pleural fluid pH is probably the single most useful test, with empyema strongly suggested by a pH <7.22.
- If there is no associated pneumonia: is the fluid a transudate or an exudate? The two are distinguished by Light's criteria (see below); causes of transudates and exudates are shown in Table 10.
- Send for microscopy and culture: both anaerobic and aerobic, and for TB.
- Send for cytology.
- Measure protein, lactate dehydrogenase (LDH) and pH.

 My colleagues and I demonstrated that with the use of simultaneously obtained serum and pleural fluid protein and lactic acid dehydrogenase (LDH) values, 99% of pleural effusions could be correctly classified as either transudates or exudates. Exudative pleural effusions meet at least one of the following criteria, whereas transudative pleural effusions meet none:
1 Pleural fluid protein divided by serum protein greater than 0.5
2 Pleural fluid LDH divided by serum LDH greater than 0.6
3 Pleural fluid LDH greater than two-thirds the upper limit of normal for the LDH.
(Light's criteria for classification of pleural effusions [1].)

 For suspected malignant effusions it can be helpful to send a large volume and have this spun in the laboratory to magnify the cellular portion.

Table 10 Causes of pleural effusions.

Classification	Example
Transudates	Congestive cardiac failure, cirrhosis, nephrotic syndrome, myxoedema, peritoneal dialysis
Exudates	Malignancy, infectious (bacterial, tuberculosis, fungal, parasitic, viral), pulmonary emboli, collagen vascular (rheumatoid, SLE, Sjögren's syndrome, Wegener's, Churg–Strauss), gastrointestinal (pancreatic disease, subphrenic abscess, oesophageal perforation), yellow-nail syndrome, haemothorax, chylothorax, drug-induced (amiodarone, dantrolene, methotrexate, practolol, nitrofurantoin)

SLE, systemic lupus eythematosus.

Pleural biopsy

Pleural biopsy should be performed in those with an exudative pleural effusion to exclude malignancy. It is reasonable to attempt this with an Abrams' needle, but it is important to remember that because this is a blind (unguided) procedure a negative result does not exclude any diagnosis.

Ultrasound of the chest

In cases of loculated effusion, it is best to aspirate the effusion under ultrasound guidance.

Computed tomographic scan of chest

This investigation quantifies the pleural fluid collection, but also examines the lung parenchyma and may identify unsuspected tumours or solid pleural disease.

Management

The treatment of the effusion depends on the cause, but three cases require special consideration:
- parapneumonic effusions
- empyema
- malignant pleural effusions.

Parapneumonic effusions

Parapneumonic effusions that resolve with appropriate antibiotics are called uncomplicated parapneumonic effusions and do not require tube drainage.

Empyema

- The patient should receive appropriate doses of parenteral antibiotics.
- A chest drain is required: delay in draining an empyema

is associated with an increase in mortality. Use at least a 28 F size drain so that it will not become obstructed with fibrin.

The presence of pleural fluid loculations can prevent complete drainage by mechanical means alone. Intrapleural streptokinase and urokinase have been used to destroy the fibrin membranes that separate the locules and facilitate drainage. Streptokinase (250 000 units) or urokinase (100 000 units) dissolved in 30–60 mL of normal saline is given intrapleurally via the drain, which is then clamped for 1–2 h. On release of the clamp, a successful response is heralded by an increase in the amount of fluid drained and improvement in the chest radiograph. Fibrinolytics can be given daily for 14 days: they do not have any effect on the systemic bleeding parameters.

In patients who remain ill and with inadequate drainage despite intrapleural fibrinolytics, decortication should be considered. This is a major surgical procedure: all fibrous tissue is removed and pus evacuated.

Malignant pleural effusions

Patients with large pleural effusions caused by untreatable malignancies can be very dyspnoiec. This should be treated (unless the patient's life expectancy is very short indeed) with pleurodesis, either locally via a chest drain or by a thoracoscopic approach. In the editor's experience reaccumulation rates are significantly lower after thoracosopic procedures and this approach is preferred unless the patient is expected to die within 1 month.

The indications for inserting a chest drain into a parapneumonic effusion/empyema are:
- pus in pleural cavity (empyema)
- organisms visible in pleural fluid on microscopy
- positive pleural fluid culture
- pleural fluid pH <7.20
- serial reduction in pleural fluid pH, glucose and increase in LDH.

Bouros D, Schiza S, Panagou P, Drositis J, Siafakas N. Role of streptokinase in the treatment of acute loculated parapneumonic pleural effusions and empyema. *Thorax* 1994; 49: 852–855.

Heffner JE. Diagnosis and management of thoracic empyemas. *Curr Opin Pulm Med* 1996; 2(3): 198–205.

Heffner JE, Brown LK, Barbieri C, DeLeo JM. Pleural fluid chemical analysis in parapneumonic effusion. *Am J Respir Crit Care Med* 1995; 151: 1700–1708.

Light RW. *Pleural Diseases* (2nd edn). New York: Lea and Febiger.

1 Light RW, MacGregor MI, Luchsinger PC, Ball WC. Pleural effusions: the diagnostic separation of transudates and exudates. *Ann Intern Med* 1972; 77: 507–513.

1.11 Lung cancer with asbestos exposure

Case history

A 53-year-old taxi driver presents with a chest radiograph that shows evidence of right-sided pleural thickening associated with a moderate pleural effusion. He has previously worked in numerous labouring jobs, including as a lagger.

Clinical approach

Your main concern is that this patient has asbestos-related lung disease and that this could be mesothelioma, although asbestos also causes other pathology (Table 11). It is important to take a detailed occupational history.

How to take an occupational history

- The easiest way of recording employment is by asking the patient what he or she did immediately after leaving school and then recording positions chronologically; people tend to remember their jobs most easily this way.
- Do not forget holiday jobs from school or casual employment (Steve McQueen, the American actor, worked with asbestos for 6 months before he became famous, and he died of asbestos-related lung disease).
- Did anyone in the patient's family work in an asbestos factory and bring the dust home on their clothes?
- On a more short-term basis, particularly if you are worried about the patient's current employment, say in relation to occupational asthma—do the symptoms worsen during the working week and improve at the weekend and during the holidays?

History of the presenting problem

Underlying pathology caused by asbestos exposure

In taking the occupational history, do not forget to ask the following:
- If the patient remembers working with asbestos, how long was this for? How close was the contact and for what length of the working day? For example, was the patient working in the holds of ships unloading bags of asbestos? Were the patient's clothes covered in asbestos dust?

Table 11 Possible asbestos-related lung disease.

Classification	Example
Common	Pleural plaques, pleural thickening
Consider	Asbestos-related fibrosis (asbestosis), lung cancer, mesothelioma

- Did the patient wear protective clothing or masks? Were these provided by the employers?
- Record the names of the companies that they worked for (may be helpful for later reference).

Smoking history

This is necessary because, if there is both asbestos and tobacco exposure, then—for legal purposes—it is desirable to quantify both.

 Take an accurate smoking history and record in the notes when and if the patient has stopped smoking. If patients claim for compensation at a later date, this information will be required.

Symptoms

Persistent pain or rapid progression of symptoms are poor predictive features.
- Has the patient had any chest pain? If so, how long does it last? Does it keep them awake at night?
- Has the patient been short of breath at rest or on exercise?
- Has it been more difficult of late for the patient to lie down without feeling breathless?

Relevant past history

It is important to ascertain whether there have been any previous episodes of chest problems. Did the patient suffer from chest problems as a child? Many previous chest pathologies can leave pleural thickening.

 Causes of pleural thickening

- Asbestos exposure
- Trauma
- Previous chest infection/empyema
- Previous haemothorax
- Old TB.

Examination

Full general, respiratory and cardiac examinations are needed (see Sections 1.1, p. 153 and 1.2, p. 155), but particular attention to the following is required:
- Does the patient look in good health or obviously unwell?
- Is the patient cachectic and pale?
- Is there clubbing?
- Is there lymphadenopathy?
- What are the signs in the chest?

Approach to investigations and management

 Investigations of asbestos-related disease

- Chest radiograph—posteroanterior and lateral
- High-resolution computed tomography of the chest
- Pleural biopsy and aspiration and/or thoracoscopy
- Open lung biospy.

Investigations

Chest radiograph

In this case, the patient presented with a chest film. In general, look carefully for any pleural thickening—it is easy to miss (Figs 16 and 17a). Is there any calcification, particularly over the diaphragm? Do not forget to look for areas of fibrosis.

Computed tomography scan of chest

This is invaluable when assessing the extent of disease, whether there is pleural thickening, fibrosis or malignancy (Fig. 17b). If appropriate, a CT scan may be followed by a CT-guided biopsy. In cases of bronchogenic cancer and asbestos exposure the presence of fibrosis supports the argument that the patient was exposed to significant quantities of asbestos.

Pleural biopsy and aspiration

 A pleural biopsy with an Abrams' needle can only be carried out in the presence of a moderate to large pleural effusion, otherwise you will puncture the lung and give the patient a pneumothorax.

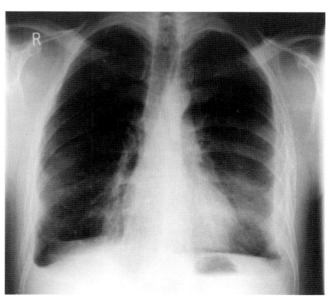

Fig. 16 Chest radiograph showing obvious left-sided pleural thickening caused by asbestos exposure. (Courtesy of Dr R. Rudd.)

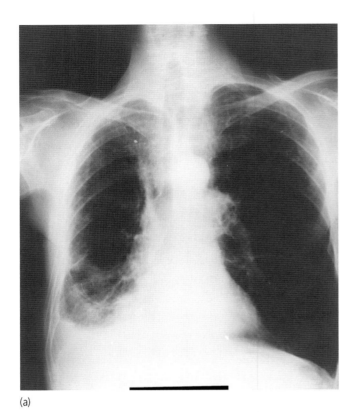

(a)

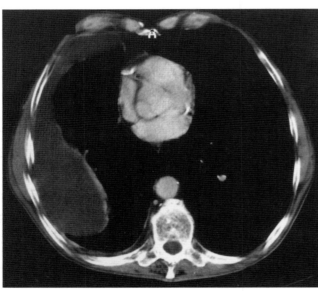

(b)

Fig. 17 (a) Chest radiograph of a patient with mesothelioma leading to right-sided pleural thickening, which has produced a volume loss and mediastinal shift. (b) Computed tomography scan of the same patient with mesothelioma showing the extent of disease invasion into the right hemithorax.

> **!** Make sure that you send pleural biopsy samples to microbiology, for microscopy and culture (including TB), as well as to histology. The diagnosis may not be malignancy, or there may be dual pathology.

Thoracoscopy

This is generally only available in specialist centres, where it can be performed by chest physicians and/or cardiothoracic surgeons. As with pleural biopsy, the presence of an abnormal amount of pleural fluid is necessary for the procedure to be carried out safely.

Management

The management is dependent on the final diagnosis:
- asbestosis: see Section 2.6.1, p. 202
- mesothelioma: see Section 2.9.2, p. 224
- lung cancer: see Section 2.9.1, p. 220.

1.12 Lobar collapse in non-smoker

Case history

A 55-year-old woman is referred with a 10-day history of productive cough, gradually increasing shortness of breath, and fever. Her symptoms have failed to resolve on oral antibiotics and her chest radiograph shows right upper lobe collapse (Fig. 18), but the same clinical approach would apply to collapse of any lobe (see Fig. 19).

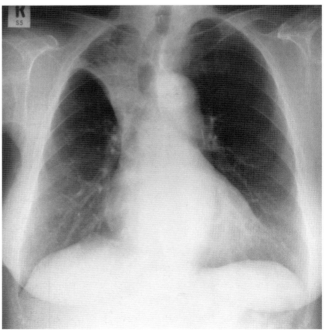

Fig. 18 Posteroanterior chest radiograph showing right upper lobe collapse. Note the tenting of the right hemidiaphragm and the raised right hilum. (Courtesy of Dr I. Vlahos.)

Clinical approach

If there is also consolidation your initial concern must be to treat the acute condition, which is likely to be a lobar pneumonia. The patient should be admitted to hospital, given oxygen (if blood gases reveal hypoxia) and appropriate antibiotics. Sputum and blood cultures should be sent for MCS.

However, collapse alone or collapse/consolidation which is slow to clear (say more than 6 weeks from the start of symptoms) requires investigation because of the possibility that there is an obstructing lesion.

History of the presenting problem

Cause of lobar collapse

A full respiratory history is essential. Be precise.
- When did the shortness of breath start? Was it before the illness that precipitated the patient's admission? If so, how long?
- How did the shortness of breath start? Was it gradual or sudden?
- Has the patient had any associated pains in the chest?
- Is there any history of haemoptysis?
- How long has the patient had the fever? What about night sweats?
- Is inhalation of a foreign body a possibility?

Bacterial infection

Patients with chronic chest problems are particularly prone to infection. In younger, non-smoking patients who are otherwise well, infection may be precipitated by colds or 'flu.

Lung cancer

Consider lung cancer in a middle-aged smoker, particularly if there is any recent history of weight loss and/or anorexia. Be aware, however, that patients with lung cancer do not have to have these symptoms, and can be asymptomatic.

Foreign body

Infants, children and patients with learning difficulties or dementia are particularly at risk. Ask for a history of choking on a peanut, losing a dental filling, or of trauma while eating food.

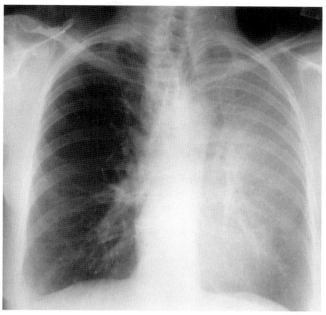

(a)

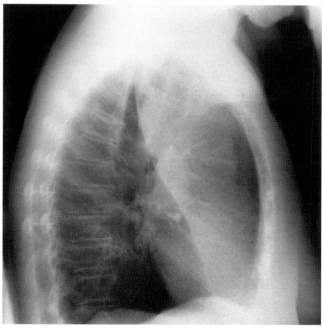

(b)

Fig. 19 (a) Posteroanterior chest radiograph and (b) lateral chest radiograph of a left upper lobe collapse. Note the veil-like opacity of the left side. (Courtesy of Dr I. Vlahos.)

Table 12 Differential diagnosis of lobar collapse.

Classification	Example
Common	Infection, i.e. bacteria, tuberculosis
Must consider	Carcinoma of the lung, foreign body
Other causes	Other tumour, e.g. carcinoid, benign adenoma, pulmonary infarct

181

Other

'Odd' symptoms such as flushing, sweats or diarrhoea may be associated with carcinoid. Bronchial adenomas frequently produce haemoptysis.

Relevant past history

Has the patient any other history to support your diagnosis?
• Is the patient a current, ex- or never-smoker?
• Has the patient ever had asthma, bronchitis or any other respiratory problems?
• Is there a personal or family history of TB?

Examination

Full general, respiratory and cardiac examinations are needed (see Sections 1.1, p. 153 and 1.2, p. 155), but particular attention to the following is required:
• Does the patient look in good health or obviously unwell?
• What is the patient's breathing like now? Comfortable or laboured?
• Is the patient cachectic and pale?
• Is there clubbing?
• Is there lymphadenopathy?
• What are the signs in the chest? Is there any evidence of consolidation (bronchial breathing)?

Approach to investigations and management

Investigations of lobar collapse
• Bronchoscopy—in anyone with persistent shadowing
• Computed tomography scan of the chest—useful in many cases.

Investigations

Bronchoscopy

This may be performed as an inpatient if symptoms are slow to resolve, or as an outpatient if persistent shadowing is seen on the chest radiograph. If an endobronchial lesion is seen, it should be biopsied and sent for histology. Bronchial washings should also be sent for cytology (even if nothing was seen) and microscopy.

 Do not forget to request specifically testing for AFB if TB is in the differential diagnosis: it is not performed routinely.

Computed tomography scan of chest

In some centres a CT scan of the chest will be performed before bronchoscopy. This has the advantage of giving the physician performing bronchoscopy a better idea of the anatomical layout of the problem and where to concentrate on taking samples, although if there is lobar collapse this is not a problem. However, a scan should certainly be requested when lung cancer is likely, and this should also include cuts of the liver and adrenals to help stage any potential tumour.

Management

• Chest infection: see *Infectious diseases*, Section 1.4
• Lung cancer: see Section 2.9.1, p. 220
• Foreign body: bronchoscopic removal if possible
• Pulmonary infarct/emboli: see Section 1.5, p. 165
• TB: see *Infectious diseases*, Section 2.6.1.

Foreign bodies

These may be seen at flexible bronchoscopy, but may be difficult to remove. If so, the patient should be given broad-spectrum antibiotics and referred immediately for rigid bronchoscopy in a specialist centre. Long-term exclusion of bronchi can lead to bronchiectasis, associated with chronic cough and repeated chest infections.

1.13 Breathlessness with a normal radiograph

Case history

A 44-year-old woman presents with a 2-year history of exertional dyspnoea. Her chest radiograph is reported as being within normal limits. Her lung function shows:
• FEV_1 83% of predicted
• vital capacity (VC) 79% predicted
• FEV_1/VC ratio 78%
• DL_{CO} 73% predicted
• PaO_2 9.6 kPa
• $PaCO_2$ 4.1 kPa.

Clinical approach

The spirometry effectively rules out obstructive lung disease. Hyperventilation (and its causes) and anaemia are excluded as primary diagnoses by the finding of hypoxia. The differential probably lies between diffuse parenchymal lung disease or a problem of the pulmonary vasculature.

History of the presenting problem

In diffuse parenchymal lung disease the patient may have a dry cough, but there may be no specific features. It will clearly be worth enquiring about systemic or iatrogenic disorders associated with lung disease (see Section 1.4, p. 160). Specific employment histories or recreational interests may also suggest diffuse parenchymal lung disease (see Section 1.11, p. 178, for details of how to take an occupational history).

A history of asthma or rhinitis may suggest the rare possibility of Churg–Strauss syndrome.

Regarding diseases of the pulmonary vasculature: in pulmonary embolus there may be a history of pleuritic chest pain or haemoptysis, but a small proportion of patients present with chronic dyspnoea alone. Ask about risk factors for pulmonary embolism (see Section 1.5, p. 163). This patient could also have primary pulmonary hypertension: hence enquire about appetite suppressants.

Examination

Full general, respiratory and cardiac examinations are needed (see Sections 1.1, p. 153 and 1.2, p. 155), but particular attention to the following is required:
- Skin and joints—may be involved in patients with diffuse parenchymal lung disease (especially sarcoid)
- Clubbing—may feature in diffuse parenchymal lung disease
- Pulse—may be atrial fibrillation in pulmonary embolism
- Cyanosis—unlikely if the PaO_2 remains 9.6 kPa
- JVP—there may be grossly elevated venous pressure or tricuspid regurgitation in chronic pulmonary embolism or primary pulmonary hypertension
- Palpable right ventricular heave—may be present in chronic pulmonary embolism or primary pulmonary hypertension
- Heart sounds—may be a loud P2 in chronic pulmonary embolism or primary pulmonary hypertension
- Auscultation—may be fine inspiratory crackles in diffuse parenchymal lung disease or pleural rubs in pulmonary embolism
- Ankle oedema—may be present in chronic pulmonary embolism or primary pulmonary hypertension.

Approach to investigations and management

Investigations

The priority is to decide whether the patient is suffering from diffuse parenchymal lung disease or a problem of the pulmonary vasculature, and the findings on clinical examination will usually indicate which of these is most likely. The investigation of specific causes follows identification of the diagnostic type, e.g. avian precipitins are measured after the diagnosis of alveolitis is made. The following investigations will each be indicated in some cases: in any particular case start with the ones most likely to give the diagnosis.

Blood tests

It is usual to measure the full blood count, inflammatory markers (CRP and ESR) and simple biochemistry (renal and liver function). A calcium and serum ACE are measured where sarcoid is a possibility.

Electrocardiogram

This may show right heart strain in pulmonary embolism or primary pulmonary hypertension.

Pulmonary function tests

In the case described some lung function tests are given, but measurement of lung volumes by body plethysmography can be useful: fibrotic lung disease should show a reduction in total lung capacity.

High-resolution computed tomography scanning

The relative efficiency of high-resolution CT scanning and chest radiography for detecting diffuse parenchymal lung disease are 94 and 80%, respectively. High-resolution CT findings can predict the histological diagnosis in 82–93% of cases. (See Section 1.4, p. 162.)

Ventilation–perfusion scanning, helical computed tomography or lower leg ultrasound

For more details on the work-up of suspected pulmonary embolism, see Section 1.5, p. 165.

Echocardiography

This is a sensitive technique for detecting primary pulmonary hypertension. However, in view of the gravity of the diagnosis, direct measurement of pulmonary arterial pressure is usually performed both to confirm the diagnosis and to assess whether the patient responds to vasodilators (see *Cardiology*, Sections 1.10, 2.12 and 2.18). Echocardiography can also detect cardiac defects that can be occult causes of secondary pulmonary hypertension.

In primary pulmonary hypertension the patient should be formally assessed to see whether they respond to vasodilating agents. If not, the prognosis is very poor and transplantation or long-term prostacyclin infusion should be considered.

A quarter of cases of hoarseness lasting for more than 2–3 weeks result from cervical or thoracic neoplasm. Bronchoscopy or laryngoscopy is mandatory.

Management

Depends on diagnosis.

See *Cardiology*, Sections 1.10, 2.12 and 2.18.
British Thoracic Society. Suspected acute pulmonary embolism: a practical approach. *Thorax* 1999; 52 (Suppl. 4): S1–S24.
British Thoracic Society. The diagnosis, assessment and treatment of diffuse parenchymal lung disease in adults. *Thorax* 1999; 54 (Suppl. 1): S1–S30.
Gardner WN. The pathophysiology of hyperventilation. *Chest* 1996; 109: 516–534.
Peacock AJ. Primary pulmonary hypertension. *Thorax* 1999; 54: 1107–1118.
Rich S, Dantzker DR, Ayres SM *et al*. Primary pulmonary hypertension. *Ann Intern Med* 1987; 107: 216–223.

1.14 Upper airway obstruction

Case history

A 56-year-old woman presents with a 5-day history of stridor. She is obese and complains of recent hoarseness of her voice. She also complains of being tired all the time.

Clinical approach

• Wheeze indicates intrathoracic airflow obstruction, and is loudest on expiration.
• Stridor indicates extrathoracic airflow obstruction, and is loudest on inspiration.

This middle-aged patient has stridor, which is a musical sound best heard on inspiration as compared with wheeze, which is heard on expiration. It is caused by the turbulence of air passing through a narrow glottis or trachea, and indicates extrathoracic obstruction. The narrowing of the airway may be intrinsic or extrinsic, and it should be investigated urgently as it may be due to an underlying malignancy.

This patient also complains of a change in her voice and this demands urgent investigation.

History of the presenting problem

From the patient's story you will need to clarify the following:
• How long have the symptoms been present? Which came first—the voice change, the stridor or the tiredness?
• Is the patient also dyspnoeic?
• Although this patient is obese, has she lost any weight?
• Has the patient any history of cough or haemoptysis?
• Is there any history of dysphagia? This might be due to an underlying mediastinal tumour pressing on the oesophagus.
• Has the patient always been tired? Tiredness is a non-specific symptom, but along with a change in voice and obesity could point to hypothyroidism. Further support for this diagnosis would be obtained if the patient has gained weight recently or been constipated. (See *Endocrinology*, Sections 1.14 and 2.3.1.)
• Has the patient noticed any lymphadenopathy or fever? (suggests lymphoma).
• Are there any signs of superior vena cava obstruction? Swelling of the face and arms, dilated chest wall veins, or raised venous pressure would indicate intrathoracic disease pressing upon the superior vena cava.
• Are there any features of myasthenia gravis? (diplopia or dysphagia).

Causes of stridor
• Intrinsic narrowing of airway: tumour, stenosis or foreign body
• Extrinsic compression of airway: any neck or mediastinal mass
• Mediastinal fibrosis.

Relevant past history

Check the following:
• Has the patient ever had any thyroid disorder/surgery?
• Stridor can be due to tracheal stenosis secondary to intubation: has the patient ever been intubated, had an operation, or been on a breathing machine?
• Has the patient ever suffered from a lymphoma?
• Does the patient smoke or has she smoked in the past?

Examination

Full general, respiratory and cardiac examinations are needed (see Sections 1.1, p. 153 and 1.2, p. 155), but particular attention to the following is required.

General

- Look for any features of hypothyroidism. (See *Endocrinology*, Sections 1.14 and 2.3.1.)
- Is the thyroid visible or palpable?
- Is there clubbing?
- Look carefully for cervical and axillary lymphadenopathy. Check the abdomen and inguinal regions if you find nodes.
- Is there superior vena cava obstruction? (See *Oncology*, Section 1.8.)

Respiratory

Does she indeed have stridor? Ask her to cough and then take a deep breath with her mouth open—this exaggerates stridor. If there is tight obstruction there may be paradoxical indrawing of the upper thorax during inspiration.

Check for normal symmetrical movement of the chest and mediastinal shift.

Approach to investigations and management

Investigations

Blood tests

Thyroid function tests, full blood count, serum calcium, renal and liver function tests, acetylcholine receptor antibodies if suspicion of myasthenia.

Flow–volume loops

These can be helpful if the picture is not acute. An example of upper airway obstruction is shown in Fig. 20.

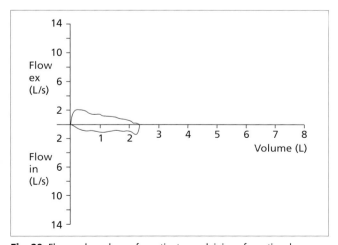

Fig. 20 Flow–volume loop of a patient complaining of exertional dyspnoea. Diagnosis: tracheal stenosis.

Bronchoscopy or laryngoscopy

Mandatory in undiagnosed upper airway obstruction. If the patient is unwell it is prudent to have anaesthetic assistance for this examination.

Tensilon test

This is indicated in suspected myasthenia gravis with underlying thymoma. (See *Neurology*, Section 2.2.5.)

Chest radiograph

This may show mediastinal mass (including thymoma) or lymphadenopathy.

Computed tomography

This is only helpful if intrathoracic disease is identified, or for the staging of localized head and neck disease.

Radionuclide scanning

Thyroid scans can be used to look for retrosternal goitre. Mediastinal thyroid tissue can be of two origins: usually cervical goitre, which extends substernally and brings its blood supply from the neck; more rarely primary intrathoracic goitre, which has its own blood supply (helpful to plan surgery).

Management

As always, the treatment is of the problem diagnosed.
- Laser therapy or stenting can be used for postintubation stenosis.
- If the problem is at the level of the vocal cords, then tracheostomy can be helpful if the problem itself cannot be treated.
- If there is tracheal stenosis that cannot be treated, then the use of a helium–oxygen mixture (which has a low resistance to flow) may provide palliation.

1.15 Difficult decisions

Case history

A 73-year-old man with COPD is admitted with an acute hypercapnic exacerbation. He has previously been confined to his home because of exertional dyspnoea despite the use of domiciliary oxygen and nebulized bronchodilators. He fails to improve with conventional therapy and non-invasive ventilation. Should he be treated with endotracheal ventilation?

Clinical approach

This is an example of a classical difficulty in clinical medicine in which you are deciding whether to offer a potentially life-saving therapy. However, there is no guarantee of success, and the process may be unpleasant for the patient. Moreover, even if the therapy is successful and the patient survives this episode, he is likely to be left with even greater respiratory disability than he had prior to this illness, and there is no doubt that—whatever is done —his medium- to long-term outlook is very poor indeed.

 'Prioritizing autonomy'—this means enabling the patient to decide what treatment he or she wants; the doctor's duty being to outline available effective treatments.

In formulating the decision one has to address the following.
• Is the patient able to make an informed decision about endotracheal ventilation?
• What history can be obtained from relatives or carers?
• What are the chances of success?

Informed decisions

The best management plan would be to explain the options to the patient and allow the patient to make an informed decision. In practice, patients with acute hypercapnic respiratory failure frequently have an altered conscious level, and even if they do not, they are often unable to take part in a valid discussion about endotracheal ventilation. A useful way round this problem is to discuss the option while the patient is well (i.e. in the outpatient clinic), and this is particularly worthwhile for those who have already survived intensive care unit (ICU) admission. Have such discussions been had with this patient? Is there any record of the patient in the medical notes? Has the patient written a 'living will'?

Obtaining a history

For an adult patient the next of kin cannot give or withhold consent to treatment and, as the patient is likely to die without endotracheal ventilation (and may well do so even with it), it is unfair to place perception of this responsibility with the next of kin (see *General clinical issues*, Section 2). However, it is very helpful to spend time talking to someone (preferably the next of kin) who knows the patient: when the patient was well, he may have expressed an opinion about the future in general or 'life-support machines' in particular.

The next of kin should also be able to say whether the patient was satisfied with their pre-illness quality of life, and about exercise tolerance and symptom load.

Chances of success

Non-respiratory specialists often give a pessimistic prognosis for patients with hypercapnic exacerbation of COPD that is not justified by the data: the median survival for hypercapnic patients who subsequently become normocapnic being 2.9 years. Factors giving a worse prognosis are acidaemia, uraemia and severe co-morbidity. If the clinician feels that the chances of a successful outcome with a particular therapy are negligible, they should not offer therapy—this is the argument of futility.

History of the presenting problem

The purpose of this aspect of the history is to see whether there is a precipitating cause (e.g. pneumothorax or lobar pneumonia) that would account for the development of respiratory failure. If there is a remediable cause then the case for endotracheal ventilation is greatly strengthened.

Relevant past history

You need to determine whether:
• there is any serious comorbidity that will affect outcome (e.g. chronic renal failure)
• the patient had much, if any, respiratory reserve prior to this illness, as judged by exercise performance
• the patient had previously had treatment optimized by a specialist in respiratory medicine (likely in this case because of home oxygen and nebulizers).

Examination

You will have already examined the patient prior to forming the decision to offer conventional therapy and non-invasive ventilation. It is appropriate to examine the patient again to make sure that nothing 'surprising' has happened, e.g. development of pneumothorax, but examination at this stage is unlikely to contribute to the decision regarding endotracheal ventilation, except to assess the response to treatment (or confirm the lack of it).

Approach to investigations and management

Investigations

Investigations are unlikely to contribute, having established on clinical grounds that the patient is failing to make progress with conventional therapy and non-invasive support. The exception is where the patient has deteriorated after an initial improvement: it is then important to exclude a treatable cause, e.g. pneumothorax.

Management

A suggested algorithm is shown in Fig. 21. In general, factors favouring the use of endotracheal ventilation are:
• an identifiable remediable cause (e.g. drug overdose, lobar pneumonia, postsurgery)
• no previous ICU admissions

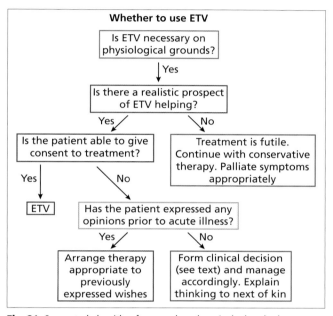

Fig. 21 Suggested algorithm for use when there is doubt whether endotracheal ventilation (ETV) should be offered.

• an acceptable domestic quality of life
• no previous advice from a respiratory specialist.
Factors likely to discourage endotracheal ventilation are:
• a poor domestic quality of life despite maximal medical therapy
• severe comorbidity.

Intubation

If the patient comes to intubation then recent data suggest that the outcome can be improved by an early transition [1], in the ICU environment, to non-invasive ventilation. If the patient stabilizes but fails to improve then, very occasionally, they may request withdrawal of ventilatory support. Because mechanical ventilation is a medical therapy, a competent patient may do this; however, this situation presents difficult personal and ethical issues and it is prudent to obtain the input of colleagues from other disciplines including psychiatry.

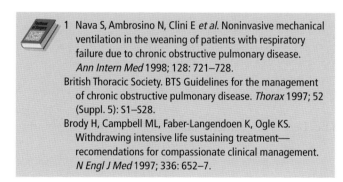

1 Nava S, Ambrosino N, Clini E *et al*. Noninvasive mechanical ventilation in the weaning of patients with respiratory failure due to chronic obstructive pulmonary disease. *Ann Intern Med* 1998; 128: 721–728.
British Thoracic Society. BTS Guidelines for the management of chronic obstructive pulmonary disease. *Thorax* 1997; 52 (Suppl. 5): S1–S28.
Brody H, Campbell ML, Faber-Langendoen K, Ogle KS. Withdrawing intensive life sustaining treatment— recomendations for compassionate clinical management. *N Engl J Med* 1997; 336: 652–7.

2 Diseases and treatments

2.1 Upper airway

2.1.1 OBSTRUCTIVE SLEEP APNOEA

Aetiology

OSA results from pharyngeal collapse during sleep, with a consequent abolition or reduction of inspiratory airflow. This process is associated with arousals from sleep and, in turn, daytime sleepiness [1].

The major predisposing factor is obesity but, independent of this, the syndrome is more common in men, perhaps because of gender differences in fat deposition. Other predisposing/exacerbating factors include:
- craniofacial abnormalities
- alcohol and sedative use
- hypothyroidism
- acromegaly
- nasal congestion.

Epidemiology

One to five per cent of adult men have the sleep apnoea syndrome, but the prevalence of OSA is a function of the prevalence of obesity. However, it should be emphasized that not all patients with OSA are sleepy and that some sleepy patients do not have OSA [2].

Clinical presentation

Common

- Snoring
- Excessive daytime somnolence
- Restless or unrefreshing sleep
- Report of witnessed apnoeas from bed partner.

Uncommon

- Nocturnal choking sensation
- Nocturia
- Reduced libido
- Morning headache.

Rare

- Insomnia
- Nocturnal cough
- Gastro-oesophageal reflux
- Polycythaemia.

 Not all patients who are sleepy have OSA. Do not forget to ask questions pertinent to other causes of hypersomnolence and check that the sleep opportunity is adequate.

Physical signs

The patient should have a full respiratory and cardiovascular examination with particular emphasis on:
- general appearance—features of hypothyroidism or acromegaly?
- the upper airway—can the patient breathe through the nose? Is there tonsillar enlargement? Is there retrognathia?
- collar size—when adjusted for height, neck circumference is predictive of OSA (for example a 17-inch collar size in a man 1.78 m tall would give a positive predictive value of >66% of OSA [3])
- evidence of hypertension or cardiac failure
- evidence of coexistent lung disease.

Investigations

Confirming the diagnosis

Some form of overnight study is required. The gold standard test is full polysomnography. The advantage of this test is that it confirms electroencephalographically that the patient is asleep and also identifies other diagnoses (e.g. narcolepsy–cataplexy or periodic limb movement) that might contribute to daytime somnolence.

However, polysomnography is expensive and many patients can be diagnosed using a limited respiratory sleep study or simple oximetry (Fig. 22). It is important to understand the limitations of the diagnostic study employed if the patient subsequently fails to respond to therapy.

Staging the disease

ECG, chest radiograph, FBC—where appropriate consider arterial blood gases, echocardiography, thyroid function tests.

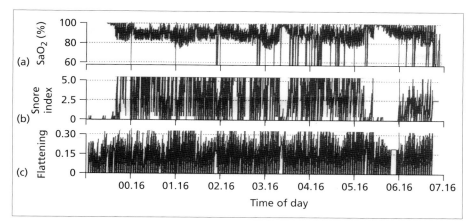

Fig. 22 Traces from a respiratory sleep study in a patient with sleep apnoea. The oximetry trace (a) shows frequent desaturation associated with snoring (b) and obstructive apnoeas (c). The apnoea–hypopnoea index was calculated to be 76/h.

Differential diagnosis

Excessive daytime somnolence

- Inadequate sleep opportunity
- Narcolepsy
- Periodic limb movement
- Idiopathic hypersomnolence.

Disturbed sleep

Chronic respiratory failure due to lung, neuromuscular or other disease.

Treatment

 The first principle of treating any sleep disorder is to establish good sleep habits (known as 'sleep hygiene').

General

- The patient's sleep habits ('hygiene') should be reviewed. The patient should have an adequate sleep opportunity and an appropriate sleeping environment; use of a patient information leaflet may be helpful.
- Where appropriate weight loss should be encouraged.
- The need for treatment is determined by symptoms (usually excessive daytime somnolence) or end-organ complication (e.g. polycythaemia).
- Patients in the UK should advise the DVLA and their motor insurer of their diagnosis.

Dental devices

These devices vary in design but are usually custom made for each patient (Fig. 23). Although they are substantially less effective in edentuluous patients this is not an absolute contraindication. They work by holding the tongue and mandible forward, enlarging the retroglossal space.

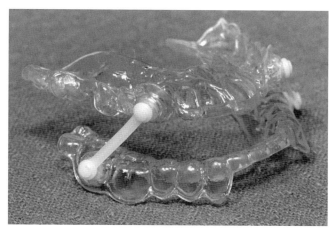

Fig. 23 Example of a mandibular advancement device.

Nasal continuous positive airways pressure

This therapy involves the application of positive pressure via a tightly fitting nasal mask which acts as a pneumatic splint to hold the airway open. This therapy has been shown in randomized trials to reduce daytime somnollence [1].

It is usual to perform a titration study to determine the optimal nasal CPAP level and, in many centres, a further study to confirm efficacy of treatment. Compliance with therapy is a function of support offered to patients [4]: it is therefore the view of the College that nasal CPAP services are centralized in specialist centres. Bilevel ventilatory support is sometimes used for OSA patients who require a high level of nasal CPAP.

Surgery

- Surgery to alleviate nasal obstruction may reduce nasal symptoms but is of limited value for OSA.
- Uvulopalatoplasty (UVPP) is sometimes recommended, but current opinion is that subsequent therapy with nasal CPAP is made more difficult by prior UVPP.
- Tracheotomy is the final option for patients with life-threatening OSA who are intolerant of nasal CPAP and other measures.

Complications

Common

- Road traffic accidents; patients with an apnoea/hypopnoea index >10/h have an odds ratio >6 for motor vehicle accidents [5]
- Hypertension [6]
- Snoring (with possible social/marital problems)
- Sexual dysfunction
- Polycythaemia
- Occasional nasal bridge ulceration from mask.

Prognosis

No controlled data on morbidity exist, but in one study 3.3% of 1211 patients with OSA died during a median follow-up of 22 months [4]. Twenty per cent of patients started on CPAP do not continue with treatment.

Prevention

Reducing the weight of the general population would reduce the incidence of OSA.

1 Bennett LS. Adult obstructive sleep apnoea syndrome. *J R Coll Physicians Lond* 1999; 33: 439–444.
2 Davies RJO, Stradling JR. The epidemiology of sleep apnoea. *Thorax* 1996; 51 (Suppl. 2): S65–S70.
3 Davies RJO, Ali NJ, Stradling JR. Neck circumference and other clinical features in the diagnosis of obstructive sleep apnoea syndrome. *Thorax* 1992; 47: 101–105.
4 McArdle N, Devereux G, Heidarnejad H, Engleman HM, Mackay TW, Douglas NJ. Long-term use of CPAP therapy for sleep apnea/hypopnea syndrome. *Am J Respir Crit Care Med* 1999; 159: 1108–1114.
5 Teran-Santos J, Jiminez-Gomez A, Cordero-Guevara J and the cooperative group Burgos-Santander. The association between sleep apnea and the risk of traffic accidents. *N Engl J Med* 1999; 340: 847–851.
6 Nieto FJ, Young TB, Lind BK *et al.* Association of sleep-disordered breathing, sleep apnea, and hypertension in a large community-based study. Sleep Heart Health Study. *JAMA* 2000; 283: 1829–1836.

2.2 Atopy and asthma

2.2.1 ALLERGIC RHINITIS

Aetiology

Allergic rhinitis can be seasonal (hayfever) or perennial, with around 10% of the population suffering from symptoms. Hayfever is found in up to 20% of young people over the summer months and is often caused by tree and grass pollen and mould spores [1]. Perennial causes include the faeces of the house-dust mite, domestic pets or occupational exposure to dust, fumes and aerosols [2]. It is therefore important to take an occupational history.

Clinical presentation

Patients present with sneezing, itching, watery rhinorrhoea and nasal obstruction.

Physical signs

Look for nasal polyps that can both cause and exacerbate rhinitis.

Investigations

The majority of patients are treated with success empirically; for patients refractory to therapy consider the differential diagnosis (below) and consider occupational history, skin-prick testing, full blood count and eosinophil count.

Differential diagnosis

Other non-allergic causes of rhinitis include infection, nasal polyps, foreign bodies or anatomical variants, nasal tumours, granulomatous diseases, vasomotor (secondary to 'over-the-counter' medication), idiopathic.

Treatment

- Allergen avoidance—not always possible.
- Topical (nasal) steroids—often very effective. Side effects are local irritation and nose bleeds. Check for compliance and technique if there is a failure to improve.
- Oral antihistamines—warn about sedative side effects of some preparations and interactions with other drugs, i.e. terfenadine with erythromycin results in prolonged QT interval.
- Cromoglycates—no major side effects, but require frequent use. Eye drops are particularly effective in allergic conjuctivitis.
- Immunotherapy—desensitization is sometimes possible in selected patients. The technique must be performed in specialist centres.

1 Furham SR. Summer hay fever. In: Durham SR, ed. *ABC of Allergies.* London: BMJ Books, 1998: 16–18.
2 Mackay IS, Durham SR. Perennial rhinitis. In Durham SR, ed. *ABC of Allergies.* London: BMJ Books, 1998: 19–22.

2.2.2 ASTHMA

Aetiology

Asthma is defined as reversible airway obstruction associated with airway inflammation and bronchial hyperresponsiveness [1]. The hyperresponsiveness of the airways is caused by a variety of local stimuli including histamine, leukotrienes and prostaglandins. This produces the reversible airflow obstruction that leads to the characteristic symptoms of shortness of breath, chest tightness and wheeze. Risk factors include:

- a genetic predisposition
- a family or personal history of atopy
- maternal smoking, ethnicity
- socioeconomic status
- male sex.

The role of other factors such as diet and pollution (black smoke, fine particulate matter, ozone and sulphates) remains controversial. While not directly linked to an increased prevalence of the disease, they certainly exacerbate asthmatic symptoms, with increased asthma mortality in areas of high industrial pollution. Other precipitants of asthma attacks include house-dust mites, pollens, moulds, fungi, cat and dog dander, aspirin and non-steroidal anti-inflammatory drugs (NSAIDs) in sensitive patients (approximately 5%), and occupational exposure [2].

Epidemiology

The prevalence of asthma continues to rise worldwide, particularly in developed countries. Approximately 10% of the adult population in the UK have asthma and, despite effective medication, there are still approximately 1600 deaths from the disease each year (these figures do not include COPD).

This continued morbidity and mortality highlights the importance of education of both patients and their doctors, with an emphasis on adequate treatment regimens, good compliance, even with maintenance regimens, and rapid access to medical help when deterioration occurs.

Patients are at particular risk of dying from asthma if they:
- are taking more than three classes of drugs
- have required hospital admission in the last year
- have psychosocial problems (compliance?)
- have ever had life-threatening asthma.

Clinical presentations

- Severe acute attacks—acute breathlessness and wheeze; hypoxia and/or carbon dioxide retention can lead to stupor and/or confusion

- Chronic asthma—shortness of breath, wheeze, chronic cough, particularly at night when associated with disturbed sleep pattern. Symptoms may be produced by exposure to cold air or exercise.

An isolated dry cough is perhaps the most overlooked symptom of mild asthma (especially in children). Particularly after colds and 'flu, patients may be left with an annoying dry cough and are frequently referred to specialists for further investigation. Bronchial hyperresponsiveness is often the cause and responds to a course of low-dose inhaled steroids. It is difficult to label such individuals as truly asthmatic (a controversial issue amongst respiratory physicians), although subsequent lung function tests may be helpful. However, patients should be warned that their symptoms may return with a subsequent cold or chest infection.

Physical signs

Life-threatening asthma

- Peak flow <33% of predicted or personal best
- Silent chest
- Cyanosis
- Altered level of consciousness; confusion; coma
- Exhaustion; inability to speak
- Hypotension or bradycardia.

Severe acute attack

- Peak flow <50% of predicted or personal best
- Tachycardia
- Increased respiratory rate: >25 breaths/min
- Cannot complete sentences in one breath
- Use of accessory muscles of respiration, intercostal recession (especially children)
- Increased pulse rate: >110 beats/min.

Moderate

- Peak flow 50–70% of predicted or personal best
- Wheeze
- Dyspnoea
- Chest tightness.

The British Guidelines on Asthma Management [3] are invaluable, but remember, the patient in front of you is an individual. If you are worried in any way about someone with asthma, especially at night—admit him or her. This is particularly so for those who have an attack that has been going on for some time, if they live alone, do not have a telephone or would find it difficult to return to the hospital. Do not feel pressurized by the patient, nursing staff or the hospital's bed state to send them home.

Investigations

Measure arterial blood gases if patient presents with life-threatening signs, or Sao_2 <94%.
Blood gas markers for life-threatening asthma are:
- Normal or high $Paco_2$ (≥5–6 kPa/36–45 mmHg)
- Low pH
- Severe hypoxia in spite of oxygen treatment (Pao_2 <8 kPa/60 mmHg).

Chest radiograph

In outpatients, a chest radiograph helps exclude other causes of wheeze, such as infiltrates resulting from eosinophilia or fibrosis. For patients presenting acutely a pneumothorax should be excluded and evidence of infection looked for.

Peak flow

This can be used diagnostically to look for morning dips. Motivated chronic asthmatics can also monitor their progress at home. In patients who clearly do not take measurements on a daily basis, make sure they know their best peak flow and encourage them to at least monitor when they get coughs and cold.

All patients should be given a management plan based on deterioration of their peak flow: credit-card-sized self-management plans are produced by the National Asthma Campaign (Fig. 24).

Lung function tests

These should be performed pre- and postbronchodilator (e.g. salbutamol). They are not helpful acutely, but important as a diagnostic tool to look for evidence of reversibility and to monitor chronic asthmatics.

Allergy testing

Skin-prick tests can help identify allergens that may precipitate asthma attacks, although in practice many of these are not easily avoided.

Differential diagnosis

This includes COPD, congestive heart failure, upper airway obstruction, i.e. foreign body, tumour; pneumothorax, bronchiectasis, pulmonary eosinophilia, Wegener's granulomatosis, Churg–Strauss syndrome.

Treatment

The stepwise approach to the treatment of chronic asthma

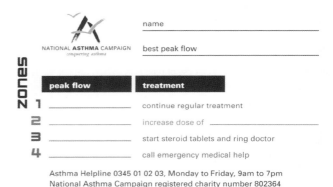

(a)

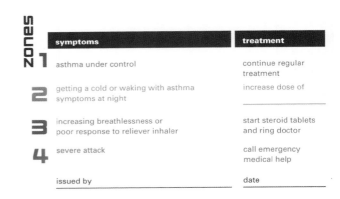

(b)

Fig. 24 Credit-card-sized self-management plan produced by the National Asthma Campaign: (a) front; (b) back. These cards are available free on request from their offices. (With permission of the National Asthma Campaign.)

remains the gold standard (Table 13). For all steps above step 1, inhaled steroids are advocated for controlling airway inflammation and therefore chronic asthma.

The management can be divided into:
- 'relievers' (short-acting β agonists)
- 'preventers' (inhaled steroids)
- 'controllers' (long-acting β agonists and leukotriene receptor antagonists).

It is important to explain to patients that the preventers and controllers must be taken regularly, while the relievers are helpful for acute symptomatic relief. Oral preparations include oral steroids, aminophylline, and the leukotriene receptor antagonists.

In acute severe asthma (Table 14), the patient should not be left sitting in a side room in accident and emergency (A&E). He or she should be in the resuscitation room and monitored for cardiac rhythm and oxygen saturation. The most senior member of the medical team in the hospital (usually the Medical Registrar) should be informed of the patient's condition and urgent anaesthetic and intensive care review should be requested if the patient does not improve rapidly or if the presenting symptoms appear life threatening. Anaesthetists would rather be called to a sick patient than one who has suffered a respiratory arrest.

Table 13 British asthma guidelines for the stepwise management of chronic asthma in adults and school children. (From *Thorax* 1997; 52 (Suppl. 1) S11, Chart 1. With permission of the BMJ Publishing Group.)

Step	Management	Discussion
Step 1	Occasional use of relief bronchodilators	Inhaled short-acting β agonists 'as required' for symptom relief are acceptable. If they are needed more than once daily move to Step 2. Before altering a treatment step ensure that the patient is having the treatment and has a good inhaler technique. Address any fears
Step 2	Regular inhaled anti-inflammatory agents	Inhaled short-acting β agonists as required, plus beclometasone or budesonide increased to 100–400 μg twice daily or fluticasone 50–200 μg twice daily. Alternatively, use cromoglycate or nedocromil sodium, but if control is not achieved start inhaled steroids
Step 3	High-dose inhaled steroids or low-dose inhaled steroids plus long-acting inhaled β agonists bronchodilator	Inhaled short-acting β agonists as required, plus either beclometasone or budesonide increased to 800–2000 μg daily or fluticasone 400–1000 μg daily via a large volume spacer; or beclometasone or budesonide increased to 100–400 μg twice daily or fluticasone 50–200 μg twice daily plus salmeterol 50 μg twice daily. In the very small number of patients who experience side effects with high-dose inhaled steroids, either the long-acting inhaled β-agonist option is used, or a sustained release theophylline may be added to Step 2 medication. Cromoglycate or nedocromil may also be tried
Step 4	High-dose inhaled steroid and regular bronchodilators	Inhaled short-acting β agonists as required with inhaled beclometasone or budesonide increased to 800–2000 μg daily or fluticasone 400–1000 μg daily via a large-volume spacer; plus a sequential therapeutic trial of one or more of: • Inhaled long-acting β agonists • Sustained release theophylline • Inhaled ipratropium or oxitropium • Long-acting β-agonist tablets • High-dose inhaled bronchodilators • Cromoglycate or nedocromil
Step 5	Addition of regular steroid tablets	Inhaled short-acting β agonists as required with inhaled beclometasone or budesonide increased to 800–2000 μg daily or fluticasone 400–1000 μg daily via a large-volume spacer and one or more of the long-acting bronchodilators; plus regular prednisolone tablets in a single daily dose
Stepping down		Review treatment every 3–6 months. If control is achieved a stepwise reduction in treatment may be possible. In patients whose treatment was recently started at Step 4 or 5 or included steroid tablets for gaining control of asthma this reduction may take place after a short interval. In other patients with chronic asthma a 3–6-month period of stability should be shown before slow stepwise reduction is undertaken

Newer treatments for asthma

The leukotriene receptor antagonists are the most recent drugs to be added to the therapeutic armamentarium for asthma [4]. They include montelukast and zafirlukast and work by reducing the production of leukotrienes which cause bronchoconstriction, mucus hypersecretion and airway oedema. They may have an anti-inflammatory action (↓ eosinophils). Side effects include abdominal discomfort, diarrhoea and headaches. Their position in the stepwise treatment of asthma has yet to be decided; they may be useful in chronic asthmatics not controlled on inhaled steroids (step 3), as well as exercise-induced and aspirin-sensitive asthma. They have no place in the treatment of acute severe asthma.

1 Rees J, Kanabar D, eds. *ABC of Asthma* (4th edn). London: BMJ Publications, 2000.
2 Jarad NA. Occupational asthma. *J R Coll Physicians Lond* 1999; 33: 537–540.
3 The British Thoracic Society, the National Asthma Campaign, the Royal College of Physicians of London, in association with the General Practitioner in Asthma Group, the British Association of Accident and Emergency Medicine, the British Paediatric Society and the Royal College of Paediatrics and Child Health. The British guidelines on asthma management 1995 review and position statement. *Thorax* 1997; 52: Supplement 1.
4 Lipworth BJ. Leukotriene-receptor antagonists. *Lancet* 1999; 353: 57–62.

Stage	Guidelines
1. Immediate treatment	Oxygen 40–60% (CO_2 retention is not usually aggravated by oxygen therapy in asthma) Salbutamol 5 mg or terbutaline 10 mg via an oxygen-driven nebulizer Prednisolone tablets 30–60 mg or intravenous hydrocortisone 200 mg or both if very ill No sedatives of any kind Chest radiograph to exclude pneumothorax
	If life-threatening features are present Add ipratropium 0.5 mg to the nebulized β agonist Give intravenous aminophylline 250 mg over 20 min or salbutamol or terbutaline 250 μg over 10 min. Do not give bolus aminophylline to patients already taking oral theophyllines
2. Subsequent management	*If patient is improving continue* 40–60% oxygen Prednisolone 30–60 mg daily or intravenous hydrocortisone 200 mg 6 hourly Nebulized β agonist 4 hourly
	If patient is not improving after 15–30 min Continue oxygen and steroids Give nebulized β agonist more frequently, up to every 15–30 min Add ipratropium 0.5 mg to nebulizer and repeat 6 hourly until patient is improving
	If patient is still not improving give Aminophylline infusion (small patient 750 mg/24 h, large patient 1500 mg/24 h); monitor blood concentrations if it is continued for over 24 h Salbutamol or terbutaline infusion as an alternative to aminophylline

3. Monitoring treatment	Repeat measurement of PEF 15–30 min after starting treatment
	Oximetry: maintain SaO_2 >92%
	Repeat blood gas measurements within 2 h of starting treatment if:
	    Initial PaO_2 <8 kPa (60 mmHg) unless subsequent SaO_2 >92%, or
	    $PaCO_2$ normal or raised, or
	    Patient deteriorates
	Chart PEF before and after giving nebulized or inhaled β agonist and at least four times daily throughout hospital stay

4. When discharged from hospital, patients should have	Been on discharge medication for 24 h and have had inhaler technique checked and recorded PEF >75% of predicted or best and PEF diurnal variability <25% unless discharge is agreed with respiratory physician Treatment with oral and inhaled steroids in addition to bronchodilators Own PEF meter and written self management plan GP follow-up arranged within 1 week Follow-up appointment in respiratory clinic within 4 weeks

Table 14 British Thoracic Society guidelines for the management of acute severe asthma in adults. (From *Thorax* 1997; 52 (Suppl. 1): S12, Chart 2. With permission of the BMJ Publishing Group.)

PEF, peak expiratory flow.

2.3 Chronic obstructive pulmonary disease

Aetiology

The major aetiologic factor is tobacco consumption. Also consider α_1-antitrypsin deficiency (exacerbated by smoking). Smokers vary in their susceptibility to COPD; only 15% developing clinically relevant disease [1]. Coal miners have increased risk.

Pathophysiology

The hallmark of COPD is expiratory flow limitation; this results in a reduced FEV_1 and other characteristic lung function abnormalities (see below). However, the disease is slowly progressive and the picture therefore depends on the severity of the disease at the time of assessment [2].

Epidemiology

Prevalence is approximately 6% in men and 3% in women, being determined by smoking rates.

Clinical presentation

Because the severity of COPD necessarily passes from mild to severe, patients who present with severe disease are those that have not been identified at an earlier stage.
- Common—recurrent respiratory infections, morning cough, exertional dyspnoea
- Uncommon—picked up because of sleep disordered breathing or need for other medical intervention (e.g. elective surgery); these patients may have tolerated the common symptoms above
- Rare—cor pulmonale, ventilatory failure.

Physical signs

May be none in early disease.
- Common—hyperinflation, wheeze, coarse crackles
- Uncommon (unless disease advanced)—cyanosis, weight loss, cor pulmonale (oedema and raised JVP). Hoover's sign refers to the paradoxical inward movement of the lower lateral rib cage during inspiration.

Investigations

Spirometric tests

Depending on severity there will be a reduction in FEV_1 that is disproportionate to the fall in VC, leading to a FEV_1/VC ratio of <70%. A normal FEV_1 effectively excludes COPD but a normal peak flow can occur in mild disease. Residual volume (RV), functional residual capacity (FRC) and total lung capacity (TLC) are elevated in COPD but these measurements are not routinely made in primary care; similarly the flow–volume loop shows characteristic scalloping of the expiratory limb (Fig. 25 and see Section 3.6.2).

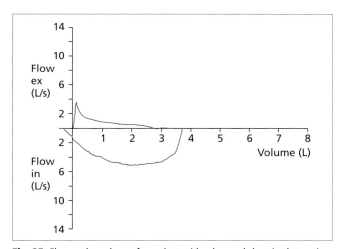

Fig. 25 Flow–volume loop of a patient with advanced chronic obstructive pulmonary disease (COPD). In this case expiratory flow limitation is severe, and marked scalloping of the curve is observed virtually throughout expiration.

Dynamic hyperinflation as a mechanism of dyspnoea in COPD

As COPD patients are flow limited during expiration, end-expiratory lung volume (EELV) has to increase when the demand placed on the respiratory system is increased (as during exercise). For a patient with severe COPD the increase in EELV could be as much as a litre.

Bronchodilator challenge

Perform this when the patient is stable. Look for improvement in FEV_1, a positive result requiring >10% and >200 mL increase. Patients can experience symptomatic relief despite a 'negative' study; if benefit needs to be documented it can be helpful to measure exercise capacity (for example by the shuttle walk test [3]).

Steroid challenge

Indicated in disease of more than moderate severity. Give prednisolone 30 mg once a day for 2 weeks; a positive result must be >10% and >200 mL increase in FEV_1.

Steroids have multiple side effects. Think which of these you are going to warn the patient about. If you are anxious that a patient is going to be susceptible to a particular side effect you may wish to give high-dose inhaled steroids instead (e.g. beclamethasone 1000 μg twice a day for 6 weeks via a spacer).

Chest radiograph

This can exclude alternative pathology. Look for bullae in advanced disease and hyperinflation (low flat diaphragms, increased number of ribs visible). An example is shown in Fig. 26.

Arterial blood gases

If SaO_2 is 92% or less, patients may benefit from domiciliary oxygen and should have their arterial/earlobe gas measured on room air. Guidelines for the administration of domiciliary oxygen are found in Section 2.12.1, p. 231.

Differential diagnosis

Because the symptoms of COPD are relatively non-specific, virtually any cardiac or pulmonary condition could feature in the differential. From a practical point of view it is important to ensure that other causes of airflow limitation, especially asthma, are not overlooked.

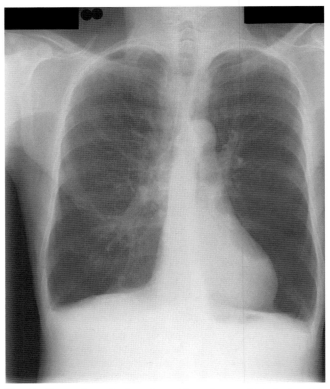

Fig. 26 Chest radiograph of a patient with emphysema. Note the low, flat diaphragms and hyperinflation. Few lung markings are seen at the bases indicating the possibility of bulbous disease.

Treatment

Emergency

See *Emergency medicine*, Section 1.10.

Stable patients

All patients with COPD should stop smoking; this is the single most important determinant of outcome. Nicotine replacement used in conjunction with a smoking cessation clinic can increase quit rates. 'Flu vaccination is recommended.

Tell patients to stop smoking when you see them for other reasons. Doctors' advice is a potent stimulus to quit.

Treatment options for COPD are stratified by stage as shown in Table 15. On-going studies examining the role of inhaled steroids in COPD may influence management in the future [4].

In patients with very advanced disease, specialist assessment is indicated if preliminary investigations suggest that lung volume reduction surgery (LVRS), transplantation or non-invasive ventilatory support is indicated.

• LVRS is a new therapy that is most effective in patients with heterogeneous lung disease predominantly involving the upper lobes. It is currently offered only at a few centres in the UK.

• Non-invasive ventilatory support is indicated (see Section 2.12.3, p. 234) in patients with daytime hypercapnia and symptoms attributable to this, particularly if they have recurrent admissions.

• Lung transplantation (see Section 2.13, p. 236) is an option for some patients.

Complications

• Common—infection (bacterial and viral), steroid side effects

• Uncommon—cor pulmonale, pneumothorax, ventilatory failure, polycythaemia, heart failure

• Rare—pulmonary hypertension, peripheral neuropathy.

Prognosis

In general is inversely related to age and postbronchodilator FEV_1 such that:

• age <60 and FEV_1 >50% predicted → 90% 3-year survival

• age >60 and FEV_1 >50% predicted → 80% 3-year survival

• age >60 and FEV_1 <50% predicted → 75% 3-year survival.

Table 15 The spectrum of chronic obstructive pulmonary disease (COPD).

Symptoms	FEV_1 (representative) (% predicted)	Management options (to consider)
Healthy	100%	Stop smoking
Smoker's cough	75%	Antibiotics for infection, inhaled bronchodilators
Exertional dyspnoea Some signs, sputum	50%	Combination BDs Steroid reversibility 'Flu vaccination Pulmonary rehabilitation
Dyspnoea on minimal exertion or rest Wheeze, cyanosis Hyperinflation	25%	Nebulized BDs Assess for domiciliary O_2 Assess for lung volume reduction surgery

BDs, bronchodilators.

The 5-year survival in patients admitted with a hypercapnic exacerbation is 28% [5].

1 British Thoracic Society. BTS Guidelines for the management of chronic obstructive pulmonary disease. *Thorax* 1997; 52: S1–S28.

2 Burrows B, Earle RH. Course and prognosis of chronic obstructive lung disease. A prospective study of 200 patients. *N Engl J Med* 1969; 280: 397–404.

3 Singh SJ, Morgan MDL, Scott S, Walters D, Hardman AE. Development of a shuttle walking test of disability in patients with chronic airways obstruction. *Thorax* 1992; 47: 1019–1024.

4 Burge, PS. EUROSCOP, ISOLDE and the Copenhagen City Lung Study. *Thorax* 1999; 54: 287–288.

5 Warren PM, Flenley DC, Millar JS, Avery A. Respiratory failure revisited: acute excerbations of chronic bronchitis between 1961 and 68 and 1970–76. *Lancet* 1980; i: 467–471.

2.4 Bronchiectasis

Aetiology

Bronchiectasis is the term used to describe abnormal irreversible dilatation of the bronchi because of the destruction of the muscular and elastic components of their wall. It was first described by Laennec in 1819 and is the end result of various pathologic processes [1–3], as listed in Table 16.

Pathology

The primary problem in bronchiectasis is subnormal respiratory defences against infections. This may be caused by:
- immunoglobulin deficiency
- impaired mucociliary clearance
- bronchial obstruction.

As a result the airway contains excess mucus and this results in bronchial infection, with recruitment of neutrophils and monocytes into the lungs. Proteolytic enzymes such as elastase and cytokines are released into the lung and result in the destruction of the elastic and muscular components of the bronchial wall. Recurrent episodes of this type finally result in bronchiectasis.

Clinical presentation

Symptoms

- Patients mildly affected may present with symptoms (Table 17) only during exacerbation.
- Severely affected patients may have some or all the symptoms continuously and may develop cor pulmonale.

Signs

See Table 18.

Table 16 Conditions associated with bronchiectasis.

Classification	Examples
Postinfectious	Tuberculosis, measles, whooping cough, bronchiolitis in infancy caused by respiratory syncytial virus, bacterial pneumonia
Bronchial obstruction	Foreign body, adenoma, enlarged external lymph nodes, middle lobe syndrome
Allergic bronchopulmonary aspergillosis	—
Impaired host defence	Hypogammaglobulinaemia, Kartagener's, Young's syndrome, primary ciliary dyskinesia (syndrome characterized by bronchiectasis, situs inversus and recurrent sinusitis)
Cystic fibrosis	—
Rare conditions	Rheumatoid arthritis (3.1% of patients), Sjögren's syndrome, relapsing polychondritis, systemic lupus erythematosus, Marfan's syndrome, ulcerative colitis, Crohn's disease, sarcoidosis, yellow-nail syndrome (lymphoedema, yellow nails and pleural effusions), toxic gas inhalation (ammonia), gastric aspiration, tracheobronchomegaly (Mounier–Kuhn syndrome), congenital cartilage deficiency (Williams—Campbell syndrome), bronchopulmonary sequestration, α_1-antitrypsin deficiency

Table 17 Symptoms of bronchiectasis.

Common
Cough
Sputum production
   Mild: <10 mL/24 h
   Moderate: 10–150 mL/24 h
   Severe: >150 mL/24 h
Dyspnoea
Haemoptysis
Fever and pleuritic chest pain during infective exacerbation

Uncommon
Sinusitis in 30%
Halitosis

Rare
Discoloured nails in yellow-nail syndrome
Infertility in Young's syndrome
Male infertility (in cystic fibrosis)
Profuse recurrent haemoptysis without purulent sputum (bronchiectasis haemorrhagica sicca)
Other features of associated conditions

Table 18 Signs of bronchiectasis.

Common
Wheeze
Crackles
Nasal polyps or sinusitis
Clubbing in 10% of patients

Uncommon
Peripheral oedema in cor pulmonale
Cyanosis in hypoxaemia

Rare (i.e. syndrome specific)
Examples include rheumatoid hands, butterfly rash, Marfanoid features

Investigations

Investigations in bronchiectasis are carried out to diagnose its presence and extent, and also to find an underlying aetiology (Figs 27 and 28, Table 19).

Treatment

Options include the following:
• Postural drainage—this should be performed at least twice daily. It helps prevent chest infections by removing secretions.
• Antibiotics—helpful during infective exacerbation. They are best used by basing choice on previous sputum culture result.
• Bronchodilators—β₂ agonists, anticholinergics and theophyllines in cases with airway obstruction.
• Oxygen/non-invasive ventilation (NIV)—the guidelines used in practice are based on data obtained from patients with COPD (qv, see Sections 2.12.1 and 2.12.3). Patients with bronchiectasis can be difficult to ventilate successfully using NIV, although this should not preclude its use for palliative purposes or as a bridge to transplantation.

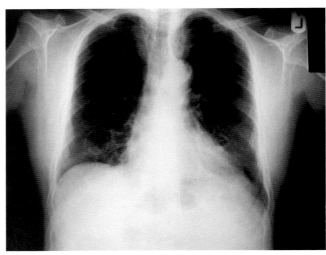

Fig. 27 Plain chest radiograph of a woman with bronchiectasis. Abnormalities are most prominent in the right lower zone.

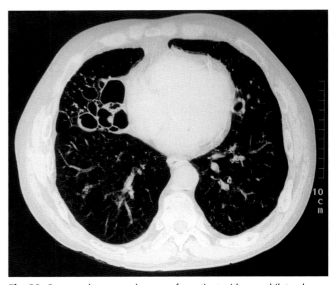

Fig. 28 Computed tomography scan of a patient with gross bilateral bronchiectasis. Many of the bronchi have a classic 'signet ring' appearance generated by an enlarged bronchus and a neighbouring vessel.

• Diuretics (with care) in the presence of cor pulmonale.
• Surgery—resection of a lobe in genuinely localized bronchiectasis or in life-threatening haemoptysis. Lung transplantation is an option (see Section 2.13, p. 236).

Specific treatments

• Regular immunoglobulin infusion in agammaglobulinaemia
• Prednisolone in allergic bronchopulmonary aspergillosis.

Complications

The complications of bronchiectasis are:
• recurrent pneumonia
• empyema and lung abscess
• pneumothorax

Table 19 Investigations in bronchiectasis.

Test type	Description	Possible finding
Generic	Chest radiograph	May be normal Tram lines, linear radioluciences (cylindrical bronchiectasis) Toothpaste lines: thick parallel markings (varicose bronchiectasis) Cysts (cystic bronchiectasis) May show features of rheumatoid arthritis, sarcoidosis, and pleural effusion in yellow-nail syndrome etc.
	High-resolution computed tomography scan	Is the investigation of choice. It is non-invasive and has a sensitivity of 84% and specificity of 82% in detecting bronchiectasis
	Lung function tests	Obstructive pattern without hyperinflation
	Arterial blood gases	In advanced disease may show hypoxia and/or hypercapnia
	Sputum cultures	May grow *Staphylococcus aureus*, *Pseudomonas aeruginosa* as well as more common respiratory pathogens
Specific (for certain diseases)	Serum immunoglobulins	May show IgG/IgG subclass/IgA deficiency
	Sweat sodium concentration	Increased in cystic fibrosis
	Eosinophils/IgE	Increased in ABPA
	ANCA/autoantibodies	If connective tissue disease is suspected
	ACE/calcium	If sarcoid is suspected

ABPA, allergic bronchopulmonary aspergillosis; ACE, angiotensin-converting enzyme; ANCA, antinuclear cytoplasmic antibodies.

- cor pulmonale
- massive haemoptysis
- brain abscess
- amyloidosis.

Prognosis

- Dismal prognosis in the preantibiotic era with patients dying from infections
- Death now mainly as a result of cor pulmonale.

Prevention

- Administration of vaccines against measles, pertussis, influenza, TB
- Prompt removal of foreign bodies and obstructing lesions
- Antibiotics in bronchopulmonary infections.

See *Rheumatology and clinical immunology*, Sections 1.1 and 2.1.1.
1 Cohen M, Sahn SA. Bronchiectasis in systemic diseases. *Chest* 1999; 116: 1063–1074.
2 Stockley RA. Bronchiectasis. *Medicine* 1999; 27 (10): 113–116.
3 Luce JM. Bronchiectasis. In: Murray, Nadel, eds. *Textbook of Respiratory Medicine* (2nd edn). W B Saunders, 1994: 1398–1417.

2.5 Cystic fibrosis

Aetiology

Cystic fibrosis (CF) is an autosomal recessive disease caused by a defect in the gene encoding an epithelial cell transmembrane protein termed the cystic fibrosis transmembrane conductance regulator (CFTR). The gene is located on the long arm of chromosome 7 and the most common mutation in the UK is ΔF508. The function of this protein is to serve as a chloride channel and also as a regulator of an epithelial sodium channel; however, the exact mechanism by which defects in CFTR-mediated ion transport cause the phenotype of cystic fibrosis (CF) is unknown [1].

The lungs of CF patients are thought not to be infected at birth, but endobronchial bacterial colonization occurs within the first months of life and usually progresses to colonization with *Pseudomonas aeruginosa*. Lung destruction follows with the development of an obstructive respiratory defect and eventually respiratory failure.

Table 20 Presentations of cystic fibrosis.

Classification	Example
Respiratory disease (40%)	Frequent infections; recurrent bronchitis/ bronchiolitis
Malabsorption (30%)	Failure to thrive, rectal prolapse, intussusception, fatty diarrhoea
Meconium ileus (20%)	
Rare	Infertility (men), cirrhosis or portal hypertension, nasal polyps, adult bronchiectasis

Epidemiology

Prevalence in Europeans is 1 in 2500; it is rare in Afro-Caribbeans (1 in 17 000) and very rare in Orientals (1 in 90 000).

Clinical presentation

Presentations of CF are shown in Table 20. The average age of newly diagnosed patients is 4.8 years, but may be up to 65 years. Diabetes occurs in 6% of adults.

 Consider CF as a potential diagnosis in adult patients with recurrent purulent chest infections.

Physical signs

These will depend on the presentation and stage of disease.

An adult patient with CF is likely to be clubbed with signs of hyperinflation. Crackles and/or wheeze may be audible. In advanced disease there may also be cyanosis or respiratory distress. The patient may appear undernourished (see below); hepatosplenomegaly may be present.

Investigations

The diagnosis of CF is based on one or more clinical features consistent with the CF phenotype (see above) plus one of:
- two CF gene mutations
- a positive sweat test
- abnormal nasal potential differences.

Gene mutations

In excess of 800 mutations are recognized: most UK laboratories only screen for 12 of these, covering an estimated 93% of the UK patients. Thus, it is possible for a patient to have CF without routine genotyping identifying a mutation. Conversely the finding of one mutation does not diagnose CF because the carrier frequency of the single gene is 1 in 25.

Sweat test

This should be performed at least twice.

Nasal potential differences

Although this can be useful for patients with a borderline sweat test, this test should not be considered diagnostic in isolation outside specialist centres.

 Investigations relevant to the management of an acutely unwell CF patient would depend on clinical presentation. In specialist CF centres all patients would undergo annual review. As well as symptomatic enquiry and a physical examination this would include, from a physician's perspective:
- chest radiograph (Fig. 29)
- full lung function tests
- full blood count (FBC), urea and electrolytes, calcium, liver function tests
- sputum microbiology
- ECG.

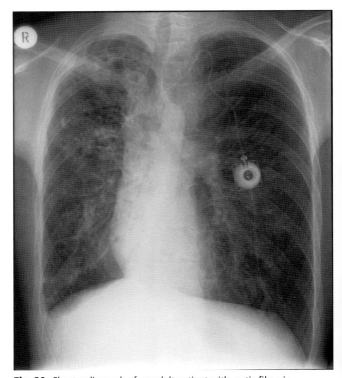

Fig. 29 Chest radiograph of an adult patient with cystic fibrosis. Hyperinflation and cystic change (most obvious in the right upper lobe) is evident. A Portacath is seen over the left lung field.

Differential diagnosis

This is the differential diagnosis of the presenting symptom.

Treatment

The best care of the CF patient requires multidisciplinary team working between a physician, nurse, social worker, physiotherapist, nutritionist, general practitioner and a genetic counsellor [2]. In CF centres all patients undergo annual review which allows assessment by this multidisciplinary team as well as the physician (see above).

Respiratory system

Respiratory symptoms should be managed aggressively with the aim being to defend pulmonary function.
• Standard therapy comprises antibiotics (both for acute infection and in colonized patients) and physiotherapy.
• Sputum clearance may be enhanced in some patients by the administration of nebulized recombinant deoxyribonuclease ('DNase').
• Bronchodilators and anti-inflammatory drugs are often helpful also.

Gastrointestinal disease

Ninety per cent of CF patients have pancreatic insufficiency and benefit from replacement of enzymes and fat-soluble vitamins. Professional dietetic assessment is indicated for all patients.

There is no specific therapy for CF liver disease, but supportive management is as for other causes of cirrhosis/portal hypertension.

Transplantation

In advanced disease lung transplantation (see Section 2.13, p. 235) offers the best chance of survival [3]. For patients awaiting a transplant, non-invasive positive pressure ventilation can be a useful bridge; endotracheal ventilation of patients with advanced CF is almost always unsuccessful.

Broadly speaking, patients may be considered suitable for transplantation if the FEV$_1$ is <30% predicted or, if rapidly declining, greater than this. Other features favouring transplantation are the development of ventilatory failure and increasing hospitalizations. Because cadaveric organs are in short supply there is increasing interest in living donor bilateral lobar lung transplantation.

 In advanced CF, respiratory failure as a result of overwhelming infection is a common cause of death. Endotracheal ventilation does not alter the outcome in this situation and hence this treatment is not usually offered.

Complications

Of pulmonary disease

The more severe complications occur in more advanced disease:
• sinusitis and nasal polyps
• bacterial respiratory infection
• pneumothorax
• haemoptysis
• aspergillosis
• respiratory failure and pulmonary hypertension.

Of gastrointestinal disease

CF adults may have abdominal pain, but the cause is seldom appendicitis or other surgically remediable problems. Although surgical advice should be sought where appropriate, most experts prefer to have a high threshold for abdominal surgery. Other complications include:
• Obstruction
• Malabsorption
• Glucose intolerance/diabetes
• Cirrhosis and portal hypertension.

Other/iatrogenic

The total list of possible complications of CF is enormous but includes:
• infertility in men
• pregnancy—represents a hazard if the FEV$_1$ is <40–50% predicted or if there is pulmonary hypertension
• ototoxicity from repeated aminoglycosides
• Portacath complications.

Prognosis

The median survival of newborns with CF is now estimated to be about 40 years; this compares with 14 years in 1969. The 5-year survival after transplantation is around 50%.

Prevention

For parents who are CF gene carriers (e.g. because a sibling with CF is already identified), prenatal diagnosis is possible. The risks of chorionic villous sampling are roughly equal to those of amniocentesis but with the advantage of giving an earlier result.

Therapy aimed at preventing the phenotypic expression of CF by gene replacement is not yet a practical clinical option [1–4].

See *Cell biology*, Section 1.
See *Gastroenterology*, Sections 1.10 and 2.4.
1 Stern M., Alton E. The pathogenesis of cystic fibrosis and progress towards gene therapy. *J R Coll Physicians Lond* 1999; 33: 434–439.
2 Varlotta L. Management and care of the newly diagnosed patient with cystic fibrosis. *Curr Opin Pulm Med* 1998; 4: 311–318.
3 Shapiro B, Veerarghaven S., Barbers RG. Lung transplantation for cystic fibrosis: an update and practical considerations for referring candidates. *Curr Opin Pulm Med* 1999; 5: 365–370.
4 Rosenstein BJ, Zeitlin PJ. Cystic fibrosis. *Lancet* 1998; 351: 277–282.

2.6 Occupational lung disease

2.6.1 ASBESTOSIS AND THE PNEUMOCONIOSES

 Prevention is better than cure.

Aetiology and pathology

The pneumoconioses are occupational lung diseases caused by inhalation of a variety of industrial dusts. Strictly speaking, asbestosis is a subtype of the pneumoconioses but, because of its relative prevalence, tends to be considered separately. Likewise, coal worker's pneumoconiosis (CWP) merits its own discussion [1–6].

CWP aside, the pneumoconioses can be divided into two subgroups (Table 21):
• benign forms—tend to be asymptomatic. Recognized by the chest radiograph appearances that they produce: small, round opacities caused by perivascular collections of dust
• fibrotic forms—produce, as the name suggests, pulmonary fibrosis associated with a restrictive lung defect. They may cause symptoms and sometimes progress to respiratory failure.

Table 21 Industrial substances whose dusts cause pneumoconiosis.

Disease type	Causative agent (disease name)
Benign disease	Iron (siderosis)
	Tin (stannosis)
	Barium (bariosis)
	Antimony
Fibrotic disease	Asbestos
	Silica (silicosis)
	Beryllium (berylliosis)
	Aluminium ores (Shaver's disease or aluminosis)

Asbestosis

The interstitial fibrosis produced by asbestos exposure is dose related, with length and level of exposure relating directly to the development and severity of symptoms. The fibrosis tends to be in the lower lobes and is frequently associated with pleural thickening and the appearance of pleural plaques on chest radiograph. Asbestos exposure can also lead to mesothelioma and lung cancer, particularly adenocarcinoma.

Coal worker's pneumoconiosis

CWP is seen in workers exposed to coal dust and accounts for 90% of claims for industrial compensation. The condition is generally divided into:
• simple CWP—based on the chest radiograph appearances of small, round opacities that represent small fibrous nodules in the lung, predominantly in the upper lobes
• complicated CWP (massive progressive fibrosis, MPF)—a patient is said to have advanced to MPF when these fibrous lesions have reached more that 3 cm in diameter. Histologically, these larger lesions commonly undergo necrosis and cavitation.

CWP associated with rheumatoid arthritis is known as Caplan's syndrome.

Clinical presentation

This may include:
• breathlessness
• cough
• jet black sputum production (CWP only).

Physical signs

Few in early disease; later:
• decreased chest expansion
• inspiratory crackles
• wheeze (CWP)
• clubbing (asbestosis, but not silicosis; rarely in CWP).

Investigations

Chest radiograph

The International Labour Office has produced a method of classification for the radiographic changes seen in pneumoconiosis. These classifications are largely based on the size and number of opacities seen on the chest radiograph and are used by medical panels when discussing compensation claims.
• For benign pneumoconiosis, small, round opacities are diagnostic of the disease.

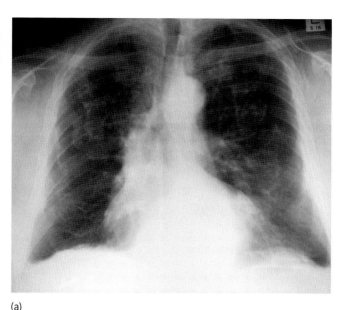

(a)

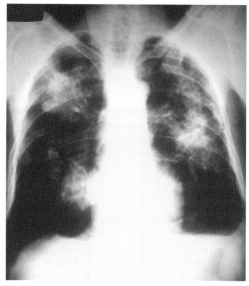

(c)

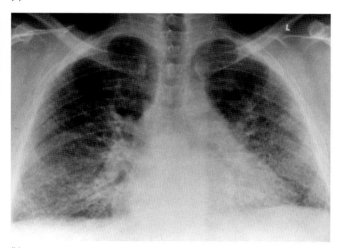

(b)

Fig. 30 (a) Chest radiograph of a patient with previous asbestos exposure with extensive pleural plaques. (Courtesy of Dr J. Moore-Gillon.) (b) Chest radiograph showing widespread pulmonary fibrosis secondary to asbestos exposure. (Courtesy of Dr R. Rudd.) (c) Chest radiograph showing the progressive massive fibrosis of coal worker's pneumoconiosis in a coal miner. (Courtesy of Dr R. Rudd.) (d) Computed tomography scan of the thorax; note the posterior changes, with pleural thickening and the adjacent early changes of asbestosis. (Courtesy of Dr J. Moore-Gillon.)

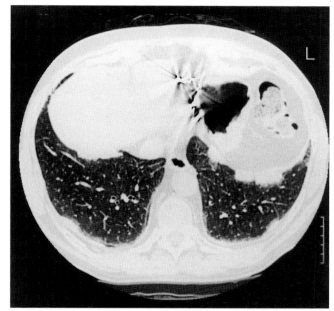

(d)

• Asbestos can produce a number of changes, including pleural thickening, pleural (holly leaf) plaques, fibrosis and evidence of tumours (Fig. 30a,b).
• Silicosis produces classical eggshell calcification around the hilar lymph nodes, as well as peripheral nodules.
• For CWP, see above (Fig. 30c).

Lung function tests

These show a restrictive picture with decreased FVC, TLC, RV and gas transfer.

High-resolution computed tomography scan

Prone and supine films will help reveal the extent of the disease, and is particularly helpful when extensive pleural disease masks the lung parenchyma (Fig. 30d).

Treatment

A priority is avoidance of further dust exposure. The workplace should, if necessary, consider review of protective equipment used by other employees. The benign pneumoconioses require no other treatment.

Fibrotic disease is normally considered resistant to therapy, excepting berylliosis, where high-dose prednisolone can produce a clinical improvement. Occasionally, courses of steroids are tried in patients with asbestosis who are showing rapid deterioration of their lung function. Treatment of CWP is largely supportive.

Complications

These may include:
- respiratory failure
- right heart failure
- TB in silicosis.

1 Waldron HA. *Lecture Notes on Occupational Medicine* (4th edn). Oxford: Blackwell Scientific Publications, 1990.
2 Jarad NA. Asbestos-related disease. *J R Coll Physicians Lond* 1999; 33: 537–540.
3 Morgan WKC, Gee JBL. Asbestos-related disease. In: Morgan WKC, Seaton A, eds. *Occupational Lung Diseases* (3rd edn). Philadelphia: W.B. Saunders, 1995.
4 Morgan WKC and Gee JBL. Coal worker's pneumoconiosis, and other pneumoconiosis. In: Morgan WKC and Seaton, eds. *Occupational Lung Diseases* (3rd edn). Philadelphia: W.B. Saunders, 1995.
5 Rudd RM. Asbestos-related disease. In: Brewis RAL, Corrin B, Geddes DM, Gibson GJ, eds. *Respiratory Medicine* (2nd edn). London: W.B. Saunders, 1998: 545–569.
6 Morgan WKC, Elmes P, McConnochie. Pneumoconiosis. In: Brewis RAL, Corrin B, Geddes DM, Gibson GJ, eds. *Respiratory Medicine* (2nd edn). London: W.B. Saunders, 1998: 570–604.

2.7 Diffuse parenchymal (interstitial) lung disease

2.7.1 CRYPTOGENIC FIBROSING ALVEOLITIS

Aetiology

Not known (by definition). More common in cigarette smokers. Speculation regarding viral or occupational aetiology. Rarely familial.

Pathophysiology

Cryptogenic fibrosing alveolitis (CFA) involves lung injury; immunological and inflammatory response; and fibrogenesis. There is evidence that the fibrogenic response becomes autonomous. Transgenic animals over-expressing transforming growth factor β develop progressive fibrosing lung disease indistinguishable histologically from CFA.

Pathology

The typical appearance is of 'usual interstitial pneumonia', where there is a patchy distribution of interstitial fibrosis, chronic inflammatory cell infiltrate and enlarged cystic air spaces.

Epidemiology

Usually age >50 years. Affects men slightly more often than women: incidence 5–10 per 100 000; prevalence 15–20 per 100 000.

Clinical presentation

Insidious (at least 3–6 months) onset of otherwise unexplained breathlessness without wheeze. There may be a dry cough, but sputum production is unusual. Haemoptysis is uncommon and suggests malignancy (see below).

Physical signs

Bibasilar fine inspiratory crackles. Clubbing in 75% of cases. In advanced cases there is cyanosis and signs of pulmonary hypertension/right ventricular failure.

Look for non-pulmonary features that would suggest alternative diagnoses, e.g. rash, arthropathy, lymphadenopathy.

Investigations

Pulmonary function studies show evidence of restriction and impaired gas exchange.

Chest radiograph shows small lung fields and reticulonodular shadowing, particularly at the bases and lung peripheries, but becoming widespread in advanced cases. Lymphadenopathy is not expected. There may be features of pulmonary hypertension.

High-resolution CT scan reveals bibasilar reticular abnormalities with honeycombing and minimal or no ground glass opacities: the appearances may be virtually pathognomonic.

Transbronchial lung biopsy or bronchiolar lavage do not support another diagnosis, i.e. there are no granulomas on biopsy and no excess lymphocytes on lavage.

Differential diagnosis

CFA is a diagnosis of exclusion. Definition (International Consensus Statement) requires: (i) the presence of a surgical biopsy (transbronchial biopsy specimens are too small to make the diagnosis, but can be useful in excluding other conditions) showing the usual interstitial pneumonia pattern of pathology; (ii) exclusion of known causes of interstitial lung disease such as drug exposures, environmental exposures and rheumatological disease; (iii) restrictive pulmonary function tests and/or impaired gas exchange; and (iv) typical features on chest radiography or high-resolution CT scans. The diagnosis is less certain in the absence of a surgical lung biopsy.

The following must be excluded:
- Diffuse rheumatological lung disease
- Occupational lung disease (asbestosis, hard metal disease)
- Chronic extrinsic allergic alveolitis
- Chronic sarcoidosis
- Various drugs (especially cytotoxics: bleomycin, busulfan, BCNU, methotrexate), inhaled agents and toxins (e.g. paraquat)
- Irradiation.

Treatment

There have been no prospective, placebo-controlled, randomized trials. As first-line treatment, most authorities recommend low-dose prednisolone (10–20 mg/day) with azathioprine (1.5–2.5 mg/kg/day, max 150 mg/day). The length of time for which treatment should be given is not known, but most recommend a minimum of 3–6 months and, if disease stabilizes or improves, continuing for at least 1 year thereafter. Many other agents have been tried, including high-dose corticosteroid (e.g. methyprednisolone 1 g i.v./day for 3 days) and cyclophosphamide for accelerated disease.

In end-stage disease, single lung transplantation is used in selected cases: the alternative is palliative treatment (oxygen, diuretics, opiates).

Complications

- Respiratory failure and cor pulmonale.
- Ten-fold increased risk of lung malignancy.

Prognosis

Median survival is <3 years: 10 years' survival is 5–10%.

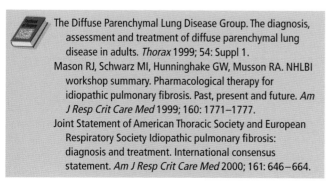

The Diffuse Parenchymal Lung Disease Group. The diagnosis, assessment and treatment of diffuse parenchymal lung disease in adults. *Thorax* 1999; 54: Suppl 1.
Mason RJ, Schwarz MI, Hunninghake GW, Musson RA. NHLBI workshop summary. Pharmacological therapy for idiopathic pulmonary fibrosis. Past, present and future. *Am J Resp Crit Care Med* 1999; 160: 1771–1777.
Joint Statement of American Thoracic Society and European Respiratory Society Idiopathic pulmonary fibrosis: diagnosis and treatment. International consensus statement. *Am J Resp Crit Care Med* 2000; 161: 646–664.

2.7.2 BRONCHIOLITIS OBLITERANS AND ORGANIZING PNEUMONIA

There is a great deal of confusion in the literature regarding these and similar terms!
- Bronchiolitis obliterans describes a condition that presents with breathlessness in which there is obliteration of the terminal bronchioles by fixed fibrosis.
- Cryptogenic organizing pneumonia (the term recommended by the American Thoracic Society/European Respiratory Society nomenclature committee) describes a disorder presenting with pneumonia-like features in which intra-alveolar histological changes spread proximally to the terminal bronchiole, which can be obliterated, but with loose fibrous tissue different from that seen in bronchiolitis obliterans.

Bronchiolitis obliterans

Aetiology

May be associated with rheumatological disease, particularly rheumatoid arthritis or Sjögren's syndrome, or after lung transplantation. Less often associated with infection, inhaled gases, drugs, or cryptogenic (cause unknown).

Pathology

Predominantly affects the terminal bronchioles, with significant narrowing and sometimes obliteration of the lumen by a mixture of cellular infiltration and fibrosis.

Clinical presentation

Progressive breathlessness, often with little wheeze. Cough is rarely productive. Haemoptysis does not occur.

Physical signs

Examination of the chest is likely to be unremarkable, excepting for evidence of respiratory failure and cor pulmonale in advanced cases.

Investigations

- Lung function tests show fixed airflow obstruction with increased residual volume. Total gas transfer for carbon monoxide is reduced, but when corrected for alveolar volume is normal.
- Chest radiograph shows large lung fields. There is no evidence of infiltration.
- High-resolution CT scan reveals patchy attenuation ('mosaicism'), which is characteristic.
- Blood tests may suggest rheumatological disease.

- Lung biopsy is not usually required to establish the diagnosis.

Differential diagnosis

Must be distinguished from other forms of chronic airflow obstruction such as COPD, asthma, and known causes/associations of bronchiolitis obliterans.

Treatment

Prednisolone 40 mg/day for 4 weeks is usually given to assess reversibility. If repeat pulmonary function testing demonstrates a significant objective response, then the dose is gradually tapered and inhaled steroid given. Azathioprine has been given without strong evidence of benefit. For end-stage disease lung transplantation is considered in selected cases.

Complications/prognosis

Respiratory failure. Treatment response is generally poor.

King TE, Jr. Bronchiolitis. In: du Bois RM and Olivieri D, (Eds). Interstitial lung disease. *European Respiratory Monograph* 2000; 14: 244–266.

Organizing pneumonia

Aetiology

Most commonly associated with rheumatological disease, especially rheumatoid arthritis and dermatomyositis/ polymyositis. Less often associated with infection, transplantation, drugs or cryptogenic (cause unknown).

Pathology

The airways distal to the terminal bronchiole and the alveoli are filled with granulation tissue.

Epidemiology

Occurs most commonly in 5th and 6th decades. Affects men and women equally.

Clinical presentation

Typically subacute with 2–3 months of cough, breathlessness and systemic features of fever, malaise and weight loss.

Physical signs

There may be a few crackles in the lung. Clubbing is rare. There may be features of systemic disease.

Investigations

- Pulmonary function tests show a restrictive defect.
- Chest radiograph shows bilateral basal and peripheral consolidation.
- High-resolution CT scan reveal more extensive changes than the chest radiograph, with peripheral air bronchograms.
- Blood tests confirm inflammatory process (raised ESR, CRP, white cell count).
- Surgical biopsy required in most cases to confirm diagnosis.

Differential diagnosis

There is a wide differential of other causes of pulmonary consolidation (e.g. infection, eosinophilic pneumonia, alveolar haemorrhage, vasculitis, alveolar proteinosis, alveolar cell carcinoma, lymphoma) hence the need for biopsy for confident diagnosis.

Treatment

Corticosteroids are usually very effective. Most would begin with prednisolone 0.75 mg/kg/day, tapering while monitoring clinical, radiological and pulmonary function test improvements.

Prognosis

Usually good: 5-year survival is about 75% for cryptogenic disease, 40–50% for that secondary to other conditions.

Cordier J-F. Organizing pneumonia. In: Thorax Rare Disease Series 8. *Thorax* 2000; 55: 318–328.

2.8 Miscellaneous conditions

2.8.1 EXTRINSIC ALLERGIC ALVEOLITIS

Aetiology

Extrinsic allergic alveolitis (EAA), also known as hypersensitivity pneumonitis, is caused by hypersensitivity to inhaled organic dusts. The best-known type is 'farmer's lung', which is associated with the presence of precipitins to antigens in spores of thermophilic actinomycetes in mouldy hay, but an enormous range of agents has been reported to cause the condition.

Epidemiology

EAA accounts for 2% of occupational lung disease: half of these cases occur in farmers.

Pathology

Histological material is rarely available, but the condition begins as a non-specific diffuse pneumonitis that later develops the characteristic feature of epithelioid non-caseating granulomata. Fibrosis and obstruction/obliteration of bronchioles arises in parallel with inflammatory changes. Honeycombing occurs in advanced cases.

Acute form of extrinsic allergic alveolitis

Clinical presentation

This can occur weeks to years after a sensitizing period of exposure. The patient develops recurrent 'flu-like illness (malaise, fever, headache, general aches and pains), with cough and breathlessness, usually starting about 6 h after exposure to the relevant organic dust. Wheeze can occur, but is not a typical feature. Breathing difficulty can range from trivial to life threatening.

Physical signs

Fever. Respiratory distress. Basal crackles. Clubbing is rare.

Investigations

Unless the patient has recently been exposed to the precipitant, pulmonary function tests are likely to be normal.

The chest radiograph may be normal, but characteristically reveals diffuse interstitial shadowing, particularly in lower and mid zones, resolving within 24–48 h after exposure has ceased.

The history is often diagnostic, but it may be necessary, particularly in circumstances not known to be associated with EAA, to make industrial hygiene measurements, e.g. with personal samplers, so that respirable agents can be identified.

The demonstration of a serum IgG antibody response to the inducing organic dust is the most widely used method of confirming hypersensitivity: a negative test effectively excludes EAA (to that antigen), but false positives are common.

When the diagnosis is in doubt, inhalational challenge tests are sometimes used in specialist centres.

Differential diagnosis

A single episode must be distinguished from other acute parenchymal lung disorders associated with systemic symptoms, the most common of these being infection. Distinction of recurrent episodes from organic dust toxic syndrome (usually caused by fungal toxins) and nitrogen dioxide pneumonitis (silo filler's disease) can be extremely difficult in those at risk of all of these conditions.

Treatment

In an acute episode, spontaneous recovery begins within 12–24 h of removal from sensitizing antigen. Steroids can hasten improvement, but there is concern that they may increase the risk of recurrence. Respiratory support (oxygen, rarely mechanical ventilation) may be needed in severe cases.

Prevention

Avoidance of exposure is the counsel of perfection, but easier said than done in many cases. Patients may be unwilling to put their livelihood (e.g. farming) or hobbies (e.g. pigeons) at risk. Exposure can be reduced by changing work practices or the use of industrial respirators. If monitoring suggests that disease is progressive despite these manoeuvres, then exposure must cease. An affected worker may be entitled to compensation.

Prognosis

Continuing exposure and repeated acute exacerbations can lead to permanent impairment of lung function, but this is relatively uncommon.

Occupational aspects

The environment that has caused illness in one individual may pose a risk to others. It may be necessary to survey the exposed population at risk, e.g. with questionnaires about respiratory symptoms and serological tests.

Chronic form of extrinsic allergic alveolitis

Clinical presentation

This presents as a gradual reduction in exercise tolerance because of worsening breathlessness. There is no systemic upset, excepting sometimes weight loss, and no acute exacerbations. Most often occurs in those exposed continuously to a low level of antigen, e.g. a patient who keeps a single budgerigar (parakeet) at home, rather than someone exposed intermittently to high levels of antigen.

Physical signs

Respiratory distress. Widespread crackles, as in cryptogenic fibrosing alveolitis, but by contrast clubbing is uncommon. Signs of pulmonary hypertension and right heart failure may develop.

Investigations

• Pulmonary function tests reveal restricted ventilation (FVC diminished in proportion to FEV_1), increased residual volume, and impaired carbon monoxide transfer factor.
• The chest radiograph can show a range of patterns, including diffuse interstitial shadowing, honeycombing and fibrotic changes (upper lobes particularly).
• High-resolution CT scanning is more sensitive than the chest radiograph, again showing a range of appearances, with a mosaic pattern being most characteristic.
• Bronchoscopy/bronchoalveolar lavage are useful in excluding other diagnoses, and lung biopsy may be needed to distinguish from cryptogenic fibrosing alveolitis in some cases.

Differential diagnosis

The main differential in many cases is from sarcoidosis, but also cryptogenic fibrosing alveolitis and other granulomatous lung conditions.

Treatment/prevention

Avoidance of exposure, as indicated above for acute EAA. There is no evidence that steroids are beneficial.

Complications/prognosis

Many patients continue their antigenic exposure despite medical advice to the contrary. Some cases develop respiratory failure, but this is relatively uncommon.

Occupational aspects

As for acute EAA.

Hendrick DJ, Faux JA, Marshall R. Budgerigar fancier's lung: the commonest variety of allergic alveolitis in Britain. *BMJ* 1978; 2: 81–84.
Grammar LC. Occupational allergic alveolitis. *Ann Allergy Asthma Immunol* 1999; 83: 602–606.

2.8.2 SARCOIDOSIS

Aetiology

Sarcoidosis is a multisystem non-caseating granulomatous disorder of unknown cause. It may result from an exaggerated cellular immune response to some antigens. Other points are:
• genetic factors—familial cases are rarely described
• increased incidence in black patients with HLA-Bw 15
• Epstein–Barr virus has been implicated
• *Mycobacterium* TB may be a trigger.

Pathology

Accumulation of T-helper (CD4) lymphocytes and mononuclear phagocytes in affected organs, driven by unknown antigens, is followed by the formation of granulomas with accumulation of macrophages and multinucleated giant cells in active disease.

The alveolar macrophages in the lungs release platelet-derived growth factor (PDGF) and fibronectin, which stimulate fibroblast proliferation and result in fibrosis, which is irreversible.

Epidemiology

• Sarcoidosis is a common disease and occurs worldwide, but there is great geographical variation. The incidence in the UK is 19 per 100 000, whilst it is uncommon in Japan.
• Maximum incidence is between 30 and 40 years.
• It is more common in females.
• In the USA, it is 10–17 times more common in black people than white.

Clinical presentation

The symptoms and signs depend on the organ involved (Table 22). In over 90% of the patients the lungs are affected. Pulmonary involvement may be asymptomatic and detected by a routine chest radiograph [1–4]. Acute or subacute sarcoidosis may develop over a period of weeks.

Investigations

Chest radiograph

The International Congress on Sarcoidosis established four stages of sarcoidosis based on the chest radiograph (Fig. 31).

Table 22 Common clinical features of sarcoidosis.

Body system involved	Symptoms	Signs
Respiratory	Cough, dyspnoea, wheeze	Crackles
Skin	Painful dusky blue nodules Shiny raised purple eruption on nose, face, hands or feet	Erythema nodosum Lupus pernio
Eyes	Gritty painful eyes, photophobia	Keratoconjunctivitis, uveitis, iridocyclitis, chorioretinitis
Musculoskeletal	Swollen digits, joint pains, proximal myopathy	Phalangeal bone cysts, proximal muscle weakness
Cardiological	Dyspnoea (cardiac failure), palpitations	Irregular pulse/rhythm disturbance, crackles at lung bases
Neurological	Headache, paraesthesia	Bell's palsy, mononeuritis, aseptic meningitis
Gastrointestinal	Abdominal pain, disordered LFTs	Pancreatitis, hepatomegaly
Endocrine–metabolic	Polyuria, polydipsia, confusion (caused by hypercalcaemia)	
Renal	Renal colic caused by calculi	
Haematological	Lymphadenopathy	Splenomegaly
Exocrine	Parotid gland enlargement	Parotid enlargement

LFT; liver function test.

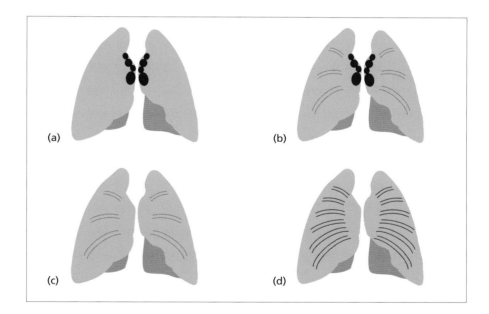

Fig. 31 Stages of sarcoidosis (International Congress on Sarcoidosis). (a) Stage I, hilar lymph node enlargement only; (b) Stage IIA, lymph node enlargement and diffuse pulmonary disease; (c) Stage IIB, diffuse pulmonary disease without lymph node enlargement; (d) Stage III, pulmonary fibrosis. NB: stage 0 is a normal chest radiograph.

Serum angiotensin-converting enzyme

- Raised levels in 41–80% of patients only.
- Raised levels also seen in hepatitis, miliary TB, HIV, histoplasmosis.

Serum calcium

Sarcoid tissue produces an abnormal hydroxylating enzyme that converts vitamin D precursors to active 1,25-dihydroxycholecalciferol and leads to hypercalcemia and hypercalciuria, which respond to corticosteroids.

Heaf or tuberculin test

Very often the main differential diagnosis is TB, either because of the finding of mediastinal lymphadenopathy, or because a biopsy obtained elsewhere (e.g. the liver) has unexpectedly shown granuloma. In this case the finding of anergy in response to Heaf or tuberculin testing would favour sarcoid. The problems with this approach are:
- prior bacille Calmette–Guérin (BCG) makes interpretation difficult
- patients with overwhelming TB can be anergic, particularly if they also have HIV.

Transbronchial biopsy

Transbronchial biopsy reveals granuloma in 85–90% of patients and these may also be seen in endobronchial specimens. In cases that are clinically clear-cut, biopsy is not required, but it is essential to obtain histological material if there is diagnostic doubt.

Tests of disease activity

These will depend on the parameters that were originally abnormal. Good examples might be:
- K_{CO} or ACE level if there is pulmonary disease
- liver function tests
- serum ACE/Ca^{2+}.

Differential diagnosis

The differential diagnosis depends on the distribution of organ involvement, but might include:
- tuberculosis
- lymphoma
- eosinophilic granuloma
- berylliosis
- interstitial fibrosis from other causes.

Treatment

Corticosteroids

The beneficial effects of corticosteroids were first reported in 1951, but many patients do not need treatment: stage 0 and 1 disease commonly resolve spontaneously. Stage 2 disease without any symptoms should be monitored for at least 6 months, with treatment offered if symptoms develop (dyspnoea and cough).

Oral prednisolone (0.5 mg/kg) daily is the treatment of choice, given for 4 weeks and then reduced in a stepwise pattern to a maintenance dose of 5–15 mg/day. The disease should be monitored by the patient's symptoms, chest radiography and TL_{CO} (see Section 3.6.2, p. 243). Relapse is common and is usually treated with an increase in the dose.

Inhaled corticosteroids

Inhaled budesonide may have a role as maintenance treatment once disease activity has been suppressed by oral steroids. Topical steroids may be used for cutaneous sarcoid, and with systemic steroids for ocular sarcoid.

Immunosuppressants and other therapies

- Choloroquine, chlorambucil, methotrexate, azathioprine, cyclophosphamide, cyclosporin and pentoxifylline have been tried in sarcoidosis, often as steroid-sparing agents
- Oxygen for hypoxemia
- Lung transplantation (see Section 2.13, p. 236).

Complications

These relate to the distribution of organ involvement:
- pulmonary fibrosis with hypoxemia resulting in cor pulmonale
- mycetoma: may grow within a lung cavity and cause severe haemoptysis
- hypercalcaemia, which can provoke renal failure
- complications related to affected organ.

Prognosis

- Stage 0 and 1 are usually self-limiting.
- Sixty to seventy per cent of patients with stage 2 disease show complete radiographic clearance within 5 years.
- Stage 3 disease is unlikely to clear and leads to cor pulmonale if untreated.

1 Flenley DC. *Respiratory Medicine* (2nd edn). Baillière Tindall, 1989: 277–284.
2 Fanburg BL, Lazarus DS. Sarcoidosis. In: Murray JF and Nadel JA, eds. *Textbook of Respiratory Medicine* (2nd edn). Nadel: W.B. Saunders, 1993: 1873–1888.
3 Crystal RG. Sarcoidosis. In: *Harrison's Principles of Internal Medicine* (12th edn). McGraw-Hill, 1991: 1463–1469.
4 The diagnosis, assessment and treatment of diffuse parenchymal lung disease in adults. British Thoracic Society recommendations. *Thorax* 1999; 54: Supplement 1.

2.8.3 PULMONARY VASCULITIS

Aetiology

This is a group of conditions characterized by antineutrophil cytoplasmic antibodies (ANCA). These antibodies are split into two types on the basis of the immunofluorescence pattern [1]:
- c-ANCA directed against proteinase-3
- p-ANCA directed against myeloperoxidase.

Some ANCA positive patterns do not fit into either category.

Many, but not all, have associated evidence of systemic vasculitis. The exact pathophysiology of vasculitides is unknown but one current hypothesis is that primed neutrophils release lysosomal enzymes and reactive oxygen species which cause endothelial damage.

Vasculitides are classified by size of vessel.

Large-vessel vasculitis

Temporal arteritis and Takayasu's arteritis cause large-vessel vasculitis. These do not generally cause pulmonary disease, excepting where there is involvement of the thoracic aorta.

Medium-vessel vasculitis

Churg–Strauss, polyarteritis nodosa and Kawasaki disease cause medium-vessel vasculitis. Churg–Strauss involves both small- and medium-sized arteries. Polyarteritis nodosa (PAN) can involve bronchial arteries.

Small-vessel vasculitis

Wegener's, Churg–Strauss and Henoch–Schönlein syndromes (rare to involve lung) cause small-vessel vasculitis. In Wegener's, involvement of the respiratory tract occurs by definition. Wegener's is c-ANCA positive in >90% of patients. p-ANCA has an association with Churg–Strauss.

For practical purposes the two conditions of greatest relevance to the lung are:
• Wegener's
• Churg–Strauss.
Some cases of Churg–Strauss syndrome have been described in patients treated for asthma with leukotriene antagonists. Opinion is divided as to whether the Churg–Strauss syndrome has been caused by these drugs or simply uncovered because of the reduction in steroid dose permitted by their use [2].

Epidemiology

• Wegener's—mean age at presentation 41 years. No gender predominance. Median time to diagnosis 5 months [3]
• Churg–Strauss—mean age of onset of asthma 35 years and of vasculitis 38 years.

Clinical presentation

Wegener's

Ninety per cent present with upper or lower respiratory tract symptoms; 73% involve nasal, sinus or tracheal airways. Respiratory symptoms include:
• cough (46%)
• haemoptysis (30%)
• pleuritis (28%).
Seventy-seven per cent develop glomerulonephritis within 2 years of onset. Fifty-two per cent develop ocular symptoms during their illness (e.g. proptosis). Sixty-seven per cent of patients experience arthralgia. Fever is present in 50% during the course of the illness. Skin involvement, mononeuritis multiplex and pericarditis are other recognized features [3].

Churg–Strauss

This has three distinct phases:
1 prodromal phase of asthma/rhinitis
2 blood and tissue eosinophilia
3 characterized by systemic vasculitis.
In the final phase cardiac (48%) and skin (67%) lesions are characteristic. Glomerulonephritis, mononeuritis, arthropathy and conjunctivitis are also recognized.

Physical signs

Depend on the clinical presentation (see above) but:
• Wegener's—pulmonary signs could include those of consolidation or pleural effusion. Upper airway ulceration may be visible on physical examination.
• Churg–Strauss—in the prodromal phase wheeze and reduced peak flow are evident. Later skin lesions (erythema, purpura ± nodules) and signs of cardiac failure can be seen.

 Consider Churg–Strauss syndrome in patients with asthma whose disease becomes more agressive and steroid dependent.

Investigations

Full blood count

In Wegener's there may be a normochromic anaemia (73%) with leucocytosis and thrombocytosis [3]. A normochromic anaemia may also occur in Churg–Strauss syndrome, but the characteristic abnormality is eosinophilia [4]. The ESR is usually high in both conditions.

Antineutrophil cytoplasmic antibodies

• Approximately 90% of patients with Wegener's are c-ANCA positive.
• Forty-eight per cent of those with Churg–Strauss syndrome are p-ANCA positive.

Histology

Except in clinically clear-cut cases histological confirmation of diagnosis is required. However, the yield of diagnostic histology by transbronchial biopsy in patients with

Wegener's is low—approximately 10% [3,5]. Alternative possibilities are:
- biopsy of upper airway lesions
- renal biopsy (if evidence of nephritis)
- open lung biopsy.

Other investigations

- Screening blood tests—renal and liver function tests, antinuclear antibodies (ANA), Rh factor, ACE and autoantibodies
- Urine—looking for proteinuria, haematuria and cellular casts as evidence of renal involvement
- Chest radiograph—may show pulmonary infiltrates, nodules, haemorrhage or a combination of these abnormalities (45% of patients)
- High-resolution CT scanning—may be a useful adjunct to diagnosis and for monitoring disease progression.

Differential diagnosis

The differential depends on the nature of the presenting symptom. The more difficult differential can be of eosinophilia. Where there is significant diagnostic doubt, the case for obtaining biopsy material is strengthened.

Treatment

- Wegener's—steroids ± cyclophosphamide ± plasmapharesis. Septrin may have a role for patients with disease confined to the upper airway. Azathioprine is often used to maintain remission
- Churg–Strauss—steroids ± cyclophosphamide ± plasmapharesis.

Complications

- Wegener's—chronic renal insufficiency (42%; a quarter of these will require dialysis), hearing loss (35%), nasal deformities (28%), tracheal stenosis (13%) and visual loss (8%)
- Churg–Strauss—essentially a more benign condition than Wegener's, but myocardial damage and gastrointestinal tract involvement are recognized.

Prognosis

- Wegener's—13% mortality
- Churg–Strauss—11% morbidity in long-term follow-up.

See *Nephrology*, Section 1.9.
See *Rheumatology and clinical immunology*, Sections 1.10, 1.20 and 2.5.
1 Burns A. Pulmonary vasculitis. *Thorax* 1998; 53: 220–227.
2 Stirling RG, Chung KF. Leukotriene antagonists and Churg–Strauss syndrome: the smoking gun. *Thorax* 1999; 54: 865–866.
3 Hoffman GS, Kerr GS, Leavitt RY *et al.* Wegener granulomatosis: an analysis of 158 patients. *Ann Intern Med* 1992; 116: 488–498.
4 Guillevin L, Cohen P, Gayraud M, Lhote F, Jarrousse B., Casassus P. Churg–Strauss syndrome. Clinical study and long-term follow up of 96 patients. *Medicine (Baltimore MD)* 1999; 78: 26–37.
5 Schnabel A, Holl-Ulrich K, Dalhoff K, Reuter M, Gross WL. Efficacy of transbronchial biopsy in pulmonary vasculitides. *Eur Resp J* 1997; 10: 2738–2743.

2.8.4 PULMONARY EOSINOPHILIA

Aetiology/pathology

Pulmonary eosinophilia is the term used for a group of disorders of different aetiology, characterized by peripheral blood eosinophilia and eosinophilic pulmonary infiltrates [1–3]. The causes of pulmonary eosinophilia are:
- allergic bronchopulmonary aspergillosis
- drug-induced pulmonary eosinophilia
- tropical pulmonary eosinophilia
- Löffler's syndrome
- Churg–Strauss syndrome
- hypereosinophilic syndrome
- eosinophilic pneumonia.

Allergic bronchopulmonary aspergillosis

This is mainly caused by *Aspergillus fumigatus*, but may be caused by other *Aspergillus* species and *Candida*. Inhaled spores are deposited in secretions and proliferate resulting in mucus plugging of the airways. There is production of IgE and IgG antibodies and eosinophilic infiltration of the lungs. Proximal bronchiectasis occurs as a result of local immune reaction.

Drug-induced pulmonary eosinophilia

Various drugs can cause pulmonary infiltrates, eosinophilia, fever and pulmonary symptoms such as wheeze and cough:
- aspirin
- methotrexate
- sulphonamides
- captopril
- naproxen
- tetracycline

- carbamazepine
- nitrofurantoin
- tolazamide
- chlorpropamide
- penicillamine
- bleomycin
- chlorpromazine
- penicillin
- gold
- imipramine
- phenytoin
- sulfasalazine.

Tropical pulmonary eosinophilia

The common causes are:
- *Wuchereria bancrofti*
- *Brugia malayi*
- *Ancylostoma duodenale*
- *Strongyloides stercoralis*
- *Toxocara canis.*

Hypereosinophilic syndrome

This is characterized by marked blood eosinophilia and eosinophilic infiltration of the heart, lungs, skin, central nervous system and other organs. It usually affects men in the fourth decade and has a high morbidity and mortality.

Chronic eosinophilic pneumonia

This is characterized by blood eosinophilia with pulmonary eosinophilic infiltration for which there is no obvious cause.

Epidemiology

- Allergic bronchopulmonary aspergillosis—the most common cause of eosinophilia. Occurs worldwide and at any age
- Drug-induced pulmonary eosinophilia—dependent on local patterns of drug use
- Tropical pulmonary eosinophilia—commonly seen in Asia, Africa and South America
- Chronic eosinophilic pneumonia—mainly affects middle-aged women with a history of asthma.

Clinical presentation

- Allergic bronchopulmonary aspergillosis—most patients present with asthma. Ten per cent have night sweats, fever or malaise.
- Drug-induced pulmonary eosinophilia—Cough, dyspnoea and fever may start within hours of taking the drug.

- Tropical pulmonary eosinophilia—most patients are young adults and present with cough, mainly nocturnal. Breathlessness, chest pain, fever, weight loss and anorexia may occur. If untreated, symptoms may persist or remit spontaneously and recur later.
- Hypereosinophilic syndrome—patients present with fever, anorexia and weight loss along with symptoms secondary to the organ affected. In 60% of cases the heart is affected with arrythmias and heart failure. In 50% of cases the lungs are involved and the patient complains of cough.
- Chronic eosinophilic pneumonia—patients present with cough, dyspnoea, fever and weight loss.

Physical signs

- Allergic bronchopulmonary aspergillosis—there may be signs of consolidation or simply wheeze
- Drug-induced pulmonary eosinophilia—wheeze and respiratory distress
- Tropical pulmonary eosinophilia—wheeze
- Hypereosinophilic syndrome—signs of mitral and tricuspid valve incompetence. Pulmonary consolidation and pleural effusions can occur.

Investigations

Allergic bronchopulmonary aspergillosis

- Blood eosinophilia is moderate (500–2000/mm^3).
- All patients show a positive immediate skin-prick test to *A. fumigatus*.
- IgG precipating antibodies to *A. fumigatus* are found in over 90% of patients.
- Total serum IgE is elevated during acute episodes, and serum IgE can be used to monitor treatment.
- Chest radiograph may show segmental or lobar collapse or bronchiectasis. In the acute phase transient pulmonary infiltrates may be seen.

Drug-induced pulmonary eosinophilia

Chest radiograph may show transient pulmonary infiltrates.

Tropical pulmonary eosinophilia

- Blood eosinophilia is high (5000–60 000/mm^3).
- IgE is markedly elevated.
- Antifilarial antibodies are present in high titre.
- Chest radiograph may be normal, but more typically shows diffuse mottling with lesions 1–3 mm in diameter.

Chronic eosinophilic pneumonia

- There is likely to be peripheral eosinophilia, anaemia, raised ESR and elevated IgE.
- Lung function tests show a restrictive or mixed defect.
- Chest radiograph shows peripheral pulmonary densities that have been described as 'photograph negative of pulmonary oedema'.

Treatment

Allergic bronchopulmonary aspergillosis

Treatment is with oral corticosteroids during acute episodes. Response to treatment can be monitored by radiologic clearing, resolution of eosinophilia or serum IgE levels.

Drug-induced pulmonary eosinophilia

Withdrawal of the drug results in resolution of the symptoms, which can be hastened by corticosteroids.

Tropical pulmonary eosinophilia

- Treatment of filarial disease is with diethylcarbamazine, building up to a dosage of 6 mg/kg per day for 3 weeks. Marked delay in treatment is associated with poor clinical response and development of pulmonary fibrosis.
- Mebendazole, albendazole or pyrantel pamoate are used if *Ascaris* or *Necator* are the cause.
- Thiabendazole is the drug of choice for *Strongyloides stercolaris*.

Hypereosinophilic syndrome

Treatment is with corticosteroids. In resistant cases, hydroxycarbamide (hydroxyurea) may be helpful.

Chronic eosinophilic pneumonia

This responds rapidly to corticosteroids, and failure to respond within 48–72 h raises the possibility of alternative diagnosis such as bronchiolitis obliterans and organizing pneumonia (BOOP, see Section 2.7.2). The dosage of corticosteroids is gradually tapered as relapses are common. Most patients regain normal lung function; a few may develop a persistent obstructive defect, and rarely pulmonary fibrosis may occur.

See *Infectious diseases*, Section 1.21.

1 Douglas NJ, Goetzl EJ. Pulmonary eosinophilia and eosinophilic granuloma. In: Murray JF, Nadel JA, eds. *Textbook of Respiratory Medicine* (2nd edn). Philadelphia: W. B. Saunders, 1994: 1913–1932.

2 Muers MF. Eosinophilic lung diseases. *Medicine* 1999; 27: 11; 167–169.

3 Harrison R. The eosinophilic lung diseases. *CME Bull Resp Med* 1998; 1(2): 27–29.

2.8.5 IATROGENIC LUNG DISEASE

Aetiology

A number of respiratory conditions may be precipitated by standard medical therapy [1], either by damage to the lung parenchyma or by disturbing the pulmonary physiology. These effects must be remembered when prescribing such treatments, and highlight the importance of taking a thorough past medical and drug history when interviewing patients. Potential mechanisms include:
- bronchoconstriction
- alveolitis
- radiotherapy.

Bronchoconstriction

Some of the drugs that can produce bronchoconstriction are:
- aspirin and the other NSAIDs
- penicillins
- tetracyclines
- cephalosporins
- cromoglycate
- β blockers
- anticholinesterases
- opiates
- iodine contrast media
- *N*-acetyl-cysteine.

Remember, drugs do not have to be given systemically to produce problems. Even eye drops such as timolol can produce wheeze and chest tightness, particularly in elderly patients.

Alveolitis

Some of the drugs that can affect the lung parenchyma are listed in Table 23. Some of these effects are potentially reversible on withdrawal of the treatment, while others may produce irreversible damage.

Table 23 Drugs that can affect the lung parenchyma.

Drug type	Drug name
Cardiac	Amiodarone Procainamide Quinidine
Antibiotics	Nitrofurantoin Sulphonamides Penicillins
Anti-inflammatory	Sulfasalazine Penicillamine Gold
Cytotoxics	Bleomycin Mitomycin Busulfan Chlorambucil Cyclophosphamide Methotrexate Carmustine

Radiotherapy

Radiation, prescribed with a view to eradicating tumour cells, also damages healthy tissues. When given to the thorax for the treatment of lymphoma, breast or lung cancer, it can produce a pneumonitis in the underlying lung. The risk of damage is proportional to the dose of radiotherapy.

Clinical presentation

The clinical presentation will be determined by the nature of the underlying pathophysiology. In general:
• bronchoconstriction presents with wheezing after drug administration
• pneumonitis or alveolitis is likely to have a slower onset with exertional dyspnoea and fine inspiratory crackles being prominent.

Investigations

In bronchoconstriction, monitoring peak flow is worthwhile to see if this improves after a couple of days. It is then worth requesting lung function testing pre- and post-bronchodilator to see if mild asthma or COPD has been unmasked.

In alveolitis there should be radiological changes visible on plain chest radiograph or high-resolution CT (Fig. 32), as well as appropriate changes in pulmonary function tests—reduced lung volumes with a reduced K_{CO}.

Radiotherapy produces more localized fibrosis that may progress to cause lung contraction. The edge is often sharply defined (Fig. 33).

Ensure that patients with radiation fibrosis are told that they have an abnormal chest radiograph, especially if the changes are persistent. This can save them unnecessary investigations in the future.

Treatment

For all suspected drug side effects it is necessary to stop the offending medication and replace with another class of drug if necessary.

Patients with bronchoconstriction may also require a bronchodilator, at least in the short term until their symptoms improve, as well as a short course of corticosteroids.

In alveolitis some patients will respond to steroid therapy; in others the damage will be irreversible, but non-progressive. Serial K_{CO} measurements are recommended by some authorities for patients taking amiodarone and other agents particularly associated with alveolitis.

1 Seaton A, Seaton D, Leitch AG. Drug-induced lung disease, oxygen toxicity and related syndromes. In: *Crofton and Douglas's Respiratory Disease.* Blackwell Scientific Publications, 1985.

2.8.6 SMOKE INHALATION

Aetiology

This term includes inhalation of a wide array of substances. In addition to the effects of toxic substances there is thermal injury to the respiratory tract, limited to the upper airways and resulting in laryngeal oedema. In fires, heat decomposition and pyrolysis causes the release of an enormous number of toxins such as carbon monoxide, cyanide, oxidants and products of preformed chemicals, which result in cytotoxic anoxia.

Studies of fire fighters and victims of fires have shown that smoke inhalation results in acute airflow obstruction and a non-specific increase in airway responsiveness after smoke inhalation.

Clinical presentation

Presentation depends on the severity of exposure, and ranges from mild airway obstruction to coma with extensive thermal injury and laryngeal oedema. In cases of severe exposure, pulmonary oedema and adult respiratory distress syndrome (ARDS) may develop immediately or following a latent period of 3–30 h. Patients may also present with symptoms of carbon monoxide poisoning (headache, confusion, clumsiness).

It is desirable to find out whether any chemicals or toxic gases were involved in the incident.

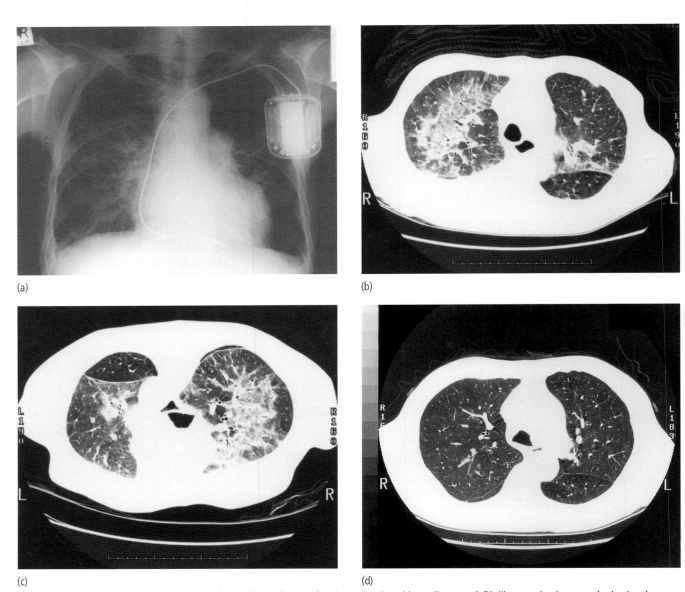

(a)　　　　　　　　　　　　　　　　(b)

(c)　　　　　　　　　　　　　　　　(d)

Fig. 32 (a) Chest radiograph of a man with ischaemic heart disease showing an implantable cardioverter defibrillator and pulmonary shadowing; he was thought to have heart failure. Computed tomography scans of the same patient (b) supine and (c) prone, taken the next day. The pulmonary shadowing does not change in position and therefore is more consistent with fibrosis secondary to amiodarone. (d) Computed tomography scan of the same patient 2 years later showing complete resolution of the fibrosis; the amiodarone had been stopped soon after the results of first scan and he was given a 6-month course of oral steroids.

 Smoke inhalation

- May include inhalation of various chemical fumes.
- Patients may be asymptomatic or gravely ill.
- It is essential to find out whether toxic chemicals were involved.
- Beware of thermal burns and possibility of laryngeal oedema. (An experienced anaesthetist should be present.)
- Smoke inhalation kills more fire victims than thermal injury.

Physical signs

Assess airway, breathing and circulation and resuscitate if necessary; otherwise look for:

- tachypnoea
- cyanosis
- thermal burns
- listen for crackles (pulmonary oedema) and wheeze
- cherry red skin, visual field defects and papilloedema of carbon monoxide poisoning.

Investigations

- Arterial blood gases—look for PaO_2, $PaCO_2$ and presence of acidosis
- Lactate level (lactic acidosis)
- Renal function (myoglobinuria secondary to muscle necrosis in carbon monoxide poisoning)

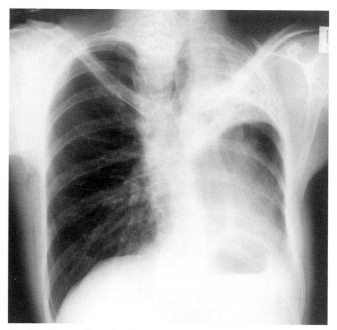

Fig. 33 Chest radiograph of a woman who had received mantel radiation for Hodgkin's lymphoma 30 years previously. The left upper lobe shows extensive tethering and fibrosis. She was referred to the chest physicians on the basis of this radiograph for bronchoscopy, with no reference to previous films. The changes had been present for many years.

• Carboxyhaemoglobin and methaemoglobin to assess the severity of inhalation
• Chest radiograph—look for pulmonary oedema and lung infiltrates
• Cardiac rhythm (arrhythmias in carbon monoxide poisoning)
• Oxygen saturation—monitor continuously.

 Carboxyhaemoglobin is detected by pulse oximeters; therefore *Sa*o$_2$ may not be an accurate reflection of oxygenation in carbon monoxide poisoning.

Treatment

Depending on exposure:
• care of thermal injury
• high-flow oxygen to correct hypoxia
• nebulized bronchodilators to relieve airway obstruction
• intravenous fluids to correct any dehydration
• hyperbaric oxygen in case of carbon monoxide levels over 40% or over 25% with seizures or arrhythmias
• intubation and ventilation if needed. Prophylactic intubation is required in severe cases
• treatment of pulmonary oedema, which can be caused by arrhythmia.

Complications

Depending on severity:
• renal failure secondary to myoglobinuria caused by rhabdomyolysis
• pulmonary oedema
• ARDS
• bronchiolitis obliterans—this usually develops 2–8 weeks after exposure, even in patients who were asymptomatic at initial presentation. It is characterized by non-productive cough and dyspnoea. It is more likely to develop in patients exposed to less soluble gases such as nitrogen dioxide and phosgene. This gradually progresses to respiratory failure.
• Increased airway responsiveness with repeated episodes of smoke inhalation (seen in fire fighters).

Prevention

Prevention will depend upon safeguard against fires in both residential buildings and chemical work places.

 Blanc PD, Schwartz DA. Acute pulmonary responses to toxic exposures. In: Murray JF, Nadel JA, eds. *Textbook of Respiratory Medicine* (2nd edn). Philadelphia: W.B. Saunders, 1994: 2056–2057.
Speizer FE. Environmental lung diseases. *Harrison's Principles of Internal Medicine* (12th edn). McGraw-Hill: 1061–1062.

2.8.7 SICKLE CELL DISEASE AND THE LUNG

Aetiology

The two major pulmonary problems that occur in sickle cell disease are:
• infection, leading to pneumonia
• veno-occulsion resulting in pulmonary emboli and infarction.
Together they make up the 'acute chest syndrome' [1].

Epidemiology

Infection is more common in children, although the risk of pneumococcal pneumonia has been reduced by the use of antibiotic prophylaxis. Adolescents and adults are more at risk of pulmonary emboli and infarction, which can lead to pulmonary hypertension and cor pulmonale.

Clinical presentation

Any 'Sickler' presenting with fever, pleuritic chest pain and shortness of breath should be carefully assessed and admitted for observation.

Aggression and/or confusion should not be mistaken for a psychotic or 'drugged-up' individual; the patient may well be hypoxic and septic.

Physical signs

These are fever, dyspnoea, crackles in lung fields, confusion, evidence of consolidation or opacities on chest radiograph.

Investigations

Emergency

For acutely ill patients obtain:
• full blood count—severe anaemia may require transfusion or exchange tranfusion
• urea and electrolytes—make sure the patient is not dehydrated
• chest radiograph—looking for pulmonary shadowing, consolidation and opacities (Fig. 34)
• arterial blood gases—looking for hypoxia; acidosis is a marker of the severity of the illness
• ECG.

Short term

Aimed at identifying reversible disease:
• ventilation–perfusion (V/Q) scan or spiral CT—look for emboli and infarction
• sputum for MCS
• echocardiographic assessment of pulmonary hypertension.

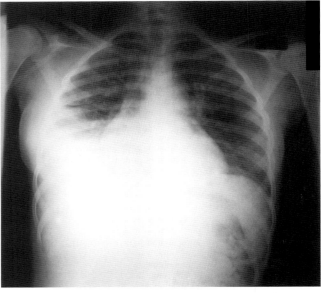

Fig. 34 Chest radiograph of a patient with sickle cell disease; there is right middle and lower lobe collapse and consolidation caused by pneumonia. Also note the cardiomegaly and small spleen. Less obvious are the surgical clips from a previous cholecystectomy. (Courtesy of Dr I. Vlahos.)

Long term

Lung function tests—note that sickle cell patients often have reduced indices even when in relative good health.

Treatment

Emergency

Try to reassure the patient, while:
• administering broad-spectrum intravenous antibiotics and fluids
• administering high-flow oxygen, humidified if possible
• giving adequate analgesia
• anticoagulating as for pulmonary emboli if veno-occlusion is suspected.

 Hypoxia in sickle disease is often ascribed to co-administration of analgesics and/or sedatives. This could be a dangerous assumption and you can check it by measurement of $Pa\text{CO}_2$. Reduction of respiratory drive should not affect the a–A gradient.

Short to long term

Close co-operation between haematologist and respiratory physician is helpful. Prophylactic antibiotics will help reduce episodes of infection. The patient may require life-long anticoagulation.

Complications

Repeated pulmonary emboli and infarction may lead to pulmonary hypertension, cor pulmonale and right heart failure in relatively young patients.

See *Haematology*, Section 1.2.
1 Serjeant GR. Pulmonary system. In: *Sickle Cell Disease*. Oxford: Oxford University Press, 1992, 150–167.

2.8.8 HUMAN IMMUNODEFICIENCY VIRUS AND THE LUNG

Aetiology/epidemiology

Lung pathology is common in patients with HIV infection and particularly in those with low CD4 counts. Like the immunocompetent, they are prone to the common viral and bacterial infections; but they are also at risk of atypical infections such as PCP [1–3]. PCP was a common cause of death in AIDS patients until the introduction of septrin prophylaxis in those with CD4 counts <200. It now tends to be seen as a first presentation of the disease in previously undiagnosed HIV.

Tuberculosis is a major cause of mortality and morbidity in HIV patients, particularly in developing countries, and non-tuberculous mycobacteria including *Mycobacterium avium intercellulare* (CD4 <100), *M. kansasii* and *M. chelonea* are also seen. Multidrug-resistant TB started to become a substantial problem in the early 1990s, with between 80 and 100% mortality. The relative numbers of patients infected with multi-drug resistant TB in Western countries remains small, but the plight of the developing world is uncertain.

Cytomegalovirus (CMV) pulmonary infection rarely occurs alone; if it is found, its presence does not affect the outcome of other lung infections. Fungal infections, e.g. *Cryptococcus neoformans*, tend to be seen as part of a disseminated syndrome.

Tumours such as Kaposi's sarcoma (KS) commonly occur in the lung as well as the skin, although lymphoma tends to arise in extrapulmonary sites in HIV patients.

Clinical presentation

The management of HIV patients with pulmonary symptoms can be difficult. Do not forget that acute shortness of breath can be caused by bacterial pneumonia, asthma or pulmonary emboli, just as in the immunocompetent. However, patients with HIV more commonly present with a history of gradually increasing breathlessness, fever, mild to moderate sputum production or just dry cough, and occasionally haemoptysis.

Physical signs

- How unwell is the patient? Are they hypoxic?
- Look for clubbing.
- Look closely in the mouth and on the skin for KS as well as other stigmata or evidence of immunodeficiency.
- Note any intercostal recession.
- Listen for crackles and wheezing.

Investigations

Chest radiograph

This may be virtually diagnostic (Fig. 35); but on the other hand it may appear normal, especially in early PCP and KS.

 Do not allow a false sense of security if the chest radiograph appears normal.

Oxygen saturation

Before and after exercise. Low postexercise oxygen saturation is almost diagnostic of PCP.

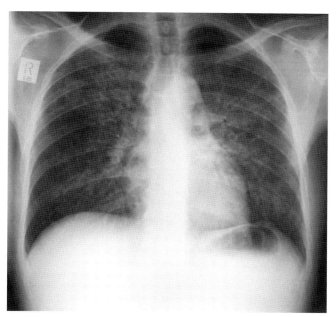

Fig. 35 Chest radiograph of a young man who presented with progressive shortness of breath, dry cough and a fever; note the classic bilateral perihilar appearance of the interstitial shadowing that is highly suggestive of *Pneumocystis carnii* pneumonia, which was later proved on bronchoscopic lavage to be the diagnosis. (Courtesy of Dr I. Vlahos.)

Arterial blood gases

Hypoxia demands explanation even if the chest radiograph seems normal.

Bronchoscopy

Because of the wide range of respiratory pathology seen in the immunosuppressed, bronchoscopy is required in this group of patients if there are new respiratory symptoms and the diagnosis is not obvious. Make sure that samples are sent for the regular investigations, but in particular:
- cytology to look for PCP
- microscopy to look for AFB
- virology to look for CMV.

Intrapulmonary KS is unusual without cutaneous KS, but not impossible.

 Sedation in HIV disease

Some newer antiretroviral agents, notably indinavir, efavirenz, nelfinavir, ritonavir and saquinavir, may greatly slow metabolism of hypnotic agents by interaction with cytochrome p450. Check what your patient is taking, or he or she may stay sleepy for several hours or longer.

Computed tomography scan of chest

Useful when other investigations are negative or disease is slow to resolve. Not essential in all patients but can be useful in unexplained hypoxia or fever (may see lymph nodes).

Treatment

Pneumocystis pneumonia

- High-dose intravenous septrin, oxygen and steroids (if PaO_2 <9.3). Do not forget to monitor bloods including FBC and liver function tests carefully. Second-line treatment in those unable to tolerate septrin is pentamidine or dapsone and trimethoprim.
- Because of the improved overall prognosis of HIV patients, full supportive care (including intubation and mechanical ventilation) is usually recommended if indicated on physiological grounds.

 In severe PCP large bullae may form. Pneumothorax could explain a sudden deterioration.

Kaposi's sarcoma

KS may improve in patients with a high viral load who are started on antiviral drugs. Otherwise, refer to an oncologist for intravenous chemotherapy.

Tuberculosis

The frequency of atypical presentations is increased but management is along conventional lines. Interactions with new-generation antivirals are a problem; specialist advice is required [4]. See *Infectious diseases*, Sections 1.39 and 2.6.

 Do not forget that drug regimens are different for atypical mycobacteria and multidrug-resistant TB.

 See *Infectious diseases*, Sections 1.26 and 2.11.
1 Miller R. AIDS and the lung. In: Adler MW, ed. *ABC of AIDS*. London: BMJ Publishing group, 1999: 26–33.
2 Miller R. Respiratory manifestations of AIDS. In: Mindel A, Miller R, eds. *AIDS, A Pocket Handbook of Diagnosis and Management* (2nd edn). Arnold, 1995.
3 Breen R, Johnson M. Respiratory infections in patients with HIV. *J R Coll Physicians Lond* 1999; 33(5): 430–433.
4 Pozniak AL, Miller R, Ormerod LP. The treatment of TB in HIV-infected persons. *AIDS* 1999; 13(4): 435–445.

2.9 Malignancy

2.9.1 LUNG CANCER

Aetiology/pathology

Smoking remains the chief cause, although other aetiological factors include asbestos, arsenic and some heavy metals. Various histological types are recognized (Table 24).

Epidemiology

Bronchial carcinoma is undoubtedly one of the leading causes of mortality in the UK with around 35 000 deaths per year [1–3]. It is more common in men, although the incidence in women continues to increase (male : female ≈ 2 : 1).

Clinical presentation

Common

Any abrupt change in respiratory symptoms in a past or current smoker merits investigation:
- cough
- haemoptysis
- shortness of breath (may represent an effusion or lobar collapse)
- chest pain.

Uncommon

Rarer presentations reflect the vagaries of anatomy or distribution of metastases:
- wheeze or stridor
- dysphagia as a result of oesophageal compression by enlarged mediastinal nodes
- nerve involvement, e.g. hoarseness secondary to recurrent laryngeal nerve palsy
- Horner's syndrome
- neuralgic pain as a result of tumour spread, e.g. Pancoast's, rib involvement

Table 24 Common histological cell types of lung cancer.

Histological classification	Types
Non-small-cell lung cancer	Squamous cell Adenocarcinoma Large cell
Small cell lung cancer	Synonym: oat cell

Table 25 Non-metastatic manifestations of lung cancer.

Syndrome	Mechanism
Cushing's syndrome	Ectopic adrenocorticotrophic hormone
SIADH	Ectopic antidiuretic hormone
Hypercalcaemia	Parathyroid hormone-like peptide
Hypertrophic pulmonary osteoarthropathy	Unknown
Eaton–Lambert syndrome	Unknown

SIADH, syndrome of inappropriate antidiuretic hormone secretion.

- loss of power and/or numbness in a limb or confusion resulting from brain metastasis
- facial swelling caused by superior vena caval obstruction
- confusion secondary to hypercalcaemia
- confusion secondary to hyponatraemia caused by syndrome of inappropriate antidiuretic hormone (SIADH) secretion
- cushingoid features and/or increased pigmentation (ectopic adrenocorticotrophic hormone secretion).

 Non-metastatic manifestations of lung cancer (Table 25).

Physical signs

Examination is often made with the benefit of a chest radiograph.

Common

Look for:
- clubbing
- tobacco-stained fingers
- cachexia
- pallor.

Uncommon

- Lymphadenopathy—feel carefully, including behind the sternomastoids
- Evidence of consolidation or pleural effusion on percussion and auscultation
- Liver edge secondary to metastases
- Bone pain caused by metastases
- Facial swelling and collateral venous circulation.

Rare

- Stridor secondary to tracheal or main bronchus involvement
- Horner's syndrome
- Pigmentation
- Skin metastases.

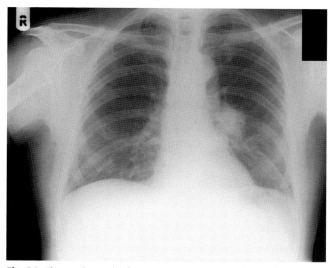

Fig. 36 Chest radiograph of a 56-year-old man presenting with cough, haemoptysis and weight loss. Note the large left hilar mass. Bronchoscopic biopsy revealed a large-cell carcinoma.

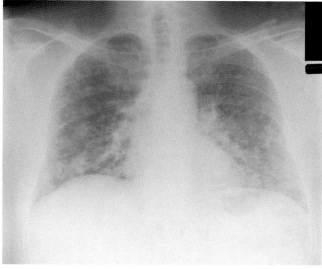

Fig. 37 Chest radiograph of a man with widespread nodular shadowing caused by diffuse adenocarcinoma of the lung.

Investigations

Chest radiograph

Posteroanterior and lateral views help to localize the lesion, especially for the bronchoscopist (Figs 36 and 37).

Bronchoscopy

If there is a visible lesion:
- biopsy for histology
- washings and brushing to cytology
- washings to microbiology for MCS and AFB (remember that infection can mimic carcinoma).

The surgeon will want to know the endobronchial anatomy.

221

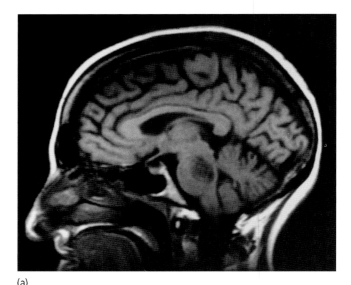

(a)

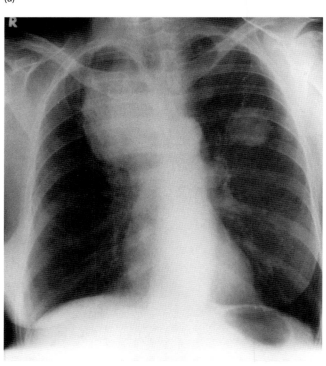

(b)

Fig. 38 This woman presented with incoordination in her left arm associated with mild loss of sensation. (a) Magnetic resonance imaging of her brain revealed a pontine lesion and (b) chest radiograph revealed left upper lobe mass associated with right paratracheal lymphadenopathy. She had a diagnosis of squamous cell carcinoma of the lung and was given palliative radiotherapy to the brain.

Computed tomography scan

For staging the tumour the scan needs to include the thorax, liver and adrenals to look for metastases, as well as the brain if there is evidence of neurological involvement (Fig. 38).

Percutaneous biopsy under computed tomography guidance

This is useful when bronchoscopy does not establish the diagnosis. The patient should be warned that there is a 10% chance of pneumothorax; they must be fit enough to tolerate such a complication.

Mediastinoscopy

Mediastinal nodes shown to be enlarged on CT/magnetic resonance imaging (MRI) are biopsied. This helps differentiate hyperplastic lymphadenopathy from tumour invasion. This can alter tumour staging and therefore operability. In some centres the nodes are sampled and analysed under frozen section before proceeding.

Positron emission tomography scans

These are becoming a useful tool in identifying tumour involvement of mediastinal nodes as well as other local spread.

Sputum cytology

This is mainly useful in patients who would not tolerate a bronchoscopy.

Blood tests

These are not diagnostic but can identify complications:
• FBC—anaemia may indicate the progression of disease and/or bone marrow involvement
• Urea and electrolytes—↓ Na may indicate SIADH; ↑ urea dehydration
• Liver function tests—if deranged may indicate metastatic disease.

Differential diagnosis

This is of the presenting problem but could include:
• infection—consolidation from a pneumonia, TB
• lung abscess
• bronchial adenoma.

Complications

The vigour with which complications are treated will depend on the patient's general performance status and local expertise (Table 26).

Table 26 Complications associated with lung cancer.

Problem	Treatment
Dyspnoea	DXT, endobronchial DXT, laser or cryotherapy, stenting, opiates
Bone metastases	DXT, non-steroidal analgesics. Prophylactic surgery is recommended if a lesion is found in a non-fractured weight-bearing bone
Brain metastases	Palliative DXT, steroids Excision occasionally recommended for single metastasis
SVC obstruction	DXT, stenting
Haemoptysis	DXT, laser bronchoscopy
Electrolyte abnormality	Correct as appropriate (see *Endocrinology*, Sections 1.1 and 1.2)

DXT, Deep X-ray therapy; SVC, superior vena cava.

Treatment

Emergency

- Radiotherapy (DXT) for superior vena caval (SVC) obstruction or tracheal/bronchial obstruction (see *Oncology*, Section 1.8)
- Laser bronchoscopy or stenting of tracheal or main bronchial obstruction—requires swift referral to specialist centre
- Pain control—early referral to Macmillan/palliative care team.

Short term

Surgery

The most important step is to decide whether the patient is a candidate for surgery or not. Age should not be a barrier for referral. Those with solitary peripheral lesions should always be referred. In general, patients presenting with central lesions, metastases or small-cell lung cancer (SCLC) are not candidates for thoracotomy. If in any doubt, always make a swift referral to your local cardio-thoracic surgeon, as in most cases resection is the only treatment likely to be curative. Make sure the patient comes back to see you immediately if they are turned down for surgery.

Non-surgical treatment

RADIOTHERAPY

High-dose DXT with curative intent may be given to patients with non-small cell lung cancer (NSCLC) without metastases who decline surgery. Patients with extrathoracic spread are generally given a palliative dose to control local symptoms as high-dose DXT has not been shown to alter prognosis but can lead to considerable morbidity.

Prophylactic cranial DXT in SCLC has been shown to improve prognosis; however, postoperative DXT following resection does not improve prognosis [4].

CHEMOTHERAPY

Oral and/or intravenous treatment is given with DXT in small-cell disease. Trials continue to evaluate its usefulness in NSCLC and before or after lung resection.

Pain and symptom control

It is essential to introduce patients and family to support teams as soon as is appropriate.

Prognosis

Overall 5-year survival is 5.5%.

Prevention

Smoking cessation

 Tomorrow, tomorrow, tomorrow … No, today.

Never underestimate your ability to counsel patients about smoking cessation—your words may just be the crucial encouragement the patient needs [5]. Particularly if you have never smoked, do not appear distant and virtuous; imagine your worst habit, even if it is not life threatening, and how difficult it would be to give up.

Recent government-sponsored initiatives in the UK may lead to increased availability of clinics to help people quit smoking. It is worth knowing what is available in your area so that you can readily advise. Although most nicotine replacement therapies (NRT) are not available on NHS hospital formularies, have an idea of what is available and encourage patients to see their general practitioners for further advice. Preparations include nicotine patches, gum, vaporizer (inhalator), sublingual tablets and nasal spray.

 Encourage patients to quit, help them set a date on which to stop and refer them to a specialist smokers' clinic if appropriate. Record your advice in their notes and general practitioner letter, and take the opportunity to ask how they are getting on if you see them again in clinic.

See *Pain Relief and Palliative Care*, Sections 2.9 and 2.10.
See *Oncology*, Section 2.9.

1 Brown JS, Spiro SG. Update on lung cancer and mesothelioma. *J R Coll Physicians Lond* 1999; 33(6): 506–512.

2 Seaton A, Seaton D, Leitch AG. Cancer in the lung. In: Seaton A, Seaton D, Leitch AG, eds. *Crofton and Douglas's Respiratory Disease*. Oxford: Blackwell Science, 1995.

3 Spiro SG. Bronchial tumours. In: Brewis RAL, Corrin B, Geddes DM, Gibson GJ, eds. *Respiratory Medicine* (2nd edn). London: W.B. Saunders, 1995: 924–961.

4 Jett JR. Is there a role for adjuvant therapy for resected non-small cell lung cancer? *Thorax* 1999; 54 (Suppl. 2): S37–S41.

5 McEwen A, West R. How to intervene against smoking. *J R Coll Physicians Lond* 1999; 33: 513–515.

2.9.2 MESOTHELIOMA

Aetiology

Asbestos fibre has been used extensively for its fire-resistant properties in the building industry, in shipbuilding and for brake and clutch lines in cars. It was mined in countries as far apart as the former USSR, Canada and South Africa, and transported to countries such as the UK by boat. The crocidolite form of asbestos is now known to be particularly hazardous in causing the associated lung diseases [1–4].

Asbestos fibres are inhaled and become lodged in the alveoli where they are incompletely phagocytosed by macrophages. The resulting inflammatory reaction leads to local tissue damage and fibrosis, and is thought to increase susceptibility to malignant change.

Epidemiology

The effects of asbestos tend to occur 20–40 years after the initial exposure. Therefore, as asbestos controls only became law in the late 1970s, it is predicted that we will continue seeing cases well into the 21st century.

Clinical presentation

- Shortness of breath (often caused by pleural effusion)
- Weight loss
- Chest wall pain.

Physical signs

Evidence of a pleural effusion and/or pleural thickening with:
- decreased expansion on the affected side
- decreased breath sounds on the affected side.

A careful occupational history is required from anyone presenting in this way (See Section 1.11).

Investigations

Despite vigorous investigation it is sometimes not possible to obtain diagnostic histology confirming mesothelioma in life. Special stains can help and it may be worth discussing this with the pathologist. See Section 1.11, p. 178.
- Pleural biopsy and aspiration
- Thoracoscopy and biopsy
- CT scan of the chest (Fig. 39).

Differential diagnosis

- Lung cancer—there is a symbiotic relationship between asbestos and smoking, with lung cancer being five times more common in smokers exposed to asbestos than smokers who have no exposure
- Sarcoma
- Benign pleural thickening.

Treatment

Emergency

- Drain associated pleural effusions if the patient is very short of breath.
- Only consider pleurodesis once you have a tissue diagnosis.

 Both pleural biopsy and thoracoscopy must be performed in the presence of a pleural effusion.

Short term

- Radical surgery, involving rib and lung resection, is attempted in a very few patients with limited disease.
- Pain can be a major problem and difficult to control, even with opiates; involve the experts, i.e. the palliative care (Macmillan) team early. Local DXT may sometime help. Cervical cordotomy can help intractable unilateral pain.
- Surgical or medical pleurodesis can help prevent recurrent pleural effusions.
- Drain sites should be irradiated to prevent recurrence; mesothelioma is notorious for seeding along tracks.

Long term

Trials with γ-interferon are underway.

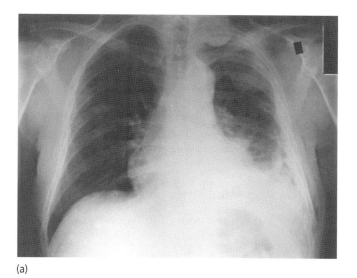

(a)

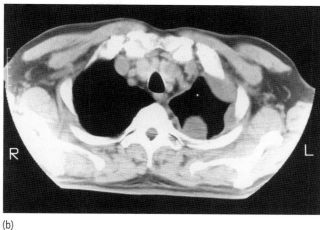

(b)

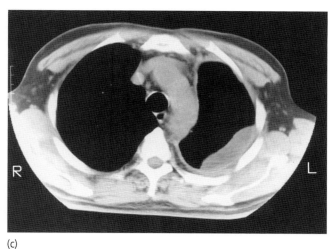

(c)

Fig. 39 (a) Chest radiograph of a man with left-sided mesothelioma; (b) computed tomography scan of the thorax shows extensive mesothelioma extending from apex, and (c) from the pleura into the thoracic cavity at the level of the left upper lobe. (Courtesy of Dr J. Moore-Gillon.)

Complications

- Repeated pleural effusions
- Severe pain.

Prognosis

Poor, with limited response to therapy. Median survival 12–18 months.

Prevention

There will continue to be a rise in the number of cases until at least 2015 as the rules controlling the use and handling of asbestos were only enforced in the late 1970s. The 20–40 years' latency from exposure to symptoms means that patients who were youngsters then will continue to present for some time.

Compensation claims

Patients with mesothelioma, asbestosis, diffuse pleural thickening and lung cancer associated with asbestosis are entitled to state compensation and receive a disability pension. Patients may also be able to make a claim against previous employers for any asbestos-related condition, including pleural plaques, and may receive compensation if the employers have been negligent in exposing them to asbestos.

If a patient wishes to pursue this course of action, the law generally allows them only 3 years in which to commence legal action after the date on which they first knew they had an asbestos-related condition. It is good practice to record that you advised the patient of this point when you diagnose an asbestos-related condition.

Similar procedures for both state benefits and claims against employers may be followed for coal worker's pneumoconiosis (CWP) and occupational asthma and a small number of other industrial lung diseases.

Disease associations

• Non-pleural mesothelioma tumours may occur as primary disease on the pericardium, usually presenting as constrictive pericarditis. Diagnosis is normally made by pericardial biopsy.

• Peritoneal mesothelioma causes vague symptoms of tiredness, lethargy and loss of appetite, followed by abdominal distension caused by ascites. Diagnosis may be made by laparoscopic omental biopsy.

See *Oncology*, Section 2.9.
1. Brown JS, Spiro SG. Update on lung cancer and mesothelioma. *J R Coll Physicians Lond* 1999; 33: 506–512.
2. Edge JR. Mesothelioma. *British Journal of Hospital Medicine* 1983; 29: 521–536.
3. Morgan WKC, Gee JBL. Asbestos-related disease. In: Morgan WKC, Seaton A, eds. *Occupational Lung Diseases* (3rd edn). W. B. Saunders, 1995.
4. Rudd RM. Asbestos-related disease. In: Brewis RAL, Corrin B, Geddes DM, Gibson GJ, eds. *Respiratory Medicine* (2nd edn). W.B. Saunders, 1995: 545–569.

2.9.3 MEDIASTINAL TUMOURS

Aetiology

The mediastinum is the part of the thorax lying between the two pleural sacs and contains the heart and various other thoracic viscera. It is a site where masses of different pathology are not uncommon: they can occur at any age and may be solid or cystic [1–3].

Based on a lateral chest radiograph, the mediastinum can be divided into three compartments (Fig. 40). Table 27 shows the normal constituents of the three compartments of the mediastinum as well as the tumours and cysts that may occur in each compartment.

Clinical presentation

Fifty per cent of all mediastinal masses are asymptomatic and 90% of these are benign. The likelihood of malignancy is higher in infants and children than in adults. The signs and symptoms of mediastinal masses depend upon the compression and invasion of nearby intrathoracic structures (Table 28). Mediastinal tumours may also be associated with various endocrine syndromes: myasthenia gravis with thymoma being particularly noteworthy (See *Neurology*, Section 2.2.5).

Investigations

The diagnostic approach to mediastinal masses can be divided into:
• imaging techniques
• techniques for obtaining tissue samples.

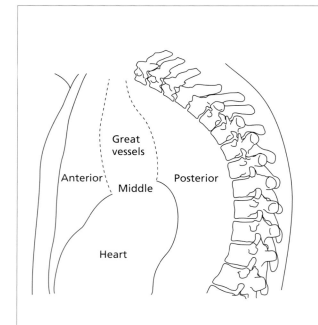
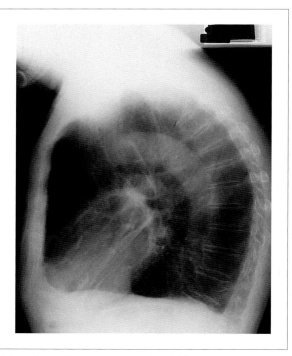

Fig. 40 Lateral chest radiograph showing division of the mediastinum into anterior, middle and posterior compartments, the middle compartment containing the heart and great vessels.

Table 27 Normal constituents of the mediastinum and tumours arising from them.

Compartment	Location	Normal contents	Examples of mediastinal mass
Anterior	Superior and anterior to the heart shadow	Thymus gland (remnant), internal mammary arterier and veins, lymph nodes, fat	Thymoma, lymphoma, retrosternal thyroid and parathyroid mass, fibroma, lipoma, teratoma, seminoma, choriocarcinoma
Middle	Posterior and inferior to the anterior compartment	Heart, pericardium, great vessels, trachea, major bronchi, phrenic nerves	Aortic arch aneurysm, pericardial cysts, left ventricular aneurysm, vascular lesions
Posterior	Lies within the margins of the thoracic vertebrae	Oesophagus, thoracic duct, descending thoracic aorta, azygos and hemiazygos veins, sympathetic chain	Oesophageal tumours, neurogenic tumours (neurofibroma, neurilemoma, neurosarcoma, ganglioneuroma, neuroblastoma, chemodectoma, phaeochromocytoma), diaphragmatic hernia, rare tumours (Adkin's tumour, Descending aortic aneurysm chordoma, mediastinal sarcoma

SVC, superior vena cava; TB, tuberculosis.

Table 28 Clinical presentation of mediastinal tumours.

Structure involved	Signs and symptoms
Trachea and main bronchus	Stridor, cough, dyspnoea, recurrent chest infections
Phrenic nerve	Diaphragmatic paralysis
Oesophagus	Dysphagia
Sympathetic trunk	Horner's syndrome
Superior vena cava	Non-pulsatile distension of neck veins, cyanosis and swelling of the face, neck and upper arm, dilated veins on chest wall
Pericardium	Pericardial effusion, pericarditis
Left recurrent laryngeal nerve	Left vocal cord palsy with hoarse voice

Imaging techniques

Chest radiograph

Most mediastinal tumours are discovered incidentally by posteroanterior or lateral chest radiographs.

Computed tomography

This helps evaluate the origin of a mediastinal mass and can also diagnose certain lesions confidently, e.g. teratoma.

Magnetic resonance imaging

This can offer superior definition to CT scanning and may be preferred prior to surgery.

Radionuclide scanning

These techniques can be used for specific lesions such as:
- radioiodine scanning for ectopic thyroid tissue
- uptake of thallium (^{201}Tl) by Hodgkin's lymphoma
- radioactive gold may be useful in localizing extra-medullary haematopoiesis.

Techniques for obtaining mediastinal tissue

- Mediastinoscopy
- Mediastinotomy.

Treatment

The treatment of a mediastinal mass would depend on the nature and location of the lesion.

1 Pierson DJ. Disorders of the pleura, mediastinum and diaphragm. In: *Harrison's Principles of Internal Medicine* (12th edn). McGraw-Hill: 1111–1116.
2 Pierson DJ. Tumours and cysts of the mediastinum. In: Murray JF, Nadel JA, eds. *Textbook of Respiratory Medicine* (2nd edn). W.B. Saunders: 2278–2290.
3 Benjamin SP, McCormack LJ, Effler DB, Groves LK. Primary tumours of the mediastinum. *Chest* 1972; 62: 297–303.

2.10 Disorders of the chest wall and diaphragm

Aetiology

A variety of chest wall disorders can lead to nocturnal hypoventilation and chronic respiratory failure, which occurs when the load placed on the respiratory muscle pump exceeds the pump's capacity. Abnormalities are initially present at night when the patient is often supine (increasing load) and drive is physiologically reduced, especially in rapid eye movement (REM) sleep.

The most common disorders are:
- post-tuberculous sequelae
- scoliosis
- kyphosis
- fibrothorax
- ankylosing spondylitis.

Post-tuberculous sequelae

Prior to the advent of combination chemotherapy, thoracoplasty was used as a treatment for pulmonary TB. Other therapies previously used (e.g. artificial pneumothoraces, phrenic nerve crush and plombage) may exacerbate load–capacity imbalance, but seldom cause ventilatory failure on their own. In the 1950s 30 000 thoracoplasties were performed in the UK.

Scoliosis

- Scoliosis is classified as congenital if there are associated spinal abnormalities (such as a hemivertebra).
- Scoliosis may also occur in association with neurological disease, notably poliomyelitis, muscular dystrophies, spinal muscular atrophy and syringomyelia.
- Most often no cause is found, when scoliosis is then termed idiopathic.

Kyphosis

When it occurs early in life (e.g. tuberculous osteomyelitis) kyphosis may cause CRF, but kyphosis alone in later life (e.g. resulting from osteoporosis or malignancy) seldom causes respiratory failure.

Fibrothorax

In fibrothorax stiffness of the thorax occurs because of pleural disease, especially after haemothorax, tuberculous empyema or asbestos exposure.

Ankylosing spondylitis

This is an unusual cause of CRF unless there is another pathology of which COPD would be the most likely.

Epidemiology

In a Swedish registry study of patients receiving home oxygen or ventilation [1] the annual demand was calculated at 3 per 10^6 population. Eighty-seven per cent of the patients had scoliosis, and half of these were as a result of previous polio.

Clinical presentation

Scoliotic patients should be regularly reviewed once their VC is less than 1.5 L.

 A minor change may precipitate respiratory failure. Consider infection or prescription of sedative drugs.

- Common—exertional dyspnoea, orthopnoea. Symptoms of nocturnal ventilatory failure (morning headache, daytime somnolence, mood or personality change)
- Uncommon—acute respiratory failure, cor pulmonale.

Physical signs

The patient should have a full respiratory, cardiac and skeletal examination looking particularly for:
- cyanosis
- carbon dioxide retention flap, dilated veins, papilloedema
- skeletal/rib-cage deformity
- presence of scars suggestive of phrenic nerve crush
- elevated JVP (may suggest pulmonary hypertension or cor pulmonale)
- respiratory signs
- ankle swelling.

Investigations

- FBC—may show polycythaemia
- arterial blood gases—may demonstrate daytime hypercapnia
- ECG—in case of rhythm disturbance and RVH
- Pulmonary function—these disorders are usually associated with a restrictive defect. Measurement of lung volumes is desirable
- Imaging—a chest radiograph is usual, although it can be almost uninterpretable in severe scoliosis. Spinal radiographs can be examined to determine the Cobb angle (Fig. 41). Angles less than 70° are seldom associated with respiratory failure unless a dual pathology exists
- Overnight transcutaneous O_2/CO_2 study—to detect incipient respiratory failure. An example of a patient with nocturnal respiratory failure despite initial normal gas tensions is shown in Fig. 42
- Echocardiography—is used to assess pulmonary artery pressure.

Differential diagnosis

There is no plausible differential diagnosis to the condition of scoliosis. Instead the clinical evaluation should seek to determine whether the magnitude of symptoms is

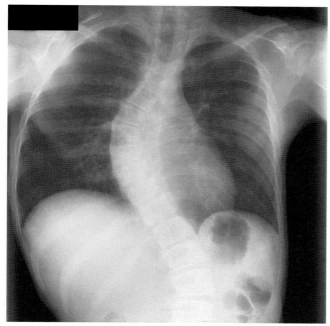

Fig. 41 Radiograph of a scoliotic patient. The Cobb angle is calculated by drawing lines parallel to the sections of spine above and below the curve. In a normal subject with a straight spine the angle is 0°, but in this case it is 66°.

appropriate for the degree of skeletal disease. If not, a second diagnosis should be sought.

Treatment

For patients who are still growing, early treatment (see below) can prevent worsening of curvature. Screening of school-age children is therefore important, as is regular review of children found to have a scoliosis.

Spinal stabilization

For children with an increasing curvature, treatment options include:

- external fixation (e.g. with a trunk brace)
- internal surgical stabilization by vertebral fusion or insertion of rods.

Although there are arguments for and against both procedures, the role of surgery is becoming increasingly important. Surgery may also be considered in adults but the main aim here is the palliation of pain.

Oxygen

Controlled oxygen therapy is indicated if the PaO_2 is <7.3 kPa. In most cases this will be combined with nocturnal nasal inspiratory pressure support (see below). Portable oxygen systems may palliate exertional dyspnoea.

Domiciliary ventilatory support

For patients with symptoms of CRF, home mechanical ventilation is effective [2]. The most commonly used technique is inspiratory pressure support delivered via a nasal mask.

Complications

See also Section 2.11, p. 230.

Common

- Musculoskeletal (relating to spinal deformity) and joint related
- Respiratory tract infection
- Hypertension.

Less common

- Chronic respiratory failure [3]
- Pulmonary artery hypertension.

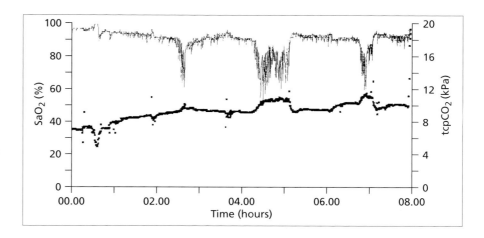

Fig. 42 Overnight O_2/CO_2 study in a patient with a scoliosis. Three dips in Sao_2 (upper line) are demonstrated with an associated rise in $tcpCO_2$, (lower line) which correspond to REM sleep. Note that this patient has gas tensions in the normal range initially and therefore probably has normal daytime blood gases.

Prognosis

Untreated patients have significant increase in mortality which becomes apparent at age 40–50. The risk is greatest for infantile onset scoliosis and least for adolescent onset scoliosis. The most common causes of death are respiratory failure and cardiovascular disease [4].

Disease associations

Idiopathic scoliosis is associated with congenital cardiac and urogenital defects.

1 Pehrsson K, Nachemson A, Olofson J, Strom K, Larsson S. Respiratory failure in scoliosis and other thoracic deformities. A survey of patients with home oxygen or ventilator therapy in Sweden. *Spine* 1992; 17: 714–718.

2 Simonds AK, Elliott MW. Outcome of domiciliary nasal intermittent positive pressure ventilation in restrictive and obstructive disorders. *Thorax* 1995; 50: 604–609.

3 Pehrsson K, Bake B, Larsson S, Nachemson A. Lung function in adult idiopathic scoliosis: a 20-year follow up. *Thorax* 1991; 46: 474–478.

4 Pehrsson K, Larsson S, Oden A, Nachemson A. Long-term follow up of patients with untreated scoliosis. A study of mortality, causes of death and symptoms. *Spine* 1992; 17: 1091–1096.

2.11 Complications of respiratory disease

2.11.1 CHRONIC RESPIRATORY FAILURE

Aetiology

CRF is a syndrome characterized by hypoxia and hypercapnia arising from pre-existing respiratory or other disease. Because the syndrome is chronic the pH is normal and bicarbonate retention occurs to compensate for the carbon dioxide retention.

CRF can complicate the following conditions:
- skeletal/chest wall disorders
- massive obesity
- COPD
- chronic lung diseases, e.g. bronchiectasis
- neuromuscular disease, especially past polio, motor neuron disease and the muscular dystrophies
- disorders of respiratory control.

Presentation

Symptoms include:

- morning headache
- unwanted daytime somnolence
- decline in daytime intellect/sharpness
- mood swings.

Physical signs

- Those of the underlying condition
- Carbon dioxide retention if acute on chronic decompensation
- Cor pulmonale (see Section 2.11.2, p. 230).

Investigations

Staging/confirming underlying diagnosis

Spirometry, chest radiograph.

Quantification of severity

This is necessary to assess the need for treatment:
- daytime arterial blood gases
- overnight O_2/CO_2 study
- FBC (for polycythaemia)
- renal and thyroid function.

Treatment

This should encompass:
- treatment of the underlying condition (where possible)
- consider REM modification by the use of protriptyline [1]
- non-invasive ventilation [2] (see Section 2.12.3, p. 233).

> **Be careful in patients with chronic respiratory failure**
>
> Sedative drugs or uncontrolled oxygen therapy may depress respiratory drive and precipitate acute respiratory failure.

1 Simonds AK, Parker RA, Branthwaite MA. Effects of protriptyline on sleep related disturbances of breathing in restrictive chest wall disease. *Thorax* 1986; 41: 586–590.

2 Clinical indications for non-invasive positive pressure ventilation in CRF due to restrictive lung disease, COPD, and nocturnal hypoventilation—a consensus conference report. *Chest* 1999; 116: 521–534.

2.11.2 COR PULMONALE

Aetiology

Cor pulmonale is the syndrome of chronic right heart

failure caused by pulmonary hypertension resulting from primary disease that serves to increase pulmonary artery pressure. CRF (see Section 2.11.1, p. 230) may coexist; long-standing hypoxia is a prerequisite. Cor pulmonale can complicate the following conditions:

- parenchymal lung disease
- asthma (severe or undertreated), COPD, bronchiectasis, CF
- obstructive vascular disease
- multiple pulmonary emboli, sickle cell disease, schistosomiasis, filariasis
- chest wall disorders
- obesity–hypoventilation
- OSA
- cardiac causes.

Clinical presentation

Symptoms may be difficult to discriminate from the underlying lung disease; dyspnoea and tiredness are frequent.

Physical signs

There are signs of pulmonary hypertension, RVH and right heart failure. Specifically it is worth looking for a sternal heave, tricuspid incompetence, elevation of the JVP, a tender (pulsatile) liver and pitting oedema. Atrial fibrillation is common.

Investigations

These should include:

- those relevant to the underlying condition
- FBC, renal and liver function
- chest radiograph—may show evidence of the cause. The pulmonary arteries may be prominent
- ECG—may show right axis deviation, p pulmonale, rhythm disturbance and right bundle-branch block
- echocardiography quantifies the pulmonary artery pressure and can demonstrate tricuspid regurgitation and occult structural cardiac abnormalities
- overnight O_2/CO_2 study and daytime arterial blood gases if CRF is suspected.

Treatment

- Optimize treatment of underlying disease
- Maximize oxygenation using controlled oxygen therapy or NIV
- Encourage diuresis using drugs (loop diuretics sometimes supplemented by thiazides) and fluid restriction but beware of inducing hypotension/low cardiac output by being over-zealous.

2.12 Treatments in respiratory disease

2.12.1 DOMICILIARY OXYGEN THERAPY

Principle

Oxygen is used to correct chronic or exercise-induced hypoxia. Oxygen can be given either:

- on a long-term basis (LTOT)
- briefly to palliate exercise-induced dyspnoea. This may be either after exertion from a fixed point or, if a portable system is used, during exertion.

Indications

Long-term oxygen therapy

This is indicated in patients in whom:

- the daytime PaO_2 is less than 7.3 kPa on two occasions during a period of clinical stability
- the daytime PaO_2 is between 7.3 and 8 kPa if there is coexistant polycythaemia, nocturnal hypoxaemia, peripheral oedema or pulmonary hypertension.

Although the evidence base is from patients with COPD [1, 2], LTOT is commonly prescribed to patients who are hypoxaemic from other causes.

The use of LTOT may cause carbon dioxide retention; it is therefore good practice to measure arterial (or ear-lobe) gases after acute administration of oxygen and after a period of LTOT use. Carbon dioxide retention is not an indication to withdraw LTOT but may suggest a requirement for NIV support.

Short burst

Oxygen from a fixed point is prescribed for patients with dyspnoea. Although logic would suggest reserving this therapy for those who have demonstrable desaturation (and who would therefore have a high probability of requiring LTOT) there are few relevant data. One reason for this may be that such patients often have very advanced pulmonary or malignant disease.

Ambulatory oxygen

This is indicated in patients with sufficient pulmonary reserve to exercise, but in whom this causes desaturation (a working definition being a >4% drop in SaO_2) that is correctable with oxygen.

Contraindications

Carbon dioxide retention

Carbon dioxide retention is not an absolute contraindication, but the clinician will need to assess the magnitude of carbon dioxide retention and weigh the risks/symptoms attributable to this against the benefit of improving hypoxia.

Smoking

Smoking in the presence of home oxygen is a fire hazard [3]. For this reason some clinicians do not prescribe oxygen to patients who admit a continued tobacco habit. Others argue that as some patients dishonestly deny continued smoking, this approach is unreasonable.

Practical details

For survival benefit LTOT needs to be used for a minimum of 15 h per day and is therefore best given via an oxygen concentrator. In England and Wales this is prescribed by the patient's general practitioner, but in Scotland this is the responsibility of the local chest physician.

Short-burst oxygen is more conveniently prescribed from a cylinder. Most of the devices for ambulatory oxygen administration are not currently available on prescription in the UK; they are either purchased by the specialist respiratory unit (often with charitable funds) or the patient themselves [4].

Outcome

For patients with COPD, LTOT reduces hospital admission and improves survival [1, 2].

Complications

- As well as smoking, oxygen presents a general fire risk [5]
- Services must be installed to locally determined standards.

1 Nocturnal Oxygen Therapy Trial Group. Continuous or nocturnal oxygen therapy in hypoxaemic chronic obstructive lung disease. *Ann Intern Med* 1980; 93: 391–398.
2 Medical Research Council. Long-term domiciliary oxygen therapy in chronic hypoxic cor pulmonale complicating chronic bronchitis and emphysema. Report of a working party. *Lancet* 1981; i: 681–686.
3 Maxwell DL, McGlashan JA, Andrews S, Gleeson MJ. Hazards of domiciliary oxygen therapy. *Respir Med* 1993; 87: 225–226.
4 Wedzicha JA. Domiciliary oxygen therapy services: clinical guidelines and advice for prescribers. *J R Coll Physicians Lond* 1999; 33: 445–447.
5 West GA, Primeau P. Nonmedical hazards of long-term oxygen therapy. *Respir Care* 1983; 28: 906–912.

2.12.2 CONTINUOUS POSITIVE AIRWAYS PRESSURE

Principle

CPAP describes the application of a constant pressure to the airway; the pressure may be applied to a cuffed endotracheal or tracheostomy tube or via a nasal or facial mask. It is important to appreciate that, by contrast to non-invasive ventilation (see Section 2.12.3, p. 233), no airflow will occur in a patient receiving CPAP in the absence of respiratory muscle activity (Fig. 43).

The increased airway pressure exerts a dilating force on the upper airway (hence its use in OSA, see Section 2.1.1, p. 188) and, if the upper airway is patent, increases EELV (hence its use in respiratory tract infection).

Indications

Acute

- Respiratory tract infection
- Pulmonary oedema (but caution in ischaemic heart disease)
- Postoperatively.

Chronic

- OSA
- Snoring
- Sleep-disordered breathing associated with congestive cardiac failure.

Contraindications

Nil.

Practical details

CPAP may be either high or low flow. High-flow CPAP is driven by piped air with room air entrained using a flow generator; flows in excess of 100 L/min may achieved in this way. Although this apparatus does not provide ventilatory assistance, the high flows mean that the work of breathing is much reduced. This mode is preferred for acute applications.

For domiciliary use, lightweight portable machines are available. Newer machines are able to sense flattening of the inspiratory flow curve and adjust the pressure level accordingly. It is hypothesized that this approach will improve patient adherence in OSA [1].

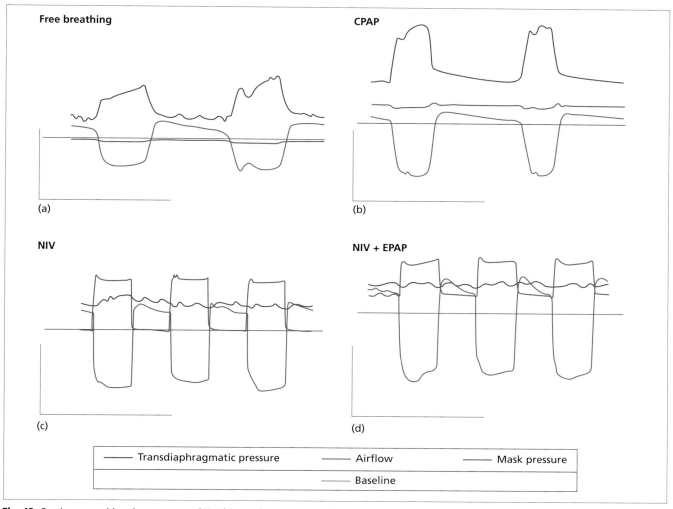

Transdiaphragmatic pressure	Airflow	Mask pressure
Baseline		

Fig. 43 Continuous positive airway pressure (CPAP) is not the same as non-invasive ventilation (NIV). In both free breathing (a) and CPAP (b) the patient still has to make an effort—shown by the large changes in transdiaphragmatic pressure. For NIV, either without expiratory positive airways pressure (EPAP) (c) or with EPAP (d), the patient's effort is minimal, but the ventilator is imposing a pressure change on the system.

Outcome

Acute

By increasing EELV *V/Q* matching is improved and, consequently, oxygenation. CPAP may not influence the course of the underlying disease so, for example, a patient developing ARDS may improve initially on CPAP but then subsequently require intubation if lung injury progresses.

Chronic

Although the effect of CPAP, if any, on cardiovascular mortality in OSA remains to be determined, randomized studies show it to be of value in improving daytime wakefulness and quality of life.

Complications

• Local—nasal bridge ulceration (Fig. 44), irritation of the nasal mucosa

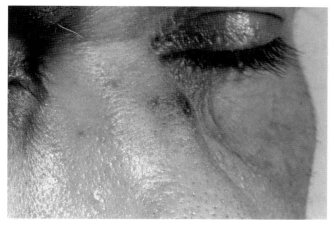

Fig. 44 This patient was receiving domiciliary ventilatory support via a nasal mask. Nasal bridge ulceration occurred and he had to switch to an alternative interface to continue his treatment.

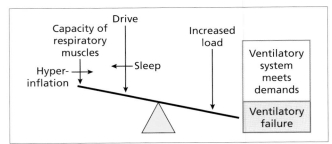

Fig. 45 As with other organ system failure, respiratory failure occurs when the load on the system exceeds capacity; this may occur acutely or chronically. During sleep the drive to the respiratory muscle pump is physiologically reduced and it is for this reason that chronic respiratory failure in its early stages demonstrates only nocturnal abnormalities.

• Systemic—may reduce cardiac preload and consequently afterload.

 1 Loube DI. Technologic advances in the treatment of obstructive sleep apnea syndrome. *Chest* 1999; 116: 1426–1433.

2.12.3 NON-INVASIVE VENTILATION

Principle

Respiratory failure results from an imbalance between the capacity of the respiratory muscle pump and the load placed upon it; this imbalance may occur chronically or acutely and for a variety of reasons (see Fig. 45). Unless treatment of the underlying cause is immediately efficacious, mechanical support is required to relieve respiratory failure. This can be given either invasively via an endotracheal tube or non-invasively.

The latter option, termed non-invasive ventilation, may be positive pressure via a nasal/facial mask or negative pressure (as for example with an 'iron lung'). In recent years the clinical uses of non-invasive positive-pressure ventilation (NIPPV) have expanded significantly.

The masks used for CPAP (see Section 2.12.2, p. 232) are also used for NIPPV and this can lead to confusion in the minds of some medical and paramedical staff. The difference between CPAP and NIPPV is not trivial and is that:
• with CPAP a constant pressure is applied to the airway
• in NIPPV a pulse of positive pressure is applied (see Fig. 43). The rate may be controlled by the machine or, more often, the patient is able to trigger the machine by initiating a breath.

If a positive pressure is applied in the expiratory phase (EPAP) in addition to the pulse delivered to support inspiration, then the machine is said to allow bilevel pressure application.

Indications

Acute

Established indications are:
• Acute NIPPV reduces intubation rate in patients with acute decompensated COPD [1]. NIPPV can also facilitate weaning [2].
• Acute respiratory failure can also be treated with NIPPV [3] but this requires the support of a specialized ICU/high-dependency unit (HDU).

 NIV treats respiratory failure. Do not be tempted to try and treat other conditions with it.

Chronic

The main indications are:
• restrictive thoracic disorders
• COPD
• neuromuscular and control of breathing disorders.
The timing of initiation of domiciliary NIV requires specialist assessment which will take into consideration the diagnosis, symptom load and physiological data [4].

Contraindications

Acute

• Patient too obtunded to co-operate
• Patient unable to protect airway
• Claustrophobia or anatomical facial deformity
• Haemodynamic instability.

Chronic

Claustrophobia or anatomical facial deformity.

Practical details

It is important that the operator is familiar with the ventilator to be used. Outside specialist units it is probably preferable to use a single model. For acute indications a full face mask is preferred, but for chronic applications a nasal mask is usually the first choice. Further detail as to how to set up a machine are beyond the scope of this work but may be found elsewhere, together with details on alternative interfaces and methods of ventilatory support such as negative pressure ventilation [5].

When using NIV for the management of acute decompensated COPD it is necessary to decide whether or not the patient is a candidate for endotracheal ventilation

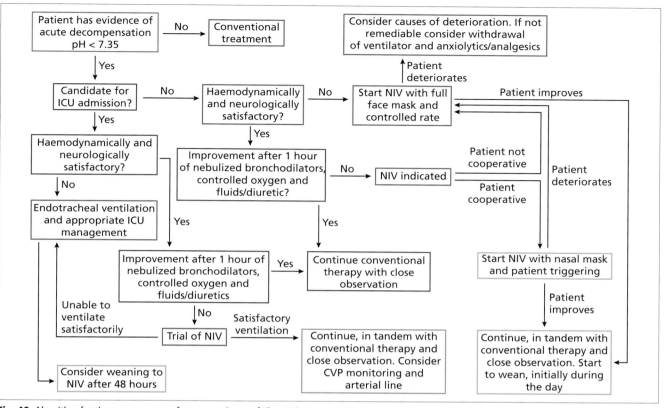

Fig. 46 Algorithm for the management of acute respiratory failure using non-invasive ventilation (NIV). CVP, central venous pressure.

(ETV) if NIV fails (see Section 1.15, p. 185). A suggested algorithm is shown in Fig. 46. If the patient is a candidate for ETV then recent data suggest that patients with a pH <7.30 after bronchodilators are best managed in an HDU/ICU environment by a physician with special expertise in NIV [6].

Outcome

Acute

In a study performed in general wards in the UK with COPD patients with a pH in the range 7.25–7.35 the mortality was 20% with standard therapy and 10% with NIV. This was stratified by pH so that for patients in the range 7.3–7.35 rates were 14.5 and 5%, respectively, and for patients with pH 7.25–7.30 were 29 and 21%, respectively [6].

Chronic

At the Brompton Hospital the 5-year chance of continuing NIV (which relates approximately to survival) was 79% for scoliosis, 94% for previous TB, 100% for past polio, 81% for neuromuscular disease, 43% for COPD. Bronchiectatics had a particularly poor prognosis; median survival 0.7 years [7].

Complications

These include:

- nasal bridge ulceration (see Fig. 44)
- aerophagy.

1 Brochard L, Mancebo J, Wysocki M *et al.* Noninvasive ventilation for acute exacerbations of chronic obstructive pulmonary disease. *N Engl J Med* 1995; 333: 817–822.

2 Nava S, Ambrosino N, Clini E *et al.* Noninvasive mechanical ventilation in the weaning of patients with respiratory failure due to chronic obstructive pulmonary disease. *Ann Intern Med* 1998; 128: 721–728.

3 Antonelli M, Conti G, Rocco M *et al.* A comparison of non-invasive positive pressure ventilation and conventional mechanical ventilation in patients with acute respiratory failure. *N Engl J Med* 1998; 339: 429–435.

4 Clinical indications for non-invasive positive pressure ventilation in chronic respiratory failure due to restrictive lung disease, COPD, and nocturnal hypoventilation—a consensus conference report. *Chest* 1999; 116: 521–534.

5 Simonds AK. *Non-Invasive Respiratory Support.* London: Chapman and Hall, 1996.

6 Plant PK, Owen JL, Elliott MW. Use of non-invasive ventilation (NIV) in acute exacerbations of COPD—Subgroup analysis of a multicentre randomised controlled trial. *Am J Respir Crit Care Med* 1999; 159: A15.

7 Simonds AK, Elliott MW. Outcome of domiciliary nasal intermittent positive pressure ventilation in restrictive and obstructive disorders. *Thorax* 1995; 50: 604–609.

2.13 Lung transplantation

Principle

The aim of transplantation is to replace a poorly functioning organ with a better one [1]. Operative procedures from cadaveric donors are:
- single (approximately 50% of the total)
- double lung transplantations (approximately 25% of the total)
- heart–lung transplantation (approximately 25% of the total).

There has been recent interest in living lobar transplantation [2], but the final position of this approach remains to be decided.

Indications

The general indication is pulmonary disease that is clinically and physiologically severe despite maximal medical therapy. As a rule of thumb the life expectancy of the condition should be less than that of the transplant recipient (see below), i.e. 2–3 years or less. The patient should be adequately nourished with an appropriate psychological state and social support.

In practice the most common diagnoses are, in order:
- COPD (including α_1-antitrypsin deficiency)
- CF
- primary pulmonary hypertension
- idiopathic pulmonary fibrosis
- pulmonary hypertension secondary to congenital cardiac disease.

There are detailed guidelines on the severity of these conditions in relation to the timing of transplantation [3].

Contraindications

Absolute contraindications are:
- unstable clinical condition
- neoplasia
- uncontrolled/untreatable infection; this does not disqualify patients with airway colonization
- significant cardiac dysfunction (unless heart–lung transplantation is considered)
- cigarette usage; drug/alcohol dependency
- serious psychological disorder.

Relative contraindications: because the supply of donor organs does not meet the demand, many units operate age restrictions.
- ventilator-dependent patients have a worse prognosis and many units feel it unethical to offer organs to these patients if non-ventilator-dependent patients also require an organ. This does not apply to patients using non-invasive ventilators.
- previous cardiac surgery, pleurectomy or pleurodesis increase operative difficulty and risk. Prior history of simple pneumothorax (and tube drainage) does not.

Practical details

Preoperative

Ideally the patient should be on as low a dose of corticosteroids as possible. Bridging strategies such as prostacyclin infusions (for primary pulmonary hypertension (PPH)) and non-invasive ventilation are of value.

Operative

Surgical details are beyond the scope of a medical text, but it should be noted that organ retrieval, preservation and assessment are crucial.

Postoperative

Regular follow-up of the patient is key. In particular repeated transbronchial biopsies are required, and the patient must perform daily spirometry.

Complications

The decline in survival is biphasic. In the first 3 months the leading causes of death are infection and primary graft failure. Later, chronic rejection becomes more important and is characterized by bronchiolitis obliterans and, physiologically, airflow obstruction.

Retransplantation is a controversial issue. While this procedure can be life saving in case of failure of the transplanted organ, many centres feel that it is unethical to offer individuals a second organ while other patients die on the transplant list because of a shortage of donor organs.

1 Thulrock EP. Lung transplantation. *Am J Respir Crit Care Med* 1997; 155: 789–818.
2 Dark JH. Lung: living related transplantation. *Br Med Bull* 1997; 53: 892–903.
3 American Society for Transplant Physicians (ASTP)/American Thoracic Society (ATS)/European Respiratory Society (ERS)/International Society for Heart and Lung Transplantation (ISHLT). International guidelines for the selection of lung transplant candidates. *Am J Respir Crit Care Med* 1998; 158: 335–339.

3 Investigations and practical procedures

3.1 Arterial blood gas sampling

Principle

To measure the oxygen and carbon dioxide tensions and acid–base status of arterial blood.

Indications

Arterial blood gas sampling was a research procedure until the mid 1960s. It is now widely performed, either by direct arterial puncture or from indwelling arterial lines. Indications include:
- respiratory failure (type I or II)
- renal failure
- hepatic failure
- cardiac failure
- drug intoxication (aspirin, narcotics)
- endogenous acid overproduction (ketoacidosis or lactic acidosis)
- severe illness, cause unknown.

For interpretation of data, see Section 3.6.1.

Contraindications

May need care in presence of bleeding disorders.

Important information for patients

The procedure should be explained to the patient. The possibility of requiring more than one attempt should be mentioned.

Practical details

Before investigation

The patient should be lying or sitting comfortably and an appropriate site selected. The radial artery of the non-dominant arm is most commonly used, but the brachial or femoral arteries can be used. Make sure you have enough sterile gauze to apply immediate pressure after the procedure.

The investigation

Clean the skin over the wrist with an antiseptic solution.

Palpate the artery between the tips of the forefinger and the middle finger of one hand.

Introduce the needle with the heparinized syringe attached to it between the fingers, at an angle of 45°, and slowly advance the needle along the line of the artery. On puncturing the artery, a small spurt of blood entering the syringe will be seen.

Withdraw 3–4 mL of blood and press a sterile pressure dressing over the site of puncture.

Expel any air bubbles and cap the syringe. The syringe should be labelled and sent to the lab immediately on ice if a blood gas machine is not available at the 'bedside'.

The role of local anaesthesia remains controversial. Although used by some, especially in paediatric practice, skilled operators maintain that it adds unnecessary complexity to the procedure.

After investigation

The pressure dressing should be kept in place for 5 min or until all bleeding stops.

Complications

In practice, complications are rare:
- haematoma
- arterial spasm leading to distal ischaemia
- femoral nerve lies lateral to the femoral artery and can be injured if femoral artery is the chosen site
- median nerve lies medial to the brachial artery and can be injured.

 Lightowler JV, Elliott MW. Local anaesthetic infiltration prior to arterial puncture for blood gas analysis: a survey of current practice and a randomised double blind placebo controlled trial. *J R Coll Physicians Lond* 1997; 31 (6): 645–646.

3.2 Aspiration of pleural effusion or pneumothorax

Principle

To aspirate fluid from a pleural effusion or air from a pneumothorax. This can be carried out using a syringe and a cannula, which is less traumatic than a chest drain (see Section 3.4), and should be considered before chest drain insertion in most cases.

Indications

- Pleural effusion—aspiration is preferred where the aim is to collect a diagnostic sample (just a few millilitres) or if the aim is simply to palliate symptoms by removing fluid where the cause is known
- Pneumothorax—aspiration is preferred unless there is respiratory embarrassment or bilateral pneumothoraces.

Contraindications

Gross abnormalities of coagulation clotting require correction. Herpes zoster or local pyoderma imply the need to choose an alternative, healthy skin area.

Important information for patients

The procedure should be explained to the patient and the possibility of developing a pneumothorax should be mentioned.

Practical details

Before procedure

A simple aspiration can be performed without local anaesthesia if the patient is co-operative. In anxious patients, lidocaine should be infiltrated into the skin and the parietal pleura. Except in the case of a diagnostic aspiration of fluid (when a 20-mL syringe and green needle suffice) the equipment required is:
- a wide-bore (grey) venflon
- a three-way tap
- a 50-mL Luer lock syringe.
In the case of an effusion, a jug and a giving set with fluid chamber cut off will also be required.

Pleural effusion technique

The patient should be seated comfortably, either on the edge of a bed resting forward onto one or more pillows on a bedside table, or 'cowboy style' on a chair (back-to-front, facing the chair back, with arms resting on the chair back).

The area of stony dullness corresponding to the radiograph should be identified and one interspace below this marked with a biro, usually in the line of the scapula.

Having cleaned the skin, the venflon is inserted while aspirating with a syringe. Remember to enter the pleural

cavity just above the rib to avoid injury to the neurovascular bundle.

When fluid is obtained, advance the cannula while removing the stylet and connect the three-way tap with the 50-mL syringe and the giving set attached.

By aspirating and then expelling into the jug, the effusion is aspirated. The purpose of the giving set is to avoid air inadvertently entering the pleural space.

Not more than 1500 mL of fluid should be aspirated in a single session as re-expansion pulmonary oedema may occur. Discontinue aspiration if the patient experiences cough, dyspnoea or faintness (signs of rapid mediastinal shift).

Pneumothorax technique

In case of a pneumothorax, with the patient in the supine position, aspirate the air from the second intercostal space in the midclavicular line. Discontinue the procedure if more than 2.5 L are aspirated (a large leak will need chest drain), if resistance is felt or if patient coughs excessively.

After procedure

Apply a dressing and request a chest radiograph.

Complications

- Entry into the pleural cavity may precipitate vasovagal syncope (give intravenous atropine)
- Rapid aspiration of effusion can lead to re-expansion pulmonary oedema
- Pneumothorax
- Haemothorax.

 Miller A. Pleural therapeutic procedures. *Medicine* 1999; 27(11): 174–176.

3.3 Pleural biopsy

Principle

Pleural biopsy is used to obtain a sample of the parietal pleura for cytological and microbiological examination.

Indications

All cases of exudative pleural effusion of undetermined cause. Discrete pleural lesions are best biopsied under radiological control because of the difficulty matching the surface landmarks to radiological anatomy.

Contraindications

- Absence of adequate pleural fluid
- Borderline respiratory function—production of a pneumothorax can precipitate respiratory failure
- Empyema—risk of development of multiple subcutaneous abscesses
- Presence of a bleeding diasthesis
- Thrombocytopenia (if platelets <50 000/mm^3, platelets should be transfused before the procedure).

Important information for patients

The procedure should be explained to the patient and the possibility of developing a pneumothorax should be mentioned.

Practical details

Before procedure

Premedication with an opiate or midazolam will help to reduce pain and anxiety.

The patient should be comfortable during the procedure and this is best achieved by having him or her sitting on the edge of the bed or on a stool with arms and head resting on one or more pillows on a bedside table. The operator stands behind the patient.

The site for the biopsy should be selected with care on the basis of a recent chest radiograph and clinical presentation. The best site is in the intercostal space below the spot where the tactile fremitus is lost and the percussion note becomes dull, superior to the rib below and hence avoiding the neurovascular bundle.

The procedure

The procedure can be performed either using the Abrams' needle or the Cope's needle. The Abrams' needle is more common and hence will be described here.

After positioning the patient and cleaning the skin with sterile solution, the skin and underlying tissues are infiltrated with 1% lidocaine. It is essential to anaesthetize the parietal pleura, which is rich in pain receptors. Do this as follows: once you have entered the pleural cavity and are aspirating pleural fluid, withdraw the needle slightly until nothing comes on aspiration. At this stage the needle is in contact with the parietal pleura: infiltrate with lidocaine, and allow 5 min for it to act.

Prepare for the biopsy by using a scalpel to make a small incision (0.5 cm) in the skin and the tissues, dissecting if necessary with forceps.

Introduce the Abrams' needle into the pleural space using constant and firm pressure. Then remove the stylet

and, with the inner cannula in the closed position, attach a syringe to the inner cannula.

Rotate the inner cannula anticlockwise in the outer cannula to open the distal notch.

Aspirate pleural fluid and withdraw the needle slowly until it hooks onto the pleura.

Rotate the inner cannula into the closed position and remove the whole needle.

A specimen of the pleura should be found in the tip of the needle. Three specimens are normally obtained at the 3 o'clock, 6 o'clock and 9 o'clock positions.

After procedure

A dressing at the site should be applied and a chest radiograph should be requested.

Complications

Although many complications are possible these are not common in practice:
- vasovagal syncope (give intravenous atropine)
- pneumothorax/haemopneumothorax
- bronchopleural fistula if the viseral pleura is damaged
- bleeding because of damage to the intercostal artery or vein
- visceral damage—spleen, liver, kidney.

3.4 Intercostal tube insertion

Principle

Intercostal tube insertion enables drainage fluid, air, blood or pus from the pleural cavity. It can be life saving, and may have to be performed rapidly and in unusual places. All doctors should be able to perform it.

Indications

- Tension pneumothorax
- Bilateral pneumothorax
- Empyema (use a tube of large diameter 28–32 F)
- Any patient with pneumothorax who is to be ventilated
- Haemothorax
- Any pleural effusion adversely affecting patients breathing (and not relieved by aspiration)
- To drain the pleural cavity dry prior to pleurodesis.

Contraindications

There are no absolute contraindications. However:
• bleeding diastheses should be corrected before chest drain insertion when possible
• it can be difficult to insert a drain if the pleura is thickened.

 Patients with COPD may have large bullae that resemble pneumothoraces. They will not be helped by intercostal tube drainage.

Important information for patients

The procedure should be explained to the patient and the possibility of developing a haemothorax should be mentioned.

Practical details

Before procedure

Premedication with an opiate or midazolam will reduce pain and anxiety; however, bear in mind the respiratory depression that can occur as a result of these drugs.

The patient should be lying supine with the head end of the bed elevated 30–45° and the arm held behind the head. A recent chest radiograph should be reviewed and the site of insertion should be marked. The drain should be inserted in the triangle of safety:
• between the anterior and posterior axillary lines, preferably anterior to the mid-axillary line
• below the axillary vessels
• in the level of or above the nipple (i.e. fifth intercostal space)
• above the rib avoiding the neurovascular bundle.

The procedure

Infiltrate the clean skin and parietal pleura with 2% lidocaine.

Incise the skin in the line of the ribs (2 cm) and dissect soft tissue with artery forceps.

Insert two strong non-absorbable sutures: one simple suture to secure the drain and one vertical mattress suture to close the wound after removal of the drain. A purse string suture results in a circular wound, which heals with a scar and should not be used.

When the pleura is breached, insert the drain with the trocar retracted so that it acts as a rigid directional guide only. Do not use excessive force as you may damage the underlying viscera.

In case of a pneumothorax aim the drain towards the apex. In case of an effusion, aim the drain inferiorly.

Once the drain is inserted, remove the trocar slowly and connect the tube to the underwater seal system.

Secure the drain and apply sterile dressing.

After procedure

• Obtain a chest radiograph to check position of the drain.
• Always maintain the level of water above the bottom of the tube in the underwater seal system.
• The bottle should be kept below the chest level.
• Never clamp the chest drain in case of pneumothorax (risk of developing a tension pneumothorax).
• Check daily if it is draining, bubbling or swinging.

Removal of chest drain

• In case of a pneumothorax, it can be removed once there is no bubbling, minimal swinging with respiration and chest radiograph shows a fully expanded lung.
• In case of a pleural effusion, it can be removed once it is draining less than 30 mL of fluid in 24 h.

The drain should be removed with the patient performing a Valsalva manoeuvre. A chest radiograph should be performed afterwards to check for pneumothorax.

Complications

These can include:
• bronchopleural fistula caused by injury to the lung
• visceral injury (liver, heart, diaphragm, spleen, stomach)
• thoracic duct injury causing chylothorax
• long thoracic nerve damage causing winging of the scapula
• haemothorax.

 American College of Surgeons Committee on Trauma, 1993. Light RW. *Pleural diseases* (2nd edn). Lea and Febiger: 311–320.

3.5 Fibreoptic bronchoscopy and transbronchial biopsy

3.5.1 FIBREOPTIC BRONCHOSCOPY

Principle

Fibreoptic bronchoscopy allows inspection of the bronchial tree and the biopsy of abnormal lesions.

Indications

The indications given under the American Thoracic Society Guidelines are:
- diagnostic
- therapeutic.

Diagnostic

- Evaluate lung lesions that appear on chest radiograph
- Assess airway patency
- Investigate unexplained haemoptysis
- Search the origin of suspicious or positive sputum cytology
- Obtain specimen for microbiological examination in suspected infections
- Investigate cause of SVC obstruction, vocal cord palsy, unexplained pleural effusion and paralysis of a hemidiaphragm
- Evaluate a suspected tracheoesophageal fistula
- Evaluate the airways for suspected bronchial tear after thoracic trauma
- Determine the extent of respiratory injury after inhalation of noxious fumes or aspiration of gastric juice.

Therapeutic

These are often performed via an endotracheal tube:
- Remove foreign bodies
- Remove secretions or mucous plugs
- Perform difficult intubations.

3.5.2 TRANSBRONCHIAL BIOPSY

Principle

To obtain diagnostic tissue, usually in cases of suspected diffuse parenchymal lung disease.

Indications

Although the samples obtained are small and sometimes crushed, transbronchial biopsy achieves a high diagnostic yield in diffuse parenchymal lung diseases that have centrilobular accentuation, such as granulomatous and metastatic diseases. These include:
- sarcoidosis—75–89% diagnostic yield
- carcinoma—64–68% diagnostic yield
- infection
- eosinophilic pneumonia
- alveolar proteinosis.

Complications

The risk of developing a pneumothorax is 10%; however, this can be reduced by avoiding the right middle lobe and the lingula and with the use of fluoroscopy.

Sokolowski RW, Burgher LW, Jones FL *et al*. Guidelines for fibreoptic bronchoscopy in adults. *Am Rev Respir Dis* 1987; 136: 1066.
British Thoracic Society. The Diagnosis, assessment and treatment of diffuse parenchymal lung disease in adults. *Thorax* 1999; 54: Supplement 1.

3.6 Interpretation of clinical data

3.6.1 ARTERIAL BLOOD GASES

What is measured

Whenever you take a set of blood gases, make sure that you clearly record the date, time, patient's name and their inspired concentration of oxygen. This is crucial for interpretation and comparison with other results: a Po_2 of 12 kPa is normal if the patient is breathing air but grossly abnormal if they are on 60% oxygen!

Blood gas machines record various data (Table 29), and many also give a value for base excess/deficit. Calculation of base excess/deficit is designed to make it easy to separate metabolic from respiratory causes of pH disturbance. Various algorithms are used in these calculations, the principles being as follows.

Table 29 Measurements made by blood gas machines.

	Normal range	Notes
Po_2	>10.6 kPa (breathing air)	Hypoxia <8 kPa
pH	pH 7.37–7.43	
H^+	37–43 nmol/L	
Pco_2	4.7–6.0 kPa	Respiratory failure: If Po_2 <8 kPa and Pco_2 <6.5 kPa = Type I If Pco_2 >6.5 kPa = Type II
HCO_3^-	22–28 mmol/L	In dealing with problems of respiratory failure or acid–base disturbance, measurement of plasma bicarbonate is often helpful

- Predict the pH that would arise in normal blood in the presence of the PCO_2 actually measured. If PCO_2 high, then predicted pH is low; if PCO_2 is low, then predicted pH is high.
- Calculate the amount of acid or base that would have to be added to the blood to change the predicted pH into the pH as actually measured. This is the base deficit/excess (in mmol/L) and a measure of the degree of 'metabolic', as opposed to 'respiratory', disturbance. A normal value is between −2 and +2.

If the blood gas machine that you have used does not provide the base deficit/excess, then a useful rule of thumb is as follows: in uncompensated metabolic disorders, the steady-state PCO_2 (measured in mmHg, where 1 kPa = 7.6 mmHg) should be numerically equal to the last two digits of the pH. For example, a normal PCO_2 is 5.3 kPa or 40 mmHg, and a normal pH is 7.40.

If this picture is not observed, then either:
- the problem is not simply metabolic—there is a primary respiratory element to the acid–base disorder
- the metabolic change is very acute and respiratory compensation has not had time to develop (unlikely, because respiratory compensation is very rapid).

Interpreting results

Low PO_2

See Section 1.6, p. 167.

Because it is not possible to specify the precise concentration of oxygen that a patient receives, unless they are intubated and ventilated, normal values for PO_2 cannot be quoted for those breathing on 24%, 28% or other oxygen masks. As a very rough guide, the 'hypoxaemia score' can be calculated as follows:

Hypoxaemia score = PO_2 (measured in mmHg, where 1 kPa = 7.6 mmHg)/FiO_2

where FiO_2 is the fraction of oxygen inspired, in air 0.21.

If the patient were breathing air, then applying the lower limit of normal PO_2 (10.6 kPa) would give a score of 384; and the value of PO_2 taken conventionally to define hypoxia (8 kPa) would score 290. In assessing a patient breathing supplementary oxygen a value of <300 is usually taken as indicating significant compromise.

High PO_2

Air has a PO_2 of 21 kPa. Allowing for the PCO_2, the highest PO_2 that can be achieved breathing air is around 15 kPa. If a value higher than this is obtained, then the patient must have been breathing supplementary oxygen.

Low PCO_2

Hyperventilation may be:
- primary—most commonly caused by anxiety
- secondary—to metabolic acidosis, which is known as respiratory compensation.

How can you tell if the patient has a metabolic acidosis? Look for reduction in pH and increased 'negative base excess', i.e. a base excess more negative than −2. For the clinical approach to metabolic acidosis, see *Emergency medicine*, Section 1.19.

High PCO_2

Hypoventilation may be caused by problems with the respiratory (airway, lungs, respiratory muscles, chest wall) or neurological (central, neuropathic) mechanisms of respiration.

How can you tell if this is acute or chronic? In chronic carbon dioxide retention the HCO_3^- rises (secondary metabolic alkalosis) and the chloride falls.

Much more rarely a high PCO_2 is secondary to metabolic alkalosis, which would be known as respiratory compensation. How can you tell if the patient has a metabolic alkalosis? Look for elevation in pH and an increased 'base excess', i.e. a base excess more positive than +2.

pH or H^+

Alterations in acid–base status can result from changes in PCO_2, bicarbonate concentration, or both:
- If the primary process affects PCO_2, then the alteration is described as a respiratory acidosis/alkalosis.
- If the primary process affects bicarbonate, then the terms metabolic acidosis/alkalosis are used.
- 'Mixed' disorders are those that arise as a result of more than one 'primary' process.

Whatever the primary process, it will usually be accompanied by secondary change in either PCO_2 or bicarbonate concentration, such that change in blood pH is minimized.

Putting the values for PCO_2, pH and bicarbonate for any particular patient on to the nomograms shown in Figs 47 and 48 will define the type of any acid–base disturbance, as is done by calculation of the base deficit/excess shown above.

Once the type of acid–base disturbance is known, consideration must be directed towards specific causes:
- respiratory acidosis—see Sections 1.8, p. 172 and 1.15, p. 185
- respiratory alkalosis—see *Emergency medicine*, Section 1.7
- metabolic acidosis—see *Emergency medicine*, Section 1.19.

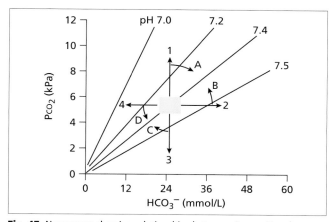

Fig. 47 Nomogram showing relationships between PCO_2, pH and bicarbonate. Shaded area depicts normal range. Perturbations: (1) respiratory acidosis, with (A) secondary metabolic alkalosis; (2) metabolic alkalosis, with (B) secondary respiratory acidosis; (3) respiratory alkalosis, with (C) secondary metabolic acidosis; (4) metabolic acidosis, with (D) secondary respiratory alkalosis.

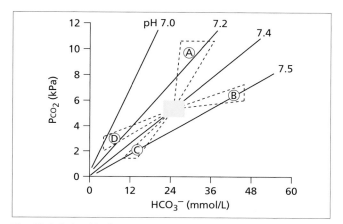

Fig. 48 Relationships between PCO_2, pH and bicarbonate seen clinically in the four simple types of acid–base disturbance. Shaded area depicts normal range. Perturbations: (A) respiratory acidosis; (B) metabolic alkalosis; (C) respiratory alkalosis; (D) metabolic acidosis.

3.6.2 LUNG FUNCTION TESTS

See Table 30.

Peak flow

This is a valuable guide to airway obstruction, but is also influenced by patient aptitude and lung volume among other factors.

Spirometry

There are portable spirometers which can be transported to the wards. The VC may be reduced by many disorders, but the FEV_1 is disproportionately reduced in obstructive conditions. This may be quantified from the FEV_1/FVC ratio (Table 31, Fig. 49). This ratio is normally 80% (range 70–85%), although the 'normal ratio' tends to decline with age.

- A decreased ratio indicates an obstructive lung defect.
- A raised ratio is suggestive of a restrictive defect.

This distinction can only be made absolutely by measurement of TLC (see *Physiology*, Section 2).

Laboratory lung function

This needs the patient to be relatively well: it is not possible for really sick patients. It records lung volumes (TLC, RV), flow–volume loops and estimates the efficiency of gas transfer into the lung using carbon monoxide (TL_{CO}, K_{CO}).

After looking at the FEV_1 and FVC, lung volumes are helpful in further interpretation of the underlying pathology.

Table 30 Lung function: definitions.

Abbreviation	Meaning and units	Description
PEF	Peak expiratory flow, L/s	Maximum rate of expiratory airflow during maximum forced expiration
FEV_1	Forced expiratory volume in 1 s, L	Volume of air expired during first second of a forced expiration
FVC	Forced vital capacity, L	Volume of air expired by a forceful expiration after taking a full inflation
FEV_1/FVC	Ratio, %	—
TLC	Total lung capacity, L	Total volume of air in the lungs after maximum inspiration
RV	Residual volume, L	Volume of air remaining in the lung after a maximum expiration
FRC	Functional residual capacity, L	Volume of air remaining in the lungs at the end of normal expiration without any muscle activity. The 'neutral point' of the respiratory system

Table 31 Causes of restrictive and obstructive lung defects.

Type of defect	Spirometric pattern	Examples
Restrictive	Increased FEV$_1$/FVC ratio	Pulmonary fibrosis, respiratory muscle weakness, obesity, pleural disease, chest wall and skeletal disorders
Obstructive	Decreased FEV$_1$/FVC ratio	COPD, asthma

COPD, chronic obstructive pulmonary disease; FEV$_1$, forced expiratory volume in 1 s; FVC, forced vital capacity.

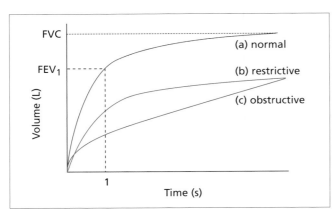

Fig. 49 Spirometry curves for (a) a normal patient; (b) patient with a restrictive lung defect; and (c) patient with an obstructive lung defect. FEV$_1$, forced expiratory volume after 1 s; FVC, forced vital capacity.

Gas transfer

TL_{CO} and K_{CO} are measurements of gas diffusion across the alveolar membrane. K_{CO} is corrected for lung volume as $K_{CO} = TL_{CO}/Va$, where Va is the alveolar volume available for gas exchange. In the laboratory, carbon monoxide is used to calculate this diffusion capacity, hence the 'CO' after the terms.

If you imagine the alveolar membrane in its healthy state as being thin and permeable, say like a sheet of tissue paper, any pathological process that causes it to become thickened and coarse will slow down the movement of carbon monoxide (or oxygen) from the lung into the blood stream. Conversely, increased levels of blood and therefore haemoglobin, either in the blood stream or in the alveoli, will cause an increase in the uptake of oxygen (Table 32).

Flow–volume loops

These measure the expiratory and inspiratory flow of air (L/s) against actual volume exhaled or inhaled. The upper, expiratory curve starts with the patient at maximum/forced inhalation (TLC) and ends at total/forced expiration (RV).

The curves have characteristic shapes according to the

Table 32 Causes of increased and decreased K_{CO}.

Change in K_{CO}	Mechanism	Examples
Increased	Reduced V_A	Skeletal deformity, pleural disease and respiratory muscle weakness
	Increased capillary blood volume	Left-to-right shunt, lung haemorrhage, polycythaemia
Reduced	Destruction of lung tissue	Emphysema
	Impairment to diffusion by disease	Fibrosing alveolitis
	Reduced blood flow to pulmonary capillaries	Pulmonary vascular disease or hypertension, right-to-left shunt
	Reduced uptake by blood	Anaemia

underlying disease process and whether the pathology is causing intra- or extrathoracic obstruction to the airflow, thus distorting the shape of the curve from the normal. The most important patterns are those of expiratory flow limitation (Fig. 50).

3.6.3 OVERNIGHT OXIMETRY

This relatively cheap and easy test can be used as a baseline investigation to screen for possible sleep apnoea patients who report disturbed sleep and/or daytime somnolence. The patient's SaO_2 is continuously recorded via a finger probe while they rest.

Analysis of the results looks for drops in the saturation and the frequency of these events, which may represent episodes of apnoea. (See Section 1.8, p. 172.) Patients with recurrent hypoxic episodes and/or large dips in their oxygen should be referred for formal assessment by a physician interested in sleep disorders.

3.6.4 CHEST RADIOGRAPH

Stand back at least 1–2 m and take a long hard look. Does anything strike you straight away? If so, fine, but do not ignore the rest. Then proceed systematically as described below.

Heart

• Is the heart size normal or does it look enlarged? Estimate the cardiac width with that of the thorax; the heart should fill less than half the thoracic width.
• Follow the contours of the heart; are there any 'bits' that should not be there? Do they correspond to enlarged ventricles or atria or are they something else?
• Is there anything sitting behind the heart that makes it look distorted, e.g. dilated oesophagus, stomach?

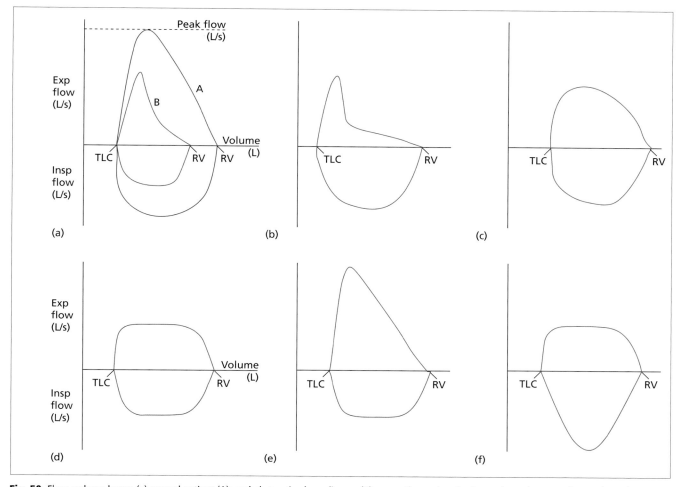

Fig. 50 Flow–volume loops: (a) normal patient (A); and obstructive lung disease (B), e.g. asthma, chronic obstructive pulmonary disease (COPD); (b) emphysema; (c) restrictive lung defect, e.g. pulmonary fibrosis; (d) fixed intra- or extrathoracic obstruction, e.g. tracheal tumour; (e) variable extrathoracic obstruction, e.g. tracheal stenosis outside the thoracic cavity, works like a one-way valve, opening on expiration while collapsing on inspiration; (f) variable intrathoracic obstruction. RV, residual volume; TLC, total lung capacity.

Lungs

• First of all, ignore the lung fields, and take a good look around the edge of the lung at the pleura—is it thickened or calcified? Are there any obvious pleural plaques? These can look surprisingly like retained self-adhesive ECG pads (and vice versa!).

• Now inspect the lung fields. Are all the pulmonary lobes and fissures present, or are they distorted, collapsed or consolidated? If there is an abnormality—where is it, how would you describe it? Shape (oval, round, wedge), size, texture (honeycomb, patchy).

Bones

• Are they of equal density throughout, or do they look 'moth-eaten'? Is there any evidence of cysts or osteolytic changes? Is there any evidence of old or new fractures, e.g. pathological fractures?

• Look carefully along the ribs for fractures or notches. Turning the chest radiograph on its side and studying the ribs often helps detract your attention from everything else.

 If a radiograph seems normal do not forget to double check the bones, the apices and the area behind the heart. Are you missing a small pneumothorax? Is there an extrathoracic abnormality (e.g. a mastectomy)? If in doubt, ask a radiologist!

Figure 51 shows in diagrammatic fashion the radiographic patterns of lobar collapse, and examples of lobar collapse.

3.6.5 COMPUTED TOMOGRAPHY SCAN OF THE THORAX

There are a number of indications for CT scans of the thorax and, as with all investigations, you need to be

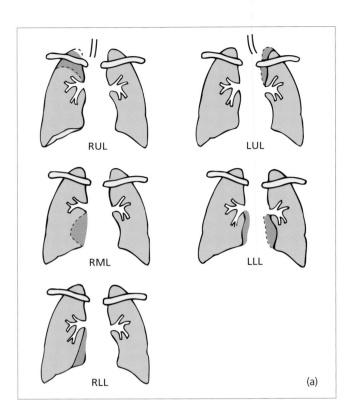

RUL

LUL

RML

LLL

RLL

(a)

Fig. 51 (a) Diagrammatic representation of the radiographic patterns of lobar collapse. Helpful information may be provided by the position of the trachea, the hilar vascular shadows and the horizontal fissure. (b) Chest radiograph of right upper lobe collapse secondary to *Mycobacterium* infection. Note the tracheal deviation and air bronchogram. Right upper lobe collapse also tends to cause elevation of the horizontal fissure, tenting (but not elevation) of the right diaphragm and a raised right hilum. (c) Potentially difficult radiograph of right middle lobe collapse. The key is the increased opacification obscuring the right cardiac border. (d) Lateral view of the right middle lobe collapse patient in (c) with a wedge of opacity in the region of the middle lobe. (e) Left lower lobe collapse; note the classic presence of 'sail sign', where the collapsed lobe lies behind the heart; also left mediastinal shift, left hilar depression and loss of the left hemidiaphragm. (See Fig. 19, p. 181 for radiographs of left upper lobe collapse, and also Fig. 18, p. 180 for another example of RUL collapse.) LLL, left lower lobe; LUL, left upper lobe; RLL, right lower lobe; RML, right middle lobe; RUL, right upper lobe. (Courtesy of Dr I. Vlahos.)

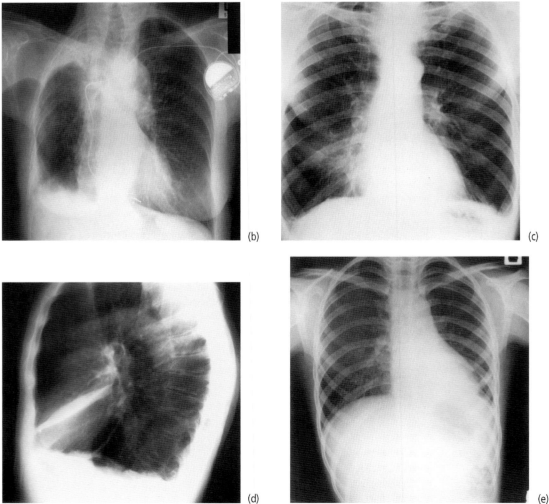

(b)

(c)

(d)

(e)

detailed on the request form as to the reasons for the test in order for the radiologists to give you the best possible service. A variety of techniques are used.

Figure 52 shows the principal mediastinal structures seen on CT scanning of the thorax.

Type of scans

High-resolution scans

Here the lung is imaged at small intervals or sections. These are often invaluable in the diagnosis of parenchymal lung disease and can be diagnostic of certain conditions, thus avoiding further more invasive investigations, e.g. sarcoidosis—beading, and pulmonary fibrosis—honeycombing of the lung.

You should also ask for the radiologist to perform prone and supine films, i.e. scan the patient lying on both back and front. This is to ensure that pulmonary interstitial fluid is not mimicking the changes of fibrosis: fluid will move downwards, while fibrosis remains in the same area of the lung on both views (Fig. 53).

Conventional scans

Staging scans for suspected lung cancer (or other discrete lesions like abcesses) involve the scanner imaging at wider intervals. The images are reproduced in two settings:
• bony or soft-tissue windows—highlight lymph node enlargement, soft-tissue involvement and bony lesions
• lung windows—concentrate on the lung parenchyma, producing images of the tumour as well as the condition of the surrounding lung, i.e. coexisting emphysema, bullae or fibrosis.

Helical computed tomography

Spiral CT is the latest technological improvement in this form of scanning. It is fast and a complete scan can be completed in one breath-hold. They are increasingly useful in the diagnosis of pulmonary emboli when contrast media is used to create a pulmonary angiogram.

Reading a scan

When you assess a CT scan, remember that you are viewing it as though you are standing at the patient's feet looking upwards, so the patient's liver is on the left of the picture and the spleen on the right, etc. Like the chest radiograph, try to follow a system through the scans.
• Follow the main vessels such as the descending and ascending aorta and its arch.
• Look carefully for enlargement of the hilar and paratracheal lymph nodes and any other soft-tissue changes (Fig. 54).
• Look at the lung windows—study the lung parenchyma and run your eye carefully around the pleura looking for any thickening, plaques and/or adjacent fibrosis.
• Finally, show a radiologist and, for your education, ask them to talk you through the scan.

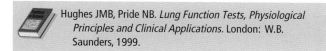

Hughes JMB, Pride NB. *Lung Function Tests, Physiological Principles and Clinical Applications.* London: W.B. Saunders, 1999.

Acknowledgements

The authors and editor would like to thank the following people for their help in the preparation of this module: Professor M. Green, Imperial College of Science Medicine and Technology, Dr J. Moore-Gillon, Department of Respiratory Medicine, Barts and The London NHS Trust, London, Dr L. Kuitert, Department of Respiratory Medicine, Barts and The London NHS Trust, London and Dr I. Vlahos, Academic Department of Radiology, Barts and The London NHS Trust, London.

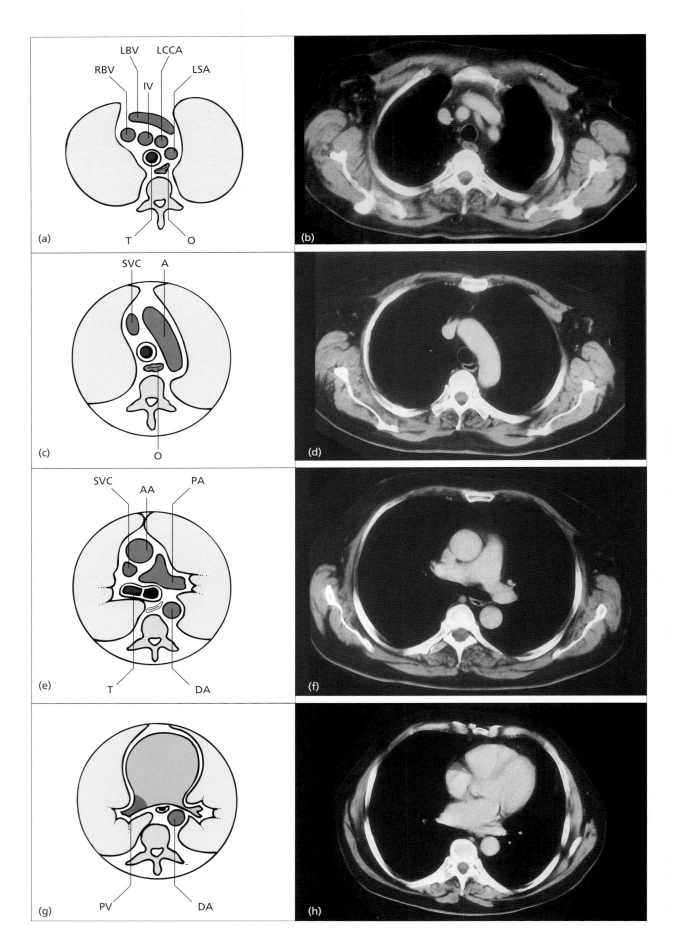

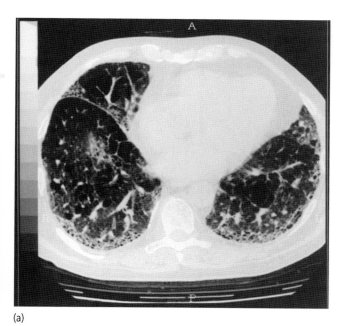

(a)

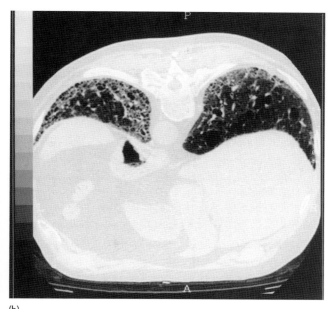

(b)

Fig. 53 Computed tomography scan of the thorax (a) supine and
(b) prone, of a man with pulmonary fibrosis. Note the different positioning
of the patient on the scanning table (at the bottom of both films). The
honeycombing appearance of the lungs remains posterior in both views.

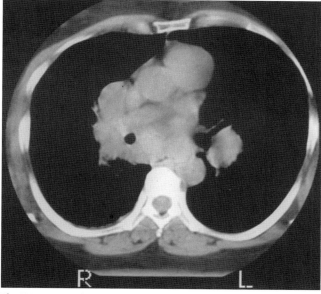

Fig. 54 Computed tomography of the thorax; note the mass of lymph
nodes that is distorting the normal architecture of the mediastinum. This
patient was subsequently diagnosed as having sarcoidosis.

Fig. 52 (*Opposite*) Principal mediastinal structures on computed tomography scanning of the thorax. Remember that you are viewing the sections from
below, i.e. the left of the thorax is on the right of the figure. (a and b) Section above the aortic arch. The trachea (T), oesophagus (O), right brachiocephalic
vein (RBV), left brachiocephalic vein (LBV), innominate vein (IV), left common carotid artery (LCCA), and left subclavian artery (LSA) are visible. (c and d)
Section at the level of the aortic arch (A). The superior vena cava (SVC) is visible. (e and f) Section below aortic arch. Both ascending (AA) and descending
(DA) aortas are visible. The trachea (T) is bifurcated and pulmonary arteries (PA) are seen. Note in (f) that the bifurcation of the trachea is present behind
the pulmonary arteries, but difficult to see in cross-section. (g and h) Section at the level of the pulmonary veins (PV). Lower lobe intrapulmonary arteries
and bronchi are not shown in the diagram. (Computed tomography scans courtesy of Dr I. Vlahos.)

4 Self-assessment

Answers are on pp. 260–262.

Question 1
A 28-year-old man presents with breathlessness. He appears anxious, but physical examination is otherwise normal. His chest radiograph is shown (Figure 55). The diagnosis is:
A normal chest radiograph
B pulmonary oligaemia suggesting pulmonary embolism
C pneumothorax
D left lower lobe collapse
E right lower lobe collapse

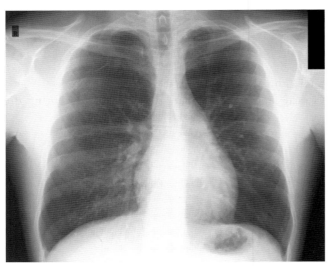

Fig. 55 Question 1.

Question 2
A 52-year-old woman presents with breathlessness that has been getting gradually worse for a couple of months. She smokes 10 cigarettes per day, which she has done for many years, has long-standing atrial fibrillation (AF), presumed ischaemic in origin, and takes furosemide, amiodarone, aspirin and atorvastatin as regular medications. On examination her pulse is 80/min (AF), blood pressure 120/80 mmHg, jugular venous pressure elevated 3 cm above the sternal angle and there are fine inspiratory crackles to mid zones bilaterally. Heart sounds are normal, and she does not have peripheral oedema. Her chest radiograph is shown (Figure 56). What is the most likely diagnosis?
A interstitial lung disease
B pulmonary oedema

C chronic pulmonary embolism
D chronic obstructive pulmonary disease
E late onset asthma

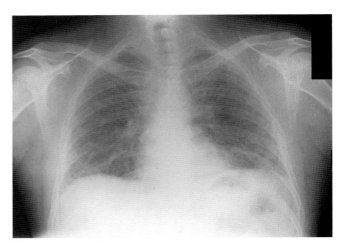

Fig. 56 Question 2.

Question 3
A 45-year-old man who smoked 15 cigarettes/day for 20 years, but stopped 3 years ago, now presents with cough and malaise. He had a deep venous thrombosis of his right leg 20 years previously after an operation to remove a cartilage from his right knee, but otherwise he has no significant past medical history, takes no regular medications, and physical examination is normal. His chest radiograph is shown (Figure 57). The most likely diagnosis is:
A lung cancer
B sarcoidosis

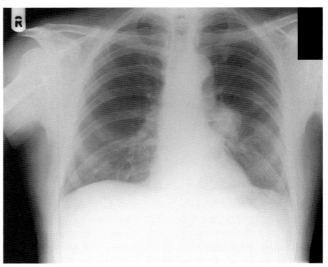

Fig. 57 Question 3.

C pulmonary hypertension
D pneumonia
E interstitial lung disease

Question 4

A 62-year-old man who smoked 10 cigarettes/day for 15 years, but stopped smoking about 30 years ago, presents with a month's history of breathlessness. He assumed that this was due to a 'chest infection', but matters have not improved, leading him to seek medical attention. He may have had a 'bit of a temperature', but he has had no other respiratory symptoms and physical examination is normal. His chest radiograph is shown (Figure 58). The diagnosis is:
A left lower lobe collapse
B right middle lobe collapse
C right upper lobe collapse
D left pneumothorax
E chronic obstructive pulmonary disease

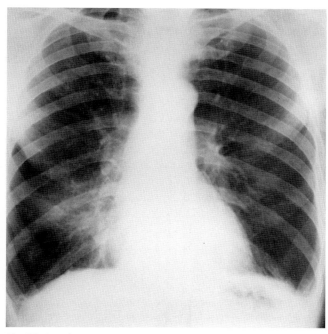

Fig. 58 Question 4.

Question 5

A 35-year-old man presents with a first episode of haemoptysis. He has felt a bit feverish for the last few days, but has not had sweats or rigors. He is generally fit and well and gives no history of previous respiratory problems. On examination his temperature is 37.8°C and his chest is clear. Which two of the following are the most likely diagnoses?
A pulmonary tuberculosis
B bronchiectasis
C pneumonia
D lung cancer

E benign bronchial tumour
F pulmonary arteriovenous malformation
G asthma
H chronic obstructive pulmonary disease
I Goodpasture's syndrome
J pulmonary embolism

Question 6

A 27-year-old woman with asthma is admitted with an acute attack. Her symptoms started around 8.00 am, but by 10.00 am she was so unwell that she needed admission to hospital. Shortly after arriving at the Accident and Emergency department she was transferred to the Intensive Care Unit. Similar incidents had occurred twice in the past. Which two of the following statements regarding near fatal asthma are correct?
A previous severe asthma attacks are a risk factor
B the short time lag between the start of symptoms and hospital admission is a risk factor
C females are especially at risk
D the risk increases in obese patients
E family history of asthma is common
F allergy to peanut is commoner in patients with near fatal asthma
G near fatal asthma occurs more frequently during the winter season
H long acting beta-2 agonists are beneficial in preventing asthma attacks
I childhood eczema is a risk factor
J parental smoking is a risk factor.

Question 7

A 35-year-old postman presents with a history of breathlessness that has been getting gradually worse over 6 months. He coughs up sputum regularly, but is otherwise well, with no significant past medical history. He smoked five to ten cigarettes per day from the age of 18 to 26 years. The two most likely diagnoses are:
A cystic fibrosis
B emphysema
C congestive cardiac failure
D alpha-1 antitrypsin deficiency
E pneumoconiosis
F asbestosis
G hypogammaglobulinaemia
H chronic obstructive pulmonary disease
I bronchial asthma
J postman's lung

Question 8

A 38-year-old woman presents with a two-year history of worsening breathlessness. Results of preliminary investigation are as follows: spirometry—Forced Expiratory Volume in one second (FEV1) 83% predicted, Vital

Capacity (VC) 79% predicted, FEV1/VC ratio 78%; chest radiograph reported as being within normal limits; blood gases (breathing air)—PaO_2 9.6 kPa, $PaCO_2$ 4.1 kPa. What are the two most likely diagnoses?

A chronic obstructive pulmonary disease

B cardiac failure

C diffuse parenchymal lung disease

D pneumocystis carinii pneumonia

E anaemia

F bronchiectasis

G asthma

H pulmonary vascular disease

I diabetes mellitus

J primary hyperventilation

Question 9

A 36-year-old woman is admitted with a history of cough and shortness of breath of 8 weeks' duration. Her chest radiograph shows bilateral mid-zone infiltrates and blood count shows a raised eosinophil count. Which two of the following drugs might be responsible for her condition?

A bleomycin

B amiodarone

C calcium tablets

D prednisolone

E heroin

F insulin

G cyclophosphamide

H busulfan

I sulfasalazine

J paracetamol

Question 10

A 37-year-old man with asthma comes to your clinic. His current medication consists of a low dose of inhaled corticosteroids and inhaled short-acting beta-2 agonist that he takes, on average, three to four times a day. What would you do?

A advise him to continue with his current medication

B commence a high dose of inhaled corticosteroid

C add an inhaled long-acting beta-2 agonist

D add a leucotriene receptor antagonist

E add a long-acting anticholinergic

Question 11

A 43-year-old woman with long-standing asthma is admitted with an exacerbation. She is cyanosed and unable to speak more than three words at a time. She is using her accessory muscles, chest expansion is reduced but the same on both sides, and a wheeze can be heard bilaterally. Which one of the following is the best initial treatment?

A maximum inspired oxygen by face mask; nebulised salbutamol (5 mg) driven by oxygen

B nebulised salbutamol (5 mg) driven by air

C nebulised salbutamol (50 mg) driven by oxygen

D oxygen 35% by face mask; nebulised salbutamol (10 mg) driven by 35% oxygen

E maximum inspired oxygen by face mask; decompress both sides of the chest by inserting venflons into the second intercostal spaces in the mid-clavicular line bilaterally.

Question 12

A 74-year-old man is treated in hospital for exacerbation of chronic obstructive pulmonary disease (COPD). His condition improves significantly and he is keen to go home. His repeated arterial blood gas (ABG) analysis (on air) shows a pH of 7.35, pCO_2 of 4.5 kPa, pO_2 of 7.1 kPa, HCO_3 of 26 mmol/L. What action would be most appropriate?

A prescribe the patient an oxygen cylinder on discharge

B discharge the patient once his ABG analysis returns to normal

C request an oxygen concentrator and discharge the patient once an oxygen concentrator is fitted

D discharge the patient and arrange a follow up in 6 weeks' time with a repeated ABG

E discharge the patient and advise a follow up by his GP

Question 13

A 58-year-old man, a smoker for many years despite repeated advice that he should stop, has chronic obstructive pulmonary disease (COPD) that is increasingly limiting his exercise capacity. You wish to conduct a trial of steroid therapy. Which of the following is the correct way of giving oral prednisolone and interpreting the outcome?

A 60 mg daily for 4 weeks, regarding a clear statement of subjective improvement by the patient as a positive response

B 10 mg daily for 2 weeks, regarding a clear statement of subjective improvement by the patient as a positive response if accompanied by a rise in FEV1

C 60 mg daily for 4 weeks, regarding a clear statement of subjective improvement by the patient as a positive response if accompanied by a rise in FEV1 of >10%

D 30 mg daily for 2 weeks, regarding an increase in FEV1 of >10% and >200 ml as a positive response

E 30 mg daily for 2 weeks, regarding a clear statement of subjective improvement by the patient as a positive response

Question 14

A 24-year-old man presents with fever, breathlessness, cough and sputum production. His only medical history of note is long-standing heavy alcohol consumption, but he had no respiratory complaint whatever until 6 weeks ago when he developed breathing difficulty with high fever and rigors. He was given antibiotics by his general practitioner and began to improve, but this improvement has not been sustained. The most likely diagnosis is:

A lung abscess
B bronchiectasis
C chronic obstructive pulmonary disease (COPD)
D asthma precipitated by chest infection
E empyema

Question 15

A 40-year-old woman, generally fit and well, is admitted with malaise and fever. Four weeks previously she had suffered a chest infection for which she was given a course of oral antibiotics. She felt better initially, but never recovered fully and is now getting worse. Her chest radiograph shows a right-sided pleural effusion. The most likely diagnosis is:
A connective tissue disorder
B lung cancer
C tuberculosis
D pulmonary embolism
E pneumonia with effusion/empyema

Question 16

A 56-year-old woman, a smoker of 20 cigarettes daily, presents with a 6-month history of progressive shortness of breath. Her past medical history is unremarkable apart from Raynaud's syndrome for which she takes a calcium channel blocker. On examination no significant abnormality is found apart from telangiectasia. Her chest radiograph shows clear lung fields, prominent pulmonary arteries and mildly enlarged heart. Spirometry is normal, but gas transfer is reduced to 50% predicted. What is the most likely diagnosis?
A cor pulmonale secondary to chronic obstructive pulmonary disease
B multiple pulmonary emboli
C pulmonary arterial hypertension
D sarcoidosis
E congestive cardiac failure

Question 17

A 63-year-old man attends the hospital with a history of proximal muscle weakness. He also gives a history of a cough of 8 weeks duration and complains of pain in the small joints of the hands. On examination he has small haemorrhages in the nail folds, but is not clubbed. There are bi-basal crackles, and a chest radiograph reveals diffuse reticular infiltrates. Lung function tests confirm a restrictive pattern. What is the underlying cause of his interstitial lung disease?
A cryptogenic fibrosing alveolitis
B ankylosing spondylitis
C polymyositis/dermatomyositis
D rheumatoid arthritis
E mixed connective tissue disorder

Question 18

A 26-year-old man is admitted with a history of 4–6 weeks of breathlessness. He initially had flu-like symptoms and was treated by his doctor with a 10-day course of ciprofloxacin. However, he then started coughing up blood, leading to urgent referral. On examination he is breathless at rest, with bilateral crackles in the lungs. Investigation reveals anaemia and impaired renal function (creatinine 220 µmol/l). Pulmonary function tests are normal apart from an abnormally high transfer factor. Urine dipstick testing shows the presence of red blood cells. What is the most likely diagnosis?
A pneumococcal pneumonia with post-streptococcal nephritis
B Goodpasture's syndrome
C chronic eosinophilic pneumonia
D bronchiolitis obliterans
E Churg-Strauss

Question 19

A 35-year-old woman is referred with a history of red, painful legs of 3 weeks duration that have not responded to a course of amoxycillin and flucloxacillin given for presumed cellulitis. She is afebrile, does not have any other symptoms, and has never smoked. Examination reveals tender purple/red nodules on her shins. Her full blood count, kidney and liver function tests are normal. A chest radiograph shows prominent hilae. What is the appropriate management?
A arrange bronchoscopy and bronchoalveolar lavage to exclude malignancy
B start azathioprine and prednisolone; follow up in clinic
C start prednisolone; follow up in clinic
D start simple analgesics; follow up in clinic
E arrange CT scan of the lungs and lung biopsy

Question 20

A 65-year-old woman is admitted with left sided pneumonia and pleural effusion. Pleural fluid is aspirated and sent for testing. Which of the following is an indication for inserting a chest drain?
A pleural fluid pH < 7.2
B serous pleural fluid
C blood stained pleural fluid
D pleural fluid glucose >2 mmol/l
E pleural fluid lactate dehydrogenase >200 IU/l

Question 21

A 78-year-old man is referred to the chest clinic with history of dyspnoea for over 3 months. He is a retired teacher and has never smoked. He has a past medical history of atrial fibrillation, which is well controlled on digoxin. He also takes warfarin and the occasional paracetamol. He is clubbed and hypoxic on air with a

SaO_2 of 89%. He has bilateral crackles and a chest radiograph confirms fibrosing alveolitis. Which of the following combination of lung function is typical of this condition?

A reduced FEV1 & FVC, FEV1/FVC < 70%, raised TLC & RV, reduced TLCO

B reduced FEV1 & FVC, FEV1/FVC > 70%, raised TLC & RV, reduced TLCO

C normal FEV1 & FVC, FEV1/FVC > 70%, raised TLC & RV, reduced TLCO

D reduced FEV1 & FVC, FEV1/FVC > 70%, reduced TLC & RV, reduced TLCO

E reduced FEV1 & FVC, FEV1/FVC > 70%, raised TLC & RV, normal TLCO

Question 22

A 40-year-old man, a smoker of 40 pack years, presents with a 3-month history of shortness of breath. His past medical history includes hypertension, cervical spondylosis and depression. Spirometry shows Forced Expiratory Volume in one second (FEV1) of 1.03 litres—67% predicted, Forced Vital Capacity (FVC) 1.03 litres—53% predicted, and FEV1/FVC of 96%. How would you interpret his spirometry results?

A normal for his age

B obstructive defect

C mixed defect

D restrictive defect

E unable to interpret as bronchial reversibility not done

Question 23

A 43-year-old woman presents with breathlessness that has been getting gradually worse over a few weeks and now makes it difficult for her to walk upstairs. On physical examination she is found to have a large left sided pleural effusion but no other abnormalities. The presence of the effusion is confirmed by chest radiography. The most appropriate initial investigation would be:

A CT chest

B diagnostic aspiration of pleural fluid followed by drainage of effusion to dryness

C diagnostic aspiration of pleural fluid with pleural biopsy

D sputum cytology

E diagnostic aspiration of pleural fluid

Question 24

A 65-year-old man presents with a history of worsening breathlessness and cough. His arterial blood gases (breathing air) show the following: pH 7.26, pO_2 6.5 kPa, pCO_2 9.5 kPa, bicarbonate 32 mmol/L. Which of the following is the most likely diagnosis?

A obstructive sleep apnoea

B acute asthma

C pulmonary embolism

D acute exacerbation of chronic obstructive pulmonary disease

E pulmonary oedema

Question 25

You are called to the resuscitation room to see a 25-year-old man whose condition has suddenly deteriorated. He had arrived 30 minutes earlier with a 2-hour history of central pleuritic chest pain and breathlessness. He collapsed while awaiting a chest radiograph and now is agitated and cyanosed with pulse 120/min and BP 80/40 mmHg. Oxygen saturation is reading 79%, with the patient breathing high flow oxygen via a re-breathe mask. Respiratory examination reveals reduced breath sounds in the right lung field with deviation of the trachea towards the left. Percussion is resonant bilaterally. What immediate course of action should you take?

A arrange for urgent portable chest radiograph

B contact the Intensive Care Unit to arrange for the patient to be ventilated

C insert large bore needle into left hemithorax

D insert large bore needle into right hemithorax

E check arterial blood gases and commence BiPAP if hypoxia is confirmed

Answers to
Self-assessment

Cardiology

Answer to Question 1

C

The most likely explanation for the history and physical findings is aortic dissection causing aortic regurgitation and with leakage of blood into the pericardium. The chest radiograph (Figure 115) is not diagnostic, but shows a suspicion of a widened mediastinum that would support this diagnosis. Urgent CT scan of the chest or transoesophageal echocardiography is required to make the diagnosis.

Answer to Question 2

D

The ECG (Figure 116) shows a short PR interval and δ waves, diagnostic of the Wolff-Parkinson-White syndrome.

Answer to Question 3

E

The patient had severe mitral regurgitation and the radiograph (Figure 117) shows cardiomegaly with an enlarged left atrium and pulmonary oedema.

Answer to Question 4

D

The ECG (Figure 118) shows ST segment elevation in leads V1-4(5) consistent with acute anterior myocardial infarction, and there are ventricular ectopics. There is no significant ST segment elevation in leads I, AVL or V6, as would be expected with lateral extension, and there are no features of posterior extension.

Answer to Question 5

E, I

Restoration of sinus rhythm can be achieved pharmacologically or by DC cardioversion. However, DC cardioversion is not likely to lead to permanent restoration of sinus rhythm in a patient who has had previous episodes of AF, hence in this case an attempt at 'chemical cardioversion' is appropriate. Class III agents—potassium channel blockers that prolong myocyte repolarisation—are most appropriate: sotalol or amiodarone. Digoxin can be used for rate control but does not promote return of sinus rhythm, indeed it's use may make this more unlikely. Class I agents—e.g. quinidine, procaineamide and disopyramide, which prolong the action potential—have been used to try to restore sinus rhythm, but NOT in patients with ischaemic heart disease (such as this man).

Answer to Question 6

C, F

Whenever you approach a patient with a broad complex tachycardia it is always safest to presume they have ventricular tachycardia until proven otherwise. In fact, it is most likely that they will have a ventricular tachycardia rather than one of the other possibilities above, which may produce similar traces on a Holter monitor. Patients with ventricular tachycardia are not always syncopal, indeed right ventricular outflow tract tachycardia usually presents with just palpitations. It occurs as a result of a triggered focus in the right ventricular outflow tract and generally carries an excellent prognosis. It is best treated with radiofrequency ablation. This is in contrast to ischaemic ventricular tachycardia which carries a very poor prognosis unless treated appropriately. In the context of impaired left ventricular function this invariably means with an implantable cardioverter defibrillator (ICD).

Answer to Question 7

C, I

Cardiac complications of Marfan's are relatively common. Usually they are related to aortic involvement, but Marfan's is associated with mitral valve prolapse and regurgitation, left ventricular dilatation and cardiac failure, pulmonary artery dilatation and regurgitation of the pulmonary valve.

Answer to Question 8

F, G

The patient has a non-ST-segment elevation myocardial infarction (NSTEMI) and has a high risk of further adverse cardiac events. The mainstay of initial treatment is aggressive anti-platelet therapy: aspirin with the addition of clopidogrel, and consideration of an infusion of Glycoprotein IIb/IIa receptor blocker (blocks the platelet receptor). A therapeutic dose of low molecular weight heparin should be commenced, and early angiography and percutaneous coronary intervention should be considered. Thrombolysis has not been shown to benefit patients with NSTEMI.

Answer to Question 9

G, H

All of the conditions listed, excepting hypothyroidism, might explain hypertension, but all other than essential hypertension and 'white coat' hypertension are rare (together accounting for less than 5% of cases). Although a secondary cause of hypertension is very unlikely it would be important to look for clues in history and examination that might suggest renovascular disease (ischaemic heart disease, transient ischmaemic attack (TIA) / stroke, peripheral vascular disease), renal disease (previous nephritis, results of urine testing for e.g. insurance/employment medicals). Episodes of palpitations, sweating or headache may suggest phaeochromocytoma, but a less exotic cause such as anxiety would be a much more likely explanation. The serum potassium concentration is just below the lower limit of normal, but primary hyper-aldosteronism (Conn's syndrome) remains exceedingly unlikely. In the case of an obese man it is also important to note that the blood pressure reading may be falsely elevated as a result of inadequate blood pressure cuff size, and it would be important to ensure that readings were taken with appropriate equipment.

Answer to Question 10

E

The guidelines on basic life support identify the importance of early access to defibrillation in cardiac arrest. They therefore suggest that no CPR is commenced until a call for emergency services has been made and the potential for early defibrillation is made possible. Once CPR begins the ratio of compressions to ventilations is 15 to 2. A precordial thump is not indicated in the unwitnessed collapse.

Answer to Question 11

D

This man has ischaemic cardiomyopathy, but no evidence of reversible ischaemia on functional (thallium) assessment. He has had symptomatic VT and therefore is at high risk of sudden death. Current evidence suggests that he will gain prognostic benefit from implantation of an implantable cardioverter defibrillator. Beta-blockers have also been shown to independently improve prognosis (and symptoms) in patients with impaired left ventricular function.

Answer to Question 12

B

Pacemaker types are identified by a 3 or 4 letter code. The first letter indicates the chamber paced (A = atrium; V = ventricle; D = both or dual), the second letter represents which chamber is sensed; and the third is what response the pacemaker gives to a sensed beat (I = inhibit; T = trigger; D = both). The fourth, usually R (rate responsive) is for more sophisticated technologies. In this case of complete heart block, in order to maintain AV synchrony, a dual chamber pacemaker is required (DDD). Assuming the atrial (p wave) rate is normal the function will be generally sensing the p wave and then pacing the ventricle.

Answer to Question 13

B

This man has severe aortic stenosis and concomitant coronary artery disease. Whilst it is impossible to differentiate which lesion is causing his current symptoms, symptomatic aortic stenosis is associated with significantly impaired prognosis and surgical intervention is warranted. Percutaneous aortic valvotomy is relatively unsuccessful in adults, with rapid restenosis.

Answer to Question 14

D

Clinically this man has an infected mitral valve replacement with a severe paravalvular leak. Following surgery the commonest infecting organisms (up to around 9 months) are coagulase negative staphylococci. Antibiotics alone will not cure the infection; the valve must be replaced again. In this case this should be with a metallic valve since a bioprosthetic valve would be likely to need replacing after 10–15 years due to degeneration, thereby subjecting him to a high-risk third operation. Bioprosthetic and metallic valves have similar risk for subsequent endocarditis.

Answer to Question 15

D

Given the lack of signs and family history of sudden death the most likely diagnosis is pulmonary hypertension. Further investigations would include transthoracic echocardiography and left and right cardiac catheterisation.

Answer to Question 16

B

Exercise testing has long been an established method for identifying patients with underlying coronary disease. Apart from changes in the ST segments, other features associated with underlying disease and adverse prognosis are ventricular arrhythmias, inadequate blood pressure response, inadequate heart rate response and angina.

Answer to Question 17

C

Patients with heart failure are considered for cardiac transplantation when significant symptoms persist despite maximal medical therapy. Due to the shortage of donors clinical guidelines have been established highlighting patients most suitable for transplantation. Significant impairment of renal function is generally considered to be a contraindication, assuming this is not reversible. Patients with prior history of cancer may be considered if there is no evidence recurrence (>5 years on from diagnosis of cancer).

Answer to Question 18

B

Beta-blockers have prognostic and symptomatic benefit in heart failure. In the UK only carvedilol and bisoprolol are licensed for this use. Digoxin can improve symptoms in severe heart failure. Whilst it may well slow resting heart rate in atrial fibrillation it has less benefit on exercise related increases in rate. This patient has permanent atrial fibrillation and DC cardioversion will not, by definition, restore sinus rhythm.

Answer to Question 19

B

Unless it is definitely known that a patient has a tendency to retain carbon dioxide, all patients with severe breathlessness should be given high flow oxygen via a reservoir bag once it has been established that their airway is clear. After the patient has been started on high flow oxygen, give furosemide 40–80 mg IV and diamorphine 2.5–5 mg IV. If matters do not improve consider isosorbide dinitrate 2–10 mg/hr IV. If matters worsen, then call the Intensive Care Unit (ICU) sooner rather than later (assuming that the man's condition prior to this acute presentation means that this is appropriate). Concurrently try to establish a cause for the acute deterioration: has he had a myocardial infarction? If so, would he benefit from thrombolysis?

Answer to Question 20

D

Anterior myocardial infarction is typically associated with an apical ventricular septal defect (VSD), whilst inferior myocardial infarction is more commonly associated with a basal VSD or posterior papillary muscle rupture. After confirmation of diagnosis by echocardiography or right heart catheter, which reveals a step up in oxygenation at ventricular level, urgent referral to a surgical centre is required, the outlook without surgical repair being extremely poor. Anterior myocardial infarction associated with an apical VSD carries a better surgical outlook than inferior myocardial infarction associated with basal VSD.

Answer to Question 21

C

The top priority is to achieve myocardial reperfusion. The presence of chest pain and ST segment elevation on ECG indicate that thrombolysis is needed immediately, notwithstanding the presence of Q waves.

Answer to Question 22

D

Drug treatment to lower serum cholesterol should be based on a person's risk of an ischaemic heart disease (IHD) event rather than initial cholesterol level. Any person who has had a myocardial infarction has about a 10% chance (without treatment) of dying from ischaemic heart disease in the following year, and about a 5% chance of IHD death in each year thereafter. All such people (in the absence of contraindications to the specific drugs) qualify for HMG-coenzyme A reductase inhibitor therapy (statins) regardless of their cholesterol level. There is a constant proportional relationship between serum cholesterol and disease risk, so any reduction in cholesterol level from any starting point leads to the same proportional reduction in IHD risk. Those people with the highest absolute starting risk (namely those with pre-existing IHD, such as this man who has had an AMI) stand to benefit the most. Non-pharmacological means of serum cholesterol reduction are far less effective, and whilst important are inadequate as sole treatment in this patient.

Answer to Question 23

A

The combination of a young patient and a 'flu-like illness makes acute viral pericarditis the most likely diagnosis in this case. The chest pain of pericarditis can be indistinguishable from that of myocardial infarction, excepting that sitting forward often eases it. The key physical sign to elicit would be a pericardial rub, and the key initial investigation would be the ECG, looking for widespread ST segment elevation, concave upwards.

Answer to Question 24

B

A normal lung perfusion scan has a specificity of around 98% for pulmonary embolism (PE), whilst specificity for CT is usually quoted at around 85% because small peripheral clots may be missed. CT scanning may, however, reveal an alternative explanation for a patient's symptoms. Although a negative D-dimer test is helpful in the context of a low index of clinical suspicion, some studies have indicated a false negative rate as high as 20% for patients with high clinical probability and most algorithms would not sanction the use of D-dimer testing at all in patients with high clinical probability. Neither normal chest radiograph, normal arterial blood gases, nor the absence of deep venous thrombosis (DVT) can be used in isolation to rule out pulmonary embolism, although they may all be helpful as part of an algorithm for the management of patients with breathlessness or pleuritic chest pain of uncertain cause.

Answer to Question 25

C

Breathlessness is the commonest symptom of pulmonary embolism (PE), and syncope is a less common (and often poorly recognised) presenting symptom. The patient is hypoxic with an oxygen saturation of only 92% on 40% oxygen, and he has non-specific but recognised ECG changes of PE. His recent varicose vein surgery is a risk factor.

Acute myocardial infarction rarely presents with syncope with no ECG changes, and ongoing hypoxia would not be explained with a 'normal' chest radiograph. Chronic obstructive pulmonary disease (COPD) is also unlikely as the cause of syncope with little evidence of severe airways obstruction.

Respiratory Medicine

Answer to Question 1
C

There is right-sided pneumothorax.

Answer to Question 2
A

The chest radiograph (Figure 56) shows bilateral alveolar shadowing due to amiodarone-induced interstitial lung disease. Pulmonary oedema could cause identical radiographic appearances in the lungs, but the normal heart sounds (no gallop rhythm) and normal sized heart on the radiograph are both against this diagnosis.

Answer to Question 3
A

The radiograph (Figure 57) shows a left hilar mass, which proved to be a large-cell carcinoma.

Answer to Question 4
B

There is opacification obscuring the right heart border due to right middle lobe collapse. A lateral radiograph of the same patient is shown in Figure 51(d) on page 246 of the Respiratory Module, clearly showing a wedge of opacity in the region of the right middle lobe.

Answer to Question 5
C, J

The most common cause of haemoptysis in a young patient is pulmonary infection, either with pyogenic bacteria or mycobacterium tuberculosis depending on the clinical context. The short history with previous good health makes TB unlikely in this case. A clear chest examination is not unusual in pneumonia, particularly in the context of atypical or viral pathogens. The next most common causes would be bronchiectasis (made unlikely in this case by the absence of any previous respiratory problems) or pulmonary embolism. Tumour (benign or malignant), Goodpasture's syndrome or pulmonary vasculitis (often as part of a pulmonary-renal syndrome) also need to be considered but are much less likely diagnoses.

Answer to Question 6
A, B

Near fatal asthma or brittle asthma is responsible for around 1000 deaths every year in the UK. It mainly occurs in young patients, previous attacks and a short time between the start of symptoms and hospital admission being the two main risk factors. The treatment of choice is hospitalisation with early start of nebulised bronchodilators, oxygen and intravenous corticosteroids. The recovery rate is normally quick. Long acting beta-2 agonists and leukotrine receptor antagonists are not successful in preventing near fatal asthma. There is no relationship between near fatal asthma and personal history of allergy. The incidence of the disease does not differ according to gender and there are no seasonal variations for the rate of hospitalisation.

Answer to Question 7
A, D

The most likely diagnosis to explain gradually worsening breathlessness with regular sputum production is bronchiectasis. This could arise as a consequence of childhood infection (measles, pneumonia, pertussis), cystic fibrosis, alpha 1 antitrypsin deficiency or hypogammaglobulinaemia (which would be suggested by recurrent pneumonia or sinusitis).

Answer to Question 8
C, H

The spirometry effectively rules out obstructive lung disease/asthma. Hypoxia excludes hyperventilation and anaemia as primary causes. The differential diagnosis lies between diffuse parenchymal lung disease and a problem with the pulmonary vasculature.

In diffuse parenchymal lung disease the patient may have a dry cough, but there may be no specific features. It will be important to ask about systemic / iatrogenic disorders associated with lung disease, and specific employment history / recreational interests may also be relevant. Note that the chest radiograph can appear entirely normal in patients with diffuse parenchymal lung disease. Regarding diseases of the pulmonary vasculature, a small number of patients with pulmonary embolism present with breathlessness alone, but primary pulmonary hypertension needs careful consideration in this case.

Answer to Question 9
A, I

Drug-induced pulmonary eosinophilia is the most common type of pulmonary eosinophilia seen in the western world. Drugs that can be responsible include ampicillin, aspirin, captopril, bleomycin, carbamazepine, dapsone, ethambutol, gold, methotrexate, penicillin, penicillamine, sulphonamides (including sulfasalazine), tamoxifen and tetracycline.

Answer to Question 10

C

This patient is in Step Two of asthma treatment, but his asthma is not well controlled as he needs to take his rescue medication more than twice a day. His treatment should be stepped up. In Step Three of asthma treatment, guidelines from the British Thoracic Society advise first adding inhaled long-acting beta-2 agonist (LABA) and then re-assessing the situation. If there is a good response to LABA, this medication should be continued. If there is benefit from LABA but control is still inadequate, LABA should be continued, and the inhaled corticosteroids should be increased to a high dose. If there is no response to LABA, then that treatment should be stopped and inhaled corticosteroids should be increased to a high dose.

Answer to Question 11

A

Resuscitation is the first priority. Maximum inspired oxygen should be given by facemask: this is best achieved using a reservoir bag at a flow rate of 15 l/min, which can generate an FiO_2 of about 85%. Nebulised salbutamol (5–10 mg) driven by oxygen should be given, and many would add ipatropium bromide (Atrovent, 500 µg) to the nebuliser chamber at the same time as the salbutamol. If the woman does not improve, then call for assistance from the Intensive Care Unit (ICU) sooner rather than later. Although it is always important to consider pneumothorax in any breathless patient, there is no evidence at all to suggest that this woman has bilateral pneumothoraces and she would not be well served by chest decompression.

Answer to Question 12

D

Long-term oxygen treatment is recommended if pO_2 is less than 7.3 kPa on two occasions in remission of COPD. This patient's pO_2 is likely to improve when he recovers from his current exacerbation and his ABG should be rechecked in about 6 weeks time. As he seems able to tolerate his mild hypoxia, he would not require any oxygen supplementation at home at this stage.

Answer to Question 13

D

Steroid challenge is indicated in chronic obstructive pulmonary disease (COPD) of more than moderate severity. Standard practice would be to give prednisolone 30 mg daily for 2 weeks, regarding an increase in FEV1 of >10% and >200 ml as a positive response. Given the non-specific effects and many side effects of steroids, it is crucial to demonstrate functional improvement: many patients with COPD have sustained severe complications of steroid treatment, e.g. vertebral fracture, without any evidence that the steroids were beneficial for their chest.

Answer to Question 14

A

The history strongly suggests pneumonia 6 weeks previously that has failed to clear. Empyema could cause persistent fever, malaise and breathlessness, but would not explain continued sputum production. Alcoholism is a risk factor for aspiration and cavitating pneumonia. Bronchiectasis typically causes chronic breathlessness and sputum production, often with febrile infective exacerbations, but will not be the diagnosis in a patient with a short respiratory history.

Answer to Question 15

E

Although all of the diagnoses listed could present in this way, pneumonia with effusion/empyema is much the most likely. Examination of the pleural fluid is critical. If associated with pneumonia and the effusion is opaque/turbid and smells foul then it is clearly an empyema, which would also be suggested by pH < 7.2.

Answer to Question 16

C

Normal spirometry excludes chronic obstructive pulmonary disease. Raynaud's syndrome with telangiectasia and radiological appearances suggestive of pulmonary hypertension with impaired gas transfer are most likely due to a vasculitic process in pulmonary circulation associated with an autoimmune rheumatic disorder.

Answer to Question 17

C

Polymyositis and dermatomyositis are inflammatory conditions involving the muscle and skin. Patients often complain of proximal muscle weakness and of pain in the small joints of the fingers. They may have ragged cuticles and haemorrhages at the finger nail folds. Interstitial lung disease can occur. Underlying malignancy (lungs, ovaries, breasts and stomach) is present in 5–8% of cases.

Answer to Question 18

B

The patient has both lung and kidney involvement typical of a 'pulmonary renal syndrome'. Goodpasture described the association of pulmonary haemorrhage with renal failure (Goodpasture's syndrome) in 1919, and the 'classic' cause of this, where the condition is due to the presence of circulating anti-glomerular basement membrane antibodies (anti-GBM antibodies) is termed Goodpasture's disease (although this wasn't the cause of the cases he described). Other causes of pulmonary hae-morrhage and renal failure include Wegener's granulo-matosis, microscopic polyangiitis and systemic lupus erythematous (SLE).

Answer to Question 19
D

The combination of bilateral hilar lymphadenopathy and erythema nodosum is diagnostic of sarcoidosis. This is usually self-limiting. She should however be followed up in clinic with full lung function tests including transfer factor and lung volumes. Serum angiotensin-converting enzyme (ACE) level and lung function can be used to monitor disease. Worsening disease should be treated with prednisolone.

Answer to Question 20
A

Infected pleural effusions should be drained. In this clinical context a pleural effusion should be drained if the pH < 7.2, Gram stain shows organisms, the fluid is frankly purulent, or if clinical improvement is slow despite antibiotics.

Answer to Question 21
D

Restrictive lung disorders are characterised by reduced FEV1 & FVC, FEV1/FVC > 70%, reduced TLC & RV and reduced TLCO.

Obstructive disorders are characterised by reduced FEV1 & FVC, FEV1/FVC < 70%, raised TLC & RV (gas trapping) and reduced TLCO (emphysema) or normal or raised TLCO (non-smoking asthmatics).

Mixed disorders may have reduced FEV1 & FVC, FEV1/FVC < 70% and raised TLC & RV, reduced, normal or raised TLCO depending on whether the obstructive disorder is due to emphysema or asthma.

Answer to Question 22
D

Reduced FEV1 and FVC with normal FEV1 ratio is compatible with restrictive defect.

Answer to Question 23
E

The first investigation should be diagnostic aspiration of pleural fluid for biochemical, microbiological and cyto-logical analysis. Light's criteria can be used to distinguish transudates from exudates: in exudates at least one of the following three criteria are met—pleural fluid protein concentration greater than 50% of that in plasma; pleural fluid LDH greater than 60% of that in plasma; pleural fluid LDH more that two thirds the upper limit of normal in plasma. Transudative pleural effusions are most commonly due to congestive cardiac failure but are sometimes associated with hypoproteinaemic states such as cirrhosis or nephrotic syndrome. Most other causes of pleural effusion are exudative.

Answer to Question 24
D

Although obtructive sleep apnoea can cause chronic respiratory failure, it is unusual to have chronic type 2 respiratory failure except in combination with some other cardiopulmonary illness. This blood gas would be most compatible with a patient with severe chronic obstructive pulmonary disease and chronic type 2 respiratory failure with an acute exacerbation.

Answer to Question 25
D

Initially the history might suggest a number of diagnoses, including cardiac tamponade, massive pulmonary embo-lism, haemothorax or aortic dissection, but the respira-tory examination findings indicate that he almost certainly has sustained a spontaneous pneumothorax that has now developed into a tension pneumothorax. The scenario indicates that the man is about to suffer a cardi-orespiratory arrest: there is no time to arrange for port-able chest radiograph before attempting to reduce the pressure in the right hemithorax with the insertion of a large bore needle. If the diagnosis is correct, insertion may be accompanied by a loud 'hiss'. Positive pressure ventilation is relatively contraindicated in this situation, and will probably not be required once the lung has re-inflated.

The Medical Masterclass series

Scientific Background to Medicine 1

Genetics and Molecular Medicine

1 Nucleic acids and chromosomes
2 Techniques in molecular biology
3 Molecular basis of simple genetic traits
4 More complex issues

Biochemistry and Metabolism

1 Requirement for energy
2 Carbohydrates
3 Fatty acids and lipids
4 Cholesterol and steroid hormones
5 Amino acids and proteins
6 Haem
7 Nucleotides

Cell Biology

1 Ion transport
2 Receptors and intracellular signalling
3 Cell cycle and apoptosis
4 Haematopoiesis

Immunology and Immunosuppression

1 Overview of the immune system
2 The major histocompatibility complex, antigen presentation and transplantation
3 T cells
4 B cells
5 Tolerance and autoimmunity
6 Complement
7 Inflammation
8 Immunosuppressive therapy

Anatomy

1 Heart and major vessels
2 Lungs
3 Liver and biliary tract
4 Spleen
5 Kidney
6 Endocrine glands
7 Gastrointestinal tract
8 Eye
9 Nervous system

Physiology

1 Cardiovascular system
  1.1 The heart as a pump
  1.2 The systemic and pulmonary circulations
  1.3 Blood vessels
  1.4 Endocrine function of the heart
2 Respiratory system
  2.1 The lungs
3 Gastrointestinal system
  3.1 The gut
  3.2 The liver
  3.3 The exocrine pancreas
4 Brain and nerves
  4.1 The action potential
  4.2 Synaptic transmission
  4.3 Neuromuscular transmission
5 Endocrine physiology
6 Renal physiology
  6.1 Blood flow and glomerular filtration
  6.2 Function of the renal tubules
  6.3 Endocrine function of the kidney

Scientific Background to Medicine 2

Statistics, Epidemiology, Clinical Trials, Meta-analyses and Evidence-based Medicine

1 Statistics
2 Epidemiology
  2.1 Observational studies
3 Clinical trials and meta-analyses
4 Evidence-based medicine

Clinical Pharmacology

1 Introducing clinical pharmacology
  1.1 Preconceived notions versus evidence
  1.2 Drug interactions and safe prescribing
2 Pharmacokinetics
  2.1 Introduction
  2.2 Drug absorption
  2.3 Drug distribution
  2.4 Drug metabolism
  2.5 Drug elimination
  2.6 Plasma half-life and steady-state plasma concentrations
  2.7 Drug monitoring
3 Pharmacodynamics
  3.1 How drugs exert their effects
  3.2 Selectivity is the key to the therapeutic utility of an agent
  3.3 Basic aspects of a drug's interaction with its target
  3.4 Heterogeneity of drug responses, pharmacogenetics and pharmacogenomics
4 Adverse drug reactions
  4.1 Introduction
  4.2 Definition and classification of adverse drug reactions
  4.3 Dose-related adverse drug reactions

4.4 Non-dose-related adverse drug reactions
4.5 Adverse reactions caused by long-term effects of drugs
4.6 Adverse reactions caused by delayed effects of drugs
4.7 Teratogenic effects
5 Prescribing in special circumstances
 5.1 Introduction
 5.2 Prescribing and liver disease
 5.3 Prescribing in pregnancy
 5.4 Prescribing for women of child-bearing potential
 5.5 Prescribing to lactating mothers
 5.6 Prescribing in renal disease
6 Drug development and rational prescribing
 6.1 Drug development
  6.1.1 Identifying molecules for development as drugs
  6.1.2 Clinical trials: from drug to medicine
 6.2 Rational prescribing
  6.2.1 Clinical governance and rational prescribing
  6.2.2 Rational prescribing, irrational patients?

Clinical Skills

General Clinical Issues

1 The importance of general clinical issues
2 History and examination
3 Communication skills
4 Being a doctor
 4.1 Team work and errors
 4.2 The 'modern' health service
 4.3 Rationing beds
 4.4 Stress

Pain Relief and Palliative Care

1 Clinical presentations
 1.1 Back pain
 1.2 Nausea and vomiting
 1.3 Breathlessness
 1.4 Confusion
2 Diseases and treatments
 2.1 Pain
 2.2 Breathlessness
 2.3 Nausea and vomiting
 2.4 Bowel obstruction
 2.5 Constipation
 2.6 Depression
 2.7 Anxiety
 2.8 Confusion
 2.9 The dying patient: terminal phase
 2.10 Palliative care services in the community

Medicine for the Elderly

1 Clinical presentations
 1.1 Frequent falls
 1.2 Sudden onset of confusion
 1.3 Urinary incontinence and immobility
 1.4 Collapse

1.5 Vague aches and pains
1.6 Swollen legs and back pain
1.7 Gradual decline
2 Diseases and treatments
 2.1 Why elderly patients are different
 2.2 General approach to managment
 2.3 Falls
 2.4 Urinary and faecal incontinence
  2.4.1 Urinary incontinence
  2.4.2 Faecal incontinence
 2.5 Hypothermia
 2.6 Drugs in elderly people
 2.7 Dementia
 2.8 Rehabilitation
 2.9 Aids and appliances
 2.10 Hearing impairment
 2.11 Nutrition
 2.12 Benefits
 2.13 Legal aspects of elderly care
3 Investigations and practical procedures
 3.1 Diagnosis vs common sense
 3.2 Assessment of cognition, mood and function

Emergency Medicine

1 Clinical presentations
 1.1 Cardiac arrest
 1.2 Collapse with hypotension
 1.3 Central chest pain
 1.4 Tachyarrythmia
 1.5 Nocturnal dyspnoea
 1.6 Bradydysrhythmia
 1.7 Acute severe asthma
 1.8 Pleurisy
 1.9 Community-acquired pneumonia
 1.10 Chronic airways obstruction
 1.11 Upper gastrointestinal haemorrhage
 1.12 Bloody diarrhoea
 1.13 'The medical abdomen'
 1.14 Hepatic encephalopathy/alcohol withdrawal
 1.15 Renal failure, fluid overload and hyperkalaemia
 1.16 Diabetic ketoacidosis
 1.17 Hypoglycaemia
 1.18 Hypercalcaemia and hyponatraemia
 1.19 Metabolic acidosis
 1.20 An endocrine crisis
 1.21 Another endocrine crisis
 1.22 Severe headache with meningism
 1.23 Acute spastic paraparesis
 1.24 Status epilepticus
 1.25 Stroke
 1.26 Coma
 1.27 Fever in a returning traveller
 1.28 Septicaemia
 1.29 Anaphylaxis
2 Diseases and treatments
 2.1 Overdoses

3 Investigations and practical procedures
  3.1 Femoral vein cannulation
  3.2 Central vein cannulation
  3.3 Intercostal chest drain insertion
  3.4 Arterial blood gases
  3.5 Lumbar puncture
  3.6 Pacing
  3.7 Haemodynamic monitoring
  3.8 Ventilatory support
  3.9 Airway management

Infectious Diseases and Dermatology

Infectious Diseases

1 Clinical presentations
  1.1 Fever
  1.2 Fever, hypotension and confusion
  1.3 A swollen red foot
  1.4 Fever and cough
  1.5 A cavitating lung lesion
  1.6 Fever, back pain and weak legs
  1.7 Fever and lymphadenopathy
  1.8 Drug user with fever and a murmur
  1.9 Fever and heart failure
  1.10 Still feverish after six weeks
  1.11 Persistent fever in ICU
  1.12 Pyelonephritis
  1.13 A sore throat
  1.14 Fever and headache
  1.15 Fever with reduced conscious level
  1.16 Fever in the neutropenic patient
  1.17 Fever after renal transplant
  1.18 Chronic fatigue
  1.19 Varicella in pregnancy
  1.20 Imported fever
  1.21 Eosinophilia
  1.22 Jaundice and fever after travelling
  1.23 A traveller with diarrhoea
  1.24 Malaise, mouth ulcers and fever
  1.25 Needlestick exposure
  1.26 Breathlessness in an HIV+ patient
  1.27 HIV+ and blurred vision
  1.28 Starting anti-HIV therapy
  1.29 Failure of anti-HIV therapy
  1.30 Don't tell my wife
  1.31 A spot on the penis
  1.32 Penile discharge
  1.33 Woman with a genital sore
  1.34 Abdominal pain and vaginal discharge
  1.35 Syphilis in pregnancy
  1.36 Positive blood cultures
  1.37 Therapeutic drug monitoring—antibiotics
  1.38 Contact with meningitis
  1.39 Pulmonary tuberculosis—follow-up failure
  1.40 Penicillin allergy
2 Pathogens and management

2.1 Antimicrobial prophylaxis
2.2 Immunization
2.3 Infection control
2.4 Travel advice
2.5 Bacteria
  2.5.1 Gram-positive bacteria
  2.5.2 Gram-negative bacteria
2.6 Mycobacteria
  2.6.1 *Mycobacterium tuberculosis*
  2.6.2 *Mycobacterium leprae*
  2.6.3 Opportunistic mycobacteria
2.7 Spirochaetes
  2.7.1 Syphilis
  2.7.2 Lyme disease
  2.7.3 Relapsing fever
  2.7.4 Leptospirosis
2.8 Miscellaneous bacteria
  2.8.1 *Mycoplasma* and *Ureaplasma*
  2.8.2 Rickettsiae
  2.8.3 *Coxiella burnetii* (Q fever)
  2.8.4 Chlamydiae
2.9 Fungi
  2.9.1 *Candida* SPP.
  2.9.2 *Aspergillus*
  2.9.3 *Cryptococcus neoformans*
  2.9.4 Dimorphic fungi
  2.9.5 Miscellaneous fungi
2.10 Viruses
  2.10.1 Herpes simplex virus types 1 and 2
  2.10.2 Varicella-zoster virus
  2.10.3 Cytomegalovirus
  2.10.4 Epstein–Barr virus
  2.10.5 Human herpes viruses 6 and 7
  2.10.6 Human herpes virus 8
  2.10.7 Parvovirus
  2.10.8 Hepatitis viruses
  2.10.9 Influenza virus
  2.10.10 Paramyxoviruses
  2.10.11 Enteroviruses
2.11 Human immunodeficiency virus
2.12 Travel–related viruses
  2.12.1 Rabies
  2.12.2 Dengue
  2.12.3 Arbovirus infections
2.13 Protozoan parasites
  2.13.1 Malaria
  2.13.2 Leishmaniasis
  2.13.3 Amoebiasis
  2.13.4 Toxoplasmosis
2.14 Metazoan parasites
  2.14.1 Schistosomiasis
  2.14.2 Strongyloidiasis
  2.14.3 Cysticercosis
  2.14.4 Filariasis
  2.14.5 Trichinosis
  2.14.6 Toxocariasis
  2.14.7 Hydatid disease
3 Investigations and practical procedures
  3.1 Getting the best from the laboratory
  3.2 Specific investigations

Dermatology

1 Clinical presentations
  1.1 Blistering disorders
  1.2 Acute generalized rashes
  1.3 Erythroderma
  1.4 A chronic, red facial rash
  1.5 Pruritus
  1.6 Alopecia
  1.7 Abnormal skin pigmentation
  1.8 Patches and plaques on the lower legs
2 Diseases and treatments
  2.1 Alopecia areata
  2.2 Bullous pemphigoid and pemphigoid gestationis
  2.3 Dermatomyositis
  2.4 Mycosis fungoides and Sézary syndrome
  2.5 Dermatitis herpetiformis
  2.6 Drug eruptions
  2.7 Atopic eczema
  2.8 Contact dermatitis
  2.9 Erythema multiforme, Stevens–Johnson syndrome, toxic epidermal necrolysis
  2.10 Erythema nodosum
  2.11 Lichen planus
  2.12 Pemphigus vulgaris
  2.13 Superficial fungal infections
  2.14 Psoriasis
  2.15 Scabies
  2.16 Urticaria and angio-oedema
  2.17 Vitiligo
  2.18 Pyoderma gangrenosum
  2.19 Cutaneous vasculitis
  2.20 Acanthosis nigricans
3 Investigations and practical procedures
  3.1 Skin biopsy
  3.2 Direct and indirect immunofluorescence
  3.3 Patch testing
  3.4 Topical therapy: corticosteroids
  3.5 Phototherapy
  3.6 Systemic retinoids

Haematology and Oncology

Haematology

1 Clinical presentations
  1.1 Microcytic hypochromic anaemia
  1.2 Chest syndrome in sickle cell disease
  1.3 Normocytic anaemia
  1.4 Macrocytic anaemia
  1.5 Hereditary spherocytosis and failure to thrive
  1.6 Neutropenia
  1.7 Pancytopenia
  1.8 Thrombocytopenia and purpura
  1.9 Leucocytosis
  1.10 Lymphocytosis and anaemia
  1.11 Spontaneous bleeding and weight loss
  1.12 Menorrhagia and anaemia
  1.13 Thromboembolism and fetal loss
  1.14 Polycythaemia
  1.15 Bone pain and hypercalcaemia
  1.16 Cervical lymphadenopathy and weight loss
  1.17 Isolated splenomegaly
  1.18 Inflammatory bowel disease with thrombocytosis
  1.19 Transfusion reaction
  1.20 Recurrent deep venous thrombosis
2 Diseases and treatments
  2.1 Causes of anaemia
    2.1.1 Thalassaemia syndromes
    2.1.2 Sickle cell syndromes
    2.1.3 Enzyme defects
    2.1.4 Membrane defects
    2.1.5 Iron metabolism and iron-deficiency anaemia
    2.1.6 Vitamin B_{12} and folate metabolism and deficiency
    2.1.7 Acquired haemolytic anaemia
    2.1.8 Bone-marrow failure and infiltration
  2.2 Haemic malignancy
    2.2.1 Multiple myeloma
    2.2.2 Acute leukaemia—acute lymphoblastic leukaemia and acute myeloid leukaemia
    2.2.3 Chronic lymphocytic leukaemia
    2.2.4 Chronic myeloid leukaemia
    2.2.5 Malignant lymphomas—non-Hodgkin's lymphoma and Hodgkin's disease
    2.2.6 Myelodysplastic syndromes
    2.2.7 Non-leukaemic myeloproliferative disorders
    2.2.8 Amyloidosis
  2.3 Bleeding disorders
    2.3.1 Inherited bleeding disorders
    2.3.2 Acquired bleeding disorders
    2.3.3 Idiopathic thrombocytopenic purpura
  2.4 Thrombotic disorders
    2.4.1 Inherited thrombotic disease
    2.4.2 Acquired thrombotic disease
  2.5 Clinical use of blood products
  2.6 Haematological features of systemic disease
  2.7 Haematology of pregnancy
  2.8 Iron overload
  2.9 Chemotherapy and related therapies
  2.10 Principles of bone-marrow and peripheral blood stem-cell transplantation
3 Investigations and practical procedures
  3.1 The full blood count and film
  3.2 Bone-marrow examination
  3.3 Clotting screen
  3.4 Coombs' test (direct antiglobulin test)
  3.5 Erythrocyte sedimentation rate vs plasma viscosity
  3.6 Therapeutic anticoagulation

Oncology

1 Clinical presentations
  1.1 A lump in the neck
  1.2 Breathlessness and a pelvic mass
  1.3 Breast cancer and headache
    1.3.1 Metastatic disease
  1.4 Cough and weakness
    1.4.1 Paraneoplastic conditions

1.5 Breathlessness after chemotherapy
1.6 Hip pain after stem cell transplantation
1.7 A problem in the family
   1.7.1 The causes of cancer
1.8 Bleeding, breathlessness and swollen arms
   1.8.1 Oncological emergencies
1.9 The daughter of a man with advanced prostate cancer
2 Diseases and treatments
  2.1 Breast cancer
  2.2 Central nervous system cancers
  2.3 Digestive tract cancers
  2.4 Genitourinary cancer
  2.5 Gynaecological cancer
  2.6 Head and neck cancer
  2.7 Skin tumours
  2.8 Paediatric solid tumours
  2.9 Lung cancer
  2.10 Liver and biliary tree cancer
  2.11 Bone cancer and sarcoma
  2.12 Endocrine tumours
3 Investigations and practical procedures
  3.1 Tumour markers
  3.2 Screening
  3.3 Radiotherapy
  3.4 Chemotherapy
  3.5 Immunotherapy
  3.6 Stem-cell transplantation

Cardiology and Respiratory Medicine

Cardiology

1 Clinical presentations
  1.1 Paroxysmal palpitations
  1.2 Palpitations with dizziness
  1.3 Syncope
  1.4 Stroke and a murmur
  1.5 Acute central chest pain
  1.6 Breathlessness and ankle swelling
  1.7 Hypotension following myocardial infarction
  1.8 Breathlessness and haemodynamic collapse
  1.9 Pleuritic pain
  1.10 Breathlessness and exertional presyncope
  1.11 Dyspnoea, ankle oedema and cyanosis
  1.12 Chest pain and recurrent syncope
  1.13 Fever, weight loss and new murmur
  1.14 Chest pain following a 'flu-like illness
  1.15 Elevated blood pressure at routine screening
  1.16 Murmur in pregnancy
2 Diseases and treatments
  2.1 Coronary artery disease
    2.1.1 Stable angina
    2.1.2 Unstable angina
    2.1.3 Myocardial infarction
  2.2 Cardiac arrhythmia
    2.2.1 Bradycardia
    2.2.2 Tachycardia

  2.3 Cardiac failure
  2.4 Diseases of heart muscle
    2.4.1 Hypertrophic cardiomyopathy
    2.4.2 Dilated cardiomyopathy
    2.4.3 Restrictive cardiomyopathy
    2.4.4 Acute myocarditis
  2.5 Valvular heart disease
    2.5.1 Aortic stenosis
    2.5.2 Aortic regurgitation
    2.5.3 Mitral stenosis
    2.5.4 Mitral regurgitation
    2.5.5 Tricuspid valve disease
    2.5.6 Pulmonary valve disease
  2.6 Pericardial disease
    2.6.1 Acute pericarditis
    2.6.2 Pericardial effusion
    2.6.3 Constrictive pericarditis
  2.7 Congenital heart disease
    2.7.1 Tetralogy of Fallot
    2.7.2 Eisenmenger's syndrome
    2.7.3 Transposition of the great arteries
    2.7.4 Ebstein's anomaly
    2.7.5 Atrial septal defect
    2.7.6 Ventricular septal defect
    2.7.7 Patent ductus arteriosus
    2.7.8 Coarctation of the aorta
  2.8 Infective diseases of the heart
    2.8.1 Infective endocarditis
    2.8.2 Rheumatic fever
  2.9 Cardiac tumours
  2.10 Traumatic heart disease
  2.11 Diseases of systemic arteries
    2.11.1 Aortic dissection
  2.12 Diseases of pulmonary arteries
    2.12.1 Primary pulmonary hypertension
    2.12.2 Secondary pulmonary hypertension
  2.13 Cardiac complications of systemic disease
    2.13.1 Thyroid disease
    2.13.2 Diabetes
    2.13.3 Autoimmune rheumatic diseases
    2.13.4 Renal disease
  2.14 Systemic complications of cardiac disease
    2.14.1 Stroke
  2.15 Pregnancy and the heart
  2.16 General anaesthesia in heart disease
  2.17 Hypertension
    2.17.1 Accelerated phase hypertension
  2.18 Venous thromboembolism
    2.18.1 Pulmonary embolism
  2.19 Driving restrictions in cardiology
3 Investigations and practical procedures
  3.1 ECG
    3.1.1 Exercise ECGs
  3.2 Basic electrophysiology studies
  3.3 Ambulatory monitoring
  3.4 Radiofrequency ablation and implantable cardioverter defibrillators
    3.4.1 Radiofrequency ablation
    3.4.2 Implantable cardioverter defibrillator
  3.5 Pacemakers
  3.6 The chest radiograph in cardiac disease

3.7   Cardiac biochemical markers
3.8   Cardiac catheterization, percutaneous transluminal coronary angioplasty and stenting
    3.8.1   Cardiac catheterization
    3.8.2   Percutaneous transluminal coronary angioplasty and stenting
3.9   Computed tomography and magnetic resonance imaging
    3.9.1   Computed tomography
    3.9.2   Magnetic resonance imaging
3.10 Ventilation–perfusion isotope scanning ($\dot{V}/\dot{Q}$)
3.11 Echocardiography
3.12 Nuclear cardiology
    3.12.1 Myocardial perfusion imaging
    3.12.2 Positron emission tomography

Respiratory Medicine

1 Clinical presentations
  1.1   New breathlessness
  1.2   Solitary pulmonary nodule
  1.3   Exertional dyspnoea with daily sputum
  1.4   Dyspnoea and fine inspiratory crackles
  1.5   Pleuritic chest pain
  1.6   Unexplained hypoxia
  1.7   Nocturnal cough
  1.8   Daytime sleepiness and morning headache
  1.9   Haemoptysis and weight loss
  1.10 Pleural effusion and fever
  1.11 Lung cancer with asbestos exposure
  1.12 Lobar collapse in non-smoker
  1.13 Breathlessness with a normal radiograph
  1.14 Upper airway obstruction
  1.15 Difficult decisions
2 Diseases and treatments
  2.1   Upper airway
    2.1.1   Obstructive sleep apnoea
  2.2   Atopy and asthma
    2.2.1   Allergic rhinitis
    2.2.2   Asthma
  2.3   Chronic obstructive pulmonary disease
  2.4   Bronchiectasis
  2.5   Cystic fibrosis
  2.6   Occupational lung disease
    2.6.1   Asbestosis and the pneumoconioses
  2.7   Diffuse parenchymal (interstitial) lung disease
    2.7.1   Cryptogenic fibrosing alveolitis
    2.7.2   Bronchiolitis obliterans and organizing pneumonia
  2.8   Miscellaneous conditions
    2.8.1   Extrinsic allergic alveolitis
    2.8.2   Sarcoidosis
    2.8.3   Pulmonary vasculitis
    2.8.4   Pulmonary eosinophilia
    2.8.5   Iatrogenic lung disease
    2.8.6   Smoke inhalation
    2.8.7   Sickle cell disease and the lung
    2.8.8   HIV and the lung
  2.9   Malignancy
    2.9.1   Lung cancer
    2.9.2   Mesothelioma
    2.9.3   Mediastinal tumours
  2.10 Disorders of the chest wall and diaphragm
  2.11 Complications of respiratory disease
    2.11.1 Chronic respiratory failure
    2.11.2 Cor pulmonale
  2.12 Treatments in respiratory disease
    2.12.1 Domiciliary oxygen therapy
    2.12.2 Continuous positive airways pressure
    2.12.3 Non-invasive ventilation
  2.13 Lung transplantation
3 Investigations and practical procedures
  3.1   Arterial blood gas sampling
  3.2   Aspiration of pleural effusion or pneumothorax
  3.3   Pleural biopsy
  3.4   Intercostal tube insertion
  3.5   Fibreoptic bronchoscopy and transbronchial biopsy
    3.5.1   Fibreoptic bronchoscopy
    3.5.2   Transbronchial biopsy
  3.6   Interpretation of clinical data
    3.6.1   Arterial blood gases
    3.6.2   Lung function tests
    3.6.3   Overnight oximetry
    3.6.4   Chest radiograph
    3.6.5   Computed tomography scan of the thorax

Gastroenterology and Hepatology

1 Clinical presentations
  1.1   Chronic diarrhoea
  1.2   Heartburn and dysphagia
  1.3   Melaena and collapse
  1.4   Haematemesis and jaundice
  1.5   Abdominal mass
  1.6   Jaundice and abdominal pain
  1.7   Jaundice in a heavy drinker
  1.8   Abdominal swelling
  1.9   Abdominal pain and vomiting
  1.10 Weight loss and tiredness
  1.11 Diarrhoea and weight loss
  1.12 Rectal bleeding
  1.13 Severe abdominal pain and vomiting
  1.14 Chronic abdominal pain
  1.15 Change in bowel habit
  1.16 Acute liver failure
  1.17 Iron-deficiency anaemia
  1.18 Abnormal liver function tests
  1.19 Progressive decline
  1.20 Factitious abdominal pain
2 Diseases and treatments
  2.1   Inflammatory bowel disease
    2.1.1   Crohn's disease
    2.1.2   Ulcerative colitis
    2.1.3   Microscopic colitis
  2.2   Oesophagus
    2.2.1   Barrett's oesophagus
    2.2.2   Oesophageal reflux and benign stricture

2.2.3 Oesophageal tumours
2.2.4 Achalasia
2.2.5 Diffuse oesophageal spasm
2.3 Gastric and duodenal disease
2.3.1 Peptic ulceration and *Helicobacter pylori*
2.3.2 Gastric carcinoma
2.3.3 Rare gastric tumours
2.3.4 Rare causes of gastrointestinal haemorrhage
2.4 Pancreas
2.4.1 Acute pancreatitis
2.4.2 Chronic pancreatitis
2.4.3 Pancreatic cancer
2.4.4 Neuroendocrine tumours
2.5 Biliary tree
2.5.1 Choledocholithiasis
2.5.2 Cholangiocarcinoma
2.5.3 Primary sclerosing cholangitis
2.5.4 Primary biliary cirrhosis
2.5.5 Intrahepatic cholestasis
2.6 Small bowel
2.6.1 Coeliac
2.6.2 Bacterial overgrowth
2.6.4 Other causes of malabsorption
2.7 Large bowel
2.7.1 Adenomatous polyps of the colon
2.7.2 Colorectal carcinoma
2.7.3 Diverticular disease
2.7.4 Intestinal ischaemia
2.7.5 Anorectal disease
2.8 Irritable bowel
2.9 Acute liver disease
2.9.1 Hepatitis A
2.9.2 Hepatitis B
2.9.3 Other viral hepatitis
2.9.4 Alcohol and alcoholic hepatitis
2.9.5 Acute liver failure
2.10 Chronic liver disease
2.11 Focal liver lesions
2.12 Drugs and the liver
2.12.1 Hepatic drug toxicity
2.12.2 Drugs and chronic liver disease
2.13 Gastrointestinal infections
2.13.1 Campylobacter
2.13.2 Salmonella
2.13.3 Shigella
2.13.4 Clostridium difficile
2.13.5 Giardia lamblia
2.13.6 Yersinia enterocolitica
2.13.7 Escherichia coli
2.13.8 Entamoeba histolytica
2.13.9 Traveller's diarrhoea
2.13.10 Human immunodeficiency virus (HIV)
2.14 Nutrition
2.14.1 Defining nutrition
2.14.2 Protein-calorie malnutrition
2.14.3 Obesity
2.14.4 Enteral and parenteral nutrition
2.14.5 Diets
2.15 Liver transplantation

2.16 Screening, case finding and surveillance
2.16.1 Surveillance
2.16.2 Case finding
2.16.3 Population screening
3 Investigations and practical procedures
3.1 General investigations
3.2 Rigid sigmoidoscopy and rectal biopsy
3.3 Paracentesis
3.4 Liver biopsy

Neurology, Ophthalmology and Psychiatry

Neurology

1 Clinical presentations
1.1 Numb toes
1.2 Back and leg pain
1.3 Tremor
1.4 Gait disturbance
1.5 Dementia and involuntary movements
1.6 Muscle pain on exercise
1.7 Increasing seizure frequency
1.8 Sleep disorders
1.9 Memory difficulties
1.10 Dysphagia
1.11 Weak legs
1.12 Neck/shoulder pain
1.13 Impotence and urinary difficulties
1.14 Diplopia
1.15 Ptosis
1.16 Unequal pupils
1.17 Smell and taste disorders
1.18 Facial pain
1.19 Recurrent severe headache
1.20 Funny turns
1.21 Hemiplegia
1.22 Speech disturbance
1.23 Visual hallucinations
1.24 Conversion disorders
1.25 Multiple sclerosis
2 Diseases and treatments
2.1 Peripheral neuropathies and diseases of the lower motor neurone
2.1.1 Peripheral neuropathies
2.1.2 Guillain–Barré Syndrome
2.1.3 Motor neuron disease
2.2 Diseases of muscle
2.2.1 Metabolic muscle disease
2.2.2 Inflammatory muscle disease
2.2.3 Inherited dystrophies (myopathies)
2.2.4 Channelopathies
2.2.5 Myasthenia gravis
2.3 Extrapyramidal disorders
2.3.1 Parkinson's disease
2.4 Dementias
2.4.1 Alzheimer's disease
2.5 Multiple sclerosis

2.6 Causes of headache
    2.6.1 Migraine
    2.6.2 Trigeminal neuralgia
    2.6.3 Cluster headache
    2.6.4 Tension-type headache
2.7 Epilepsy
2.8 Cerebrovascular disease
    2.8.1 Stroke
    2.8.2 Transient ischaemic attacks
    2.8.3 Intracerebral haemorrhage
    2.8.4 Subarachnoid haemorrhage
2.9 Brain tumours
2.10 Neurological complications of infection
    2.10.1 New variant Creutzfeldt–Jakob disease
2.11 Neurological complications of systemic disease
    2.11.1 Paraneoplastic conditions
2.12 Neuropharmacology
3 Investigations and practical procedures
3.1 Neuropsychometry
3.2 Lumbar puncture
3.3 Neurophysiology
    3.3.1 Electroencephalography
    3.3.2 Evoked potentials
    3.3.3 Electromyography
    3.3.4 Nerve conduction studies
3.4 Neuroimaging
    3.4.1 Computed tomography and computed tomographic angiography
    3.4.2 MRI and MRA
    3.4.3 Angiography
3.5 SPECT and PET
    3.5.1 SPECT
    3.5.2 PET
3.6 Carotid Dopplers

Ophthalmology

1 Clinical presentations
1.1 An acutely painful red eye
1.2 Two painful red eyes and a systemic disorder
1.3 Acute painless loss of vision in one eye
1.4 Acute painful loss of vision in a young woman
1.5 Acute loss of vision in an elderly man
1.6 Difficulty reading
1.7 Double vision
2 Diseases and treatments
2.1 Iritis
2.2 Scleritis
2.3 Retinal artery occlusion
2.4 Retinal vein occlusion
2.5 Optic neuritis
2.6 Ischaemic optic neuropathy in giant cell arteritis
2.7 Diabetic retinopathy
3 Investigations and practical procedures
3.1 Examination of the eye
    3.1.1 Visual acuity
    3.1.2 Visual fields
    3.1.3 Pupil responses
    3.1.4 Ophthalmoscopy
    3.1.5 Eye movements

3.2 Biopsy
    3.2.1 Temporal artery biopsy
    3.2.2 Conjunctival biopsy for diagnosis of sarcoidosis
3.3 Fluorescein angiography

Psychiatry

1 Clinical presentations
1.1 Acute confusional state
1.2 Panic attack and hyperventilation
1.3 Neuropsychiatric aspects of HIV and AIDS
1.4 Deliberate self-harm
1.5 Eating disorders
1.6 Medically unexplained symptoms
1.7 The alcoholic in hospital
1.8 Drug abuser in hospital
1.9 The frightening patient
2 Diseases and treatments
2.1 Dissociative disorders
2.2 Dementia
2.3 Schizophrenia and antipsychotic drugs
    2.3.1 Schizophrenia
    2.3.2 Antipsychotics
2.4 Personality disorder
2.5 Psychiatric presentation of physical disease
2.6 Psychological reactions to physical illness (adjustment disorders)
2.7 Anxiety disorders
    2.7.1 Generalised anxiety disorder
    2.7.2 Panic disorder
    2.7.3 Phobic anxiety disorders
2.8 Obsessive–compulsive disorder
2.9 Acute stress reactions and post-traumatic stress disorder
    2.9.1 Acute stress reaction
    2.9.2 Post-traumatic stress disorder
2.10 Puerperal disorders
    2.10.1 Maternity blues
    2.10.2 Post-natal depressive disorder
    2.10.3 Puerperal psychosis
2.11 Depression
2.12 Bipolar affective disorder
2.13 Delusional disorder
2.14 The Mental Health Act (1983)

Endocrinology

1 Clinical presentations
1.1 Hyponatraemia
1.2 Hypercalcaemia
1.3 Polyuria
1.4 Faints, sweats and palpitations
1.5 Crystals in the knee
1.6 Hirsutism
1.7 Post-pill amenorrhoea
1.8 Short girl with no periods
1.9 Young man who has 'not developed'
1.10 Depression and diabetes

1.11 Acromegaly
1.12 Postpartum amenorrhoea
1.13 Weight loss
1.14 Tiredness and lethargy
1.15 Flushing and diarrhoea
1.16 'Off legs'
1.17 Avoiding another coronary
1.18 High blood pressure and low serum potassium
1.19 Hypertension and a neck swelling
1.20 Tiredness, weight loss and amenorrhoea
2 Diseases and treatments
    2.1 Hypothalamic and pituitary diseases
        2.1.1 Cushing's syndrome
        2.1.2 Acromegaly
        2.1.3 Hyperprolactinaemia
        2.1.4 Non-functioning pituitary tumours
        2.1.5 Pituitary apoplexy
        2.1.6 Craniopharyngioma
        2.1.7 Hypopituitarism and hormone replacement
    2.2 Adrenal disease
        2.2.1 Cushing's syndrome
        2.2.2 Primary adrenal insufficiency
        2.2.3 Primary hyperaldosteronism
        2.2.4 Congenital adrenal hyperplasia
        2.2.5 Phaeochromocytoma
    2.3 Thyroid disease
        2.3.1 Hypothyroidism
        2.3.2 Thyrotoxicosis
        2.3.3 Thyroid nodules and goitre
        2.3.4 Thyroid malignancy
    2.4 Reproductive diseases
        2.4.1 Oligomenorrhoea/amenorrhoea and the
              premature menopause
        2.4.2 Polycystic ovarian syndrome
        2.4.3 Erectile dysfunction
        2.4.4 Gynaecomastia
        2.4.5 Delayed growth and puberty
    2.5 Metabolic and bone diseases
        2.5.1 Hyperlipidaemia
        2.5.2 Porphyria
        2.5.3 Haemochromatosis
        2.5.4 Osteoporosis
        2.5.5 Osteomalacia
        2.5.6 Paget's disease
        2.5.7 Primary hyperparathyroidism
        2.5.8 Hypercalcaemia
        2.5.9 Hypocalcaemia
    2.6 Diabetes mellitus
    2.7 Other endocrine disorders
        2.7.1 Multiple endocrine neoplasia
        2.7.2 Autoimmune polyglandular endocrinopathies
        2.7.3 Ectopic hormone syndromes
3 Investigations and practical procedures
    3.1 Stimulation tests
        3.1.1 Short synacthen test
        3.1.2 Corticotrophin-releasing hormone
              (CRH) test
        3.1.3 Thyrotrophin-releasing hormone test
        3.1.4 Gonadotrophin-releasing hormone test
        3.1.5 Insulin tolerance test
        3.1.6 Pentagastrin stimulation test
        3.1.7 Oral glucose tolerance test
    3.2 Suppression tests
        3.2.1 Low-dose dexamethasone suppression test
        3.2.2 High-dose dexamethasone suppression test
        3.2.3 Oral glucose tolerance test in acromegaly
    3.3 Other investigations
        3.3.1 Thyroid function tests
        3.3.2 Water deprivation test

Nephrology

1 Clinical presentations
    1.1 Routine medical shows dipstick haematuria
    1.2 Pregnancy with renal disease
    1.3 A swollen young woman
    1.4 Rheumatoid arthritis with swollen legs
    1.5 A blood test shows renal failure
    1.6 A worrying ECG
    1.7 Postoperative acute renal failure
    1.8 Diabetes with impaired renal function
    1.9 Renal impairment and a multi-system disease
    1.10 Renal impairment and fever
    1.11 Atherosclerosis and renal failure
    1.12 Renal failure and haemoptysis
    1.13 Renal colic
    1.14 Backache and renal failure
    1.15 Is dialysis appropriate?
    1.16 Patient who refuses to be dialysed
    1.17 Renal failure and coma
2 Diseases and treatments
    2.1 Major renal syndromes
        2.1.1 Acute renal failure
        2.1.2 Chronic renal failure
        2.1.3 End-stage renal failure
        2.1.4 Nephrotic syndrome
    2.2 Renal replacement therapy
        2.2.1 Haemodialysis
        2.2.2 Peritoneal dialysis
        2.2.3 Renal transplantation
    2.3 Glomerular diseases
        2.3.1 Primary glomerular disease
        2.3.2 Secondary glomerular disease
    2.4 Tubulointerstitial diseases
        2.4.1 Acute tubular necrosis
        2.4.2 Acute interstitial nephritis
        2.4.3 Chronic interstitial nephritis
        2.4.4 Specific tubulointerstitial disorders
    2.5 Diseases of renal vessels
        2.5.1 Renovascular disease
        2.5.2 Cholesterol atheroembolization
    2.6 Postrenal problems
        2.6.1 Obstructive uropathy
        2.6.2 Stones
        2.6.3 Retroperitoneal fibrosis or periaortitis
        2.6.4 Urinary tract infection
    2.7 The kidney in systemic disease
        2.7.1 Myeloma

2.7.2 Amyloidosis
2.7.3 Haemolyticuraemic syndrome
2.7.4 Sickle cell disease
2.7.5 Autoimmune rheumatic disorders
2.7.6 Systemic vasculitis
2.7.7 Diabetic nephropathy
2.7.8 Hypertension
2.7.9 Sarcoidosis
2.7.10 Hepatorenal syndrome
2.7.11 Pregnancy and the kidney
2.8 Genetic renal conditions
2.8.1 Autosomal dominant polycystic kidney disease
2.8.2 Alport's syndrome
2.8.3 X-linked hypophosphataemic vitamin D-resistant rickets
3 Investigations and practical procedures
3.1 Examination of the urine
3.1.1 Urinalysis
3.1.2 Urine microscopy
3.2 Estimation of renal function, 106
3.3 Imaging the renal tract
3.4 Renal biopsy

Rheumatology and Clinical Immunology

1 Clinical presentations
1.1 Recurrent chest infections
1.2 Recurrent meningitis
1.3 Recurrent facial swelling and abdominal pain
1.4 Fulminant septicaemia
1.5 Recurrent skin abscesses
1.6 Chronic atypical mycobacterial infection
1.7 Collapse during a restaurant meal
1.8 Flushing and skin rash
1.9 Drug induced anaphylaxis
1.10 Arthralgia, purpuric rash and renal impairment
1.11 Arthralgia and photosensitive rash
1.12 Systemic lupus erythematosus and confusion
1.13 Cold fingers and difficulty in swallowing
1.14 Dry eyes and fatigue
1.15 Breathlessness and weakness
1.16 Prolonged fever and joint pains
1.17 Back pain
1.18 Acute hot joints
1.19 Recurrent joint pain and morning stiffness
1.20 Foot drop and weight loss
1.21 Fever, myalgia, arthralgia and elevated acute phase indices
1.22 Non-rheumatoid pain and stiffness
1.23 A crush fracture
1.24 Widespread pain
1.25 Fever and absent upper limb pulses

2 Diseases and treatments
2.1 Immunodeficiency
2.1.1 Primary antibody deficiency
2.1.2 Combined T- and B-cell defects
2.1.3 Chronic granulomatous disease
2.1.4 Cytokine and cytokine receptor deficiencies
2.1.5 Terminal pathway complement deficiency
2.1.6 Hyposplenism
2.2 Allergy
2.2.1 Anaphylaxis
2.2.2 Mastocytosis
2.2.3 Nut allergy
2.2.4 Drug allergy
2.3 Rheumatology
2.3.1 Carpal tunnel syndrome
2.3.2 Osteoarthritis
2.3.3 Rheumatoid arthritis
2.3.4 Seronegative spondyloarthritides
2.3.5 Idiopathic inflammatory myopathies
2.3.6 Crystal arthritis: gout
2.3.7 Calcium pyrophosphate deposition disease
2.4 Autoimmune rheumatic diseases
2.4.1 Systemic lupus erythematosus
2.4.2 Sjögren's syndrome
2.4.3 Systemic sclerosis (scleroderma)
2.5 Vasculitides
2.5.1 Giant cell arteritis and polymyalgia rheumatica
2.5.2 Wegener's granulomatosis
2.5.3 Polyarteritis nodosa
2.5.4 Cryoglobulinaemic vasculitis
2.5.5 Behçet's disease
2.5.6 Takayasu's arteritis
3 Investigations and practical procedures
3.1 Assessing acute phase response
3.1.1 Erythrocyte sedimentation rate
3.1.2 C-reactive protein
3.2 Serological investigation of autoimmune rheumatic disease
3.2.1 Antibodies to nuclear antigens
3.2.2 Antibodies to double-stranded DNA
3.2.3 Antibodies to extractable nuclear antigens
3.2.4 Rheumatoid factor
3.2.5 Antineutrophil cytoplasmic antibody
3.2.6 Serum complement concentrations
3.3 Suspected immune deficiency in adults
3.4 Imaging in rheumatological disease
3.4.1 Plain radiography
3.4.2 Bone densitometry
3.4.3 Magnetic resonance imaging
3.4.4 Nuclear medicine
3.5 Arthrocentesis
3.6 Corticosteroid injection techniques
3.7 Intravenous immunoglobulin

Index

abciximab 54
abdominal pain with exertional dyspnoea 158
Abram's needle 239
acid-fast bacilli 171
    lobar collapse 182
    testing 157
acid reflux, chest pain 43
acromegaly
    hypertension 48
    obstructive sleep apnoea 188
actinomycetes 207
acute chest syndrome 217
adenosine 61
adult respiratory distress syndrome (ARDS)
    breathlessness and haemodynamic
        collapse 26
    smoke inhalation 215, 217
agammaglobulinaemia 198
age 115
airway obstruction in smoke inhalation 217
albendazole 214
alcohol consumption
    angina 52
    cardiac failure 65
    cardiomyopathy 7
    hypertension 46, 112
    ischaemic heart disease 20
    obstructive sleep apnoea 188
    withdrawal 46
allergens
    asthma 192
    breathlessness and haemodynamic
        collapse 26
allergic bronchopulmonary aspergillosis 198,
    212, 213, 214
allergic rhinitis 190
alveolar proteinosis 241
alveolitis
    iatrogenic lung disease 214, 215, *216*
    see also cryptogenic fibrosing alveolitis;
        extrinsic allergic alveolitis
ambulatory monitoring 127, *129–30*
aminophylline **194**
amiodarone
    adverse reaction 161
    atrial fibrillation 61
    cardiac embolic stroke 14
    dyspnoea with inspiratory crackles 160,
        161, 163
    interstitial lung disease 160, **161**, 215, *216*
    paroxysmal atrial fibrillation/flutter 6
    ventricular tachycardia 8, 9, 68
amyloidosis 199
anaemia
    breathlessness 154
    myxoma 95
    pregnancy 108
analgesia and pulmonary embolism 116
Ancylostoma duodenale 213
angina
    cardiac catheterization 136
    chest pain 16, 53
    complications 54
    coronary artery disease 51–4
    crescendo 17, 53
    disease associations 52

driving 118
    dyspnoea with inspiratory crackles 160
    investigations 51
    pectoris 51
    prevention 52
    prognosis 54
    PTCA 138
    stable 51–3
    syncope 10
    treatment 51–2
    unstable 17, *18*, 53–4
        aortic dissection differential
            diagnosis 100
        echocardiography contraindication 142
        exercise ECG contraindication 124
        troponin tests 135–6
angioplasty 138–9
    driving 118
angiotensin converting enzyme (ACE)
    myocardial infarction 23, 56, 57
    sarcoid 154, 169, 183, 209, 210
angiotensin converting enzyme (ACE)
    inhibitors
    aortic dissection 100
    aortic regurgitation 74
    cardiac failure 64, 65
    diabetes mellitus 105
    hypertension 112
    nocturnal cough 170
ankle oedema
    exertional dyspnoea 183
    pulmonary embolism 115
    secondary pulmonary hypertension 104
ankle swelling
    breathlessness 19–22, 33–4, 154
    dyspnoea with inspiratory crackles 160
ankylosing spondylitis 228
anorexia 156
antiarrhythmic drugs, Vaughan-Williams'
    classification 61, **62**
antibiotics
    bronchiectasis 198
    cystic fibrosis 201
    infective endocarditis 93, **94**
    prophylaxis
        mitral regurgitation 76–7
        pregnancy 109
    sickle cell disease 218
anticholinergics 198
anticoagulation
    atrial fibrillation 62
    cardiac embolic stroke 14
    contraindications 164
    sickle cell disease 218
antihistamines 190
antineutrophil cytoplasmic antibodies
    (ANCA) 162
    pulmonary vasculitis 210, 211
antiphospholipid syndrome 106
    pulmonary embolism 118
antitachycardia pacing 131
α_1-antitrypsin deficiency 158, 159
    chronic obstructive pulmonary disease 194
    lung transplantation 236
anxiety
    chest pain 16
    palpitations 4
aortic aneurysm
    abdominal 47

breathlessness and haemodynamic
        collapse 26
    MRI 140
aortic dissection 99–101
    accelerated phase hypertension 113, 114
    acute pericarditis 79
    aetiology 99
    aortic regurgitation 73
    breathlessness and haemodynamic
        collapse 25, 27
    cardiac catheterization 136
    chest pain 16, 42, 43, 44
    classification 99
    clinical presentation 99
    complications 101
    epidemiology 99
    investigations 100
    medial degeneration 99
    mediastinal widening 18, 134
    pathophysiology/pathology 99
    prognosis 101
    repair 15
    signs 99–100
    syncope 11
    treatment 100
aortic enlargement 134
aortic regurgitation 71, *72*–4
    aortic enlargement 134
    complications 74
    prognosis 74
    rheumatic fever 94
    traumatic heart disease 97
    treatment 73–4
aortic root dilatation 73
aortic rupture 98
aortic stenosis 71–2
    chest pain and recurrent syncope 36
    complications 72
    critical 35
    differential diagnosis 71
    exercise ECG contraindication 124
    grading **72**
    pregnancy 109
    prognosis 72
    senile 71
    treatment 72
    valve replacement 72
aortic stenosis, calcific 12
aortic valve
    bicuspid 72
    cusp support loss 73
    echocardiography *142*
aortic valve disease 73
    pregnancy 48, 49
aortitis 73
apnoea–hypopnoea index *189*
appetite suppressants 31
arterial blood gas
    interpretation 241–2, *243*
    pleuritic pain 29–30
    sampling 237
arteriovenous malformations 156, 158
arthritis 95
    see also rheumatoid arthritis
asbestos exposure
    chest radiographs *203*
    lung cancer 178–80, 202, 220, 224
    lung changes 203
    mesothelioma 224

asbestos exposure (*continued*)
  pleural thickening 178, 179
  smoking 179
asbestos-related disease
  investigations 179–80
  malignancy 180, *181*
  management 180
asbestosis 202–4
  compensation claims 225
  investigations 202–3
  treatment 203–4
Ascaris 214
Aschoff's nodules 94
aspergillosis
  allergic bronchopulmonary 198, 212,
    213, 214
  cystic fibrosis 201
aspergillus 94
Aspergillus fumigatus 212, 213
aspirin
  angina 51, 52, 54
  myocardial infarction 23, 57
  pulmonary eosinophilia 212
asthma 191–3, *194*
  acute severe **194**
  allergens 192
  breathlessness 154
    and haemodynamic collapse 26
  bronchiolitis obliterans differential
    diagnosis 206
  cardiac 19
  chronic obstructive pulmonary disease 195
  compensation claims for occupational 225
  cor pulmonale 231
  differential diagnosis 192
  epidemiology 191
  exertional dyspnoea 158, 183
  hypoxia 168
  investigations 192
  ischaemic heart disease 20
  life-threatening 191
  lobar collapse 182
  management 191, 192–3, **194**
  moderate 191
  nocturnal cough 170
  occupational 178
  pulmonary embolism differential
    diagnosis 116
  risk factors 191
  severe acute 191
  treatment 192–3, **194**
atenolol
  accelerated phase hypertension 114
  myocardial infarction 23
atherogenesis 105
atheromatous coronary artery plaque 53
atherosclerosis 134
atherosclerotic carotid disease 59
athlete's heart 68
atopy 190
atrial arrhythmias 89
atrial fibrillation 4, 59–63
  cardiac embolic stroke 12
  constrictive pericarditis 82
  cor pulmonale 231
  dyspnoea with inspiratory crackles 160
  heart block *123*
  hyperthyroidism 104, 105
  hypertrophic cardiomyopathy 68
  mitral regurgitation 76
  pleuritic pain 29
  pulmonary embolism 115
  radiofrequency ablation 130
  stroke 108
  tricuspid valve disease 77
atrial myxoma
  fever, weight loss and new murmur 39

mitral stenosis differential diagnosis 75
  surgical removal 15
atrial natriuretic peptide 3
atrial septal defect 89–90
  cardiac catheterization 22
atrial septostomy 103
atrioventricular (AV) block 3, 4, 58
  ECG *122–3*
atrioventricular nodal re-entry (AVNRT)
  tachycardia 59–63, 123
  Holter monitoring *129*
  radiofrequency ablation 130
atrioventricular (AV) node 123
atrioventricular re-entry (AVRT)
  tachycardia 59
  Holter monitoring *129*
  radiofrequency ablation 130
atropine 59
Austin Flint murmur 75
autonomic nervous system 110–11
autonomic neuropathy 105
azathioprine
  parenchymal lung disease 205
  sarcoidosis 210

β agonists 192, 193, **194**
β blockers
  accelerated phase hypertension 114
  angina 51, 54
  aortic dissection 100
  arrhythmias 6
  bradycardia *59*
  cardiac failure 65
  exercise ECG 125
  hypertension 112
  hypertrophic cardiomyopathy 68
  mitral stenosis 75
  myocardial infarction 56, 57
  overdose 132
β$_2$ agonists 198
BCNU 205
bendrofluazide 64
berylliosis 204
  sarcoidosis differential diagnosis 210
bicarbonate 242, *243*
bicuspid valve
  coarctation of aorta association 92
  degenerative 71
bird fancier's lung 160
birds, contact
  atypical pneumonia 168
  chronic extrinsic allergic alveolitis 207
Blalock–Taussig shunt *85*, 86
bleomycin
  cryptogenic fibrosing alveolitis differential
    diagnosis 205
  pulmonary eosinophilia 213
blood gas machines 241, 242
blood pressure
  elevated at routine screening 46–8
  measurement 47
  see also hypertension; hypotension
blue baby 33
bone pain
  lung cancer 221
  pulmonary nodule 156
bones, chest radiograph 245
brachial plexus 156
bradyarrhythmia
  ECG 120, 123
  electrophysiology studies 125
  management 12
bradycardia 58–9
  aetiology 58
  classification **58**
  clinical presentation 58
  hypothyroidism 104

investigations 58–9
  junctional *123*
  pathology/pathophysiology 58
  physical signs 58
  sinus 4
  treatment 59
brain
  abscess 85, 199
  CT scan 13
  metastases 221
  radiotherapy *222*, 223
breathing disorders
  non-invasive ventilation 234
  see also sleep disordered breathing
breathlessness
  ankle oedema and cyanosis 33–4
  ankle swelling 19–22
  bronchiolitis obliterans 205
  cardiac causes 19–20
  causes **153**
  chest radiograph 154, *155*
  chronic extrinsic allergic alveolitis 207
  cryptogenic fibrosing alveolitis 204
  CT of chest 22
  ECG 21
  echocardiography 21–2
  examination 20, 154
  exertional presyncope 30–3
    history 30–1
    investigations 32
    management 32–3
  haemodynamic collapse 25–8
    investigations 27
    management 27–8
  HIV infection 219
  hypertrophic cardiomyopathy 68
  hypotension after myocardial infarction 23
  increasing 153–5
  inspiratory crackles 160–3
    examination 161
    investigations 162–3
    management 163
  investigations 20–2, 154–5
  left ventricular function 22
  lobar collapse 180, *181*
  lung cancer 220
  management 22
  mitral regurgitation 76
  myxoma 95
  normal radiograph 182–4
  occupation 153
  pleuritic pain 163
  pneumothorax 154, *155*
  pulmonary causes **19**, 20
  pulmonary embolism 115
    differential diagnosis 116
  pulmonary hypertension 20, 22
    secondary 104
  pulmonary nodule 156
  respiratory causes 20
  ventricular septal defect 90
  see also dyspnoea
bronchial adenoma 222
bronchial carcinoma 220
bronchial obstruction
  bronchiectasis 197
  radiotherapy 223
bronchial tear investigation 241
bronchiectasis 197–9
  aetiology 197
  associated conditions **197**
  asthma differential diagnosis 192
  breathlessness with ankle oedema and
    cyanosis 33, 34
  chronic respiratory failure 230
  clinical presentation 197, **198**
  complications 198–9

cor pulmonale 198, 199
dyspnoea with inspiratory crackles 160
exertional dyspnoea 158, 159
foreign body 199
haemoptysis 198, 199
    with weight loss 175
investigations 198, **199**
lung lobe resection 198
lung transplantation 198
nocturnal cough 170
non-invasive ventilation 235
pathology 197
prevention 199
prognosis 199
treatment 198
tuberculosis 33
bronchiolitis obliterans 205–6, 214
lung transplantation 236
smoke inhalation 217
bronchitis
exertional dyspnoea 158
ischaemic heart disease 20
lobar collapse 182
bronchoconstriction 214, 215
bronchodilators
bronchiectasis 198
cystic fibrosis 201
bronchopleural fistula 239, 240
bronchoscopy
fibreoptic 240–1
laser 223
Brugia malayi 213
budesonide 210
bundle branch block 123
burns, thermal 216
busulfan 205

cachexia 82
calcification
intracardiac in myxoma 96
pulmonary artery 135
valve 107
calcium antagonists
angina 52
aortic dissection 100
hypertension 112
hypertrophic cardiomyopathy 68
mitral stenosis 75
primary pulmonary hypertension 103
calcium serum levels in sarcoid 154, 169, 183,
    209, 210
Candida 212
cannon waves 3
Caplan's syndrome 202
captopril 212
carbamazepine 213
carbon dioxide
partial pressure 242, *243*
retention 230, 232
carbon monoxide poisoning 215
smoke inhalation 216, 217
carboxyhaemoglobin 217
carcinoid syndrome
lobar collapse 182
pulmonary stenosis 78
tricuspid regurgitation 77
cardiac abscess 41
cardiac arrhythmia 58–63
benign 6
bradycardia 58–9, 104, *123*
chest pain and recurrent syncope 35, 36
driving 118, 119
life-threatening 6
malignancy 96
management 27
tachycardia 59–63
cardiac asthma 19

cardiac biochemical markers 135–6
cardiac catheterization 16, 136–8
angina 52
breathlessness 22
complications 138
contraindications 136
cardiac cycle 120
cardiac disease
chest radiograph 134–5
general anaesthesia 110
nocturnal cough 170
pregnancy 108–10
systemic complications 107–8
see also congenital heart disease; heart;
    ischaemic heart disease; rheumatic heart
    disease; valvular heart disease
cardiac failure 63–6
aetiology 63
arterial blood gas sampling 237
chronic progressive 65
clinical presentation 63–4
complications 65
driving 118, 119
dyspnoea with inspiratory crackles
    161, 162
epidemiology 63
hypertension 47
investigations 64
malignancy 96
obstructive sleep apnoea 188
pathology/pathophysiology 63
physical signs 64
prevention 65
prognosis 65
salt consumption 64
treatment 64–5
see also congestive heart failure; right
    heart failure
cardiac hypertrophy, hypertensive 67
cardiac ischaemia 15, 16
cardiac revascularization 16
cardiac silhouette 134
cardiac tamponade 23, 24
acute pericarditis 79
breathlessness and haemodynamic
    collapse 27
chest pain 44
echocardiography 45
pericardial effusion 80, 81
presentation 81
pulmonary embolism differential
    diagnosis 116
cardiac tumours 41, 95–7
cardiac valve regurgitation
breathlessness and haemodynamic
    collapse 27
fever, weight loss and new murmur 41
cardiac valves, prosthetic 109
cardiogenic shock 56
cardiomegaly 18, 134
aortic stenosis 71
exertional dyspnoea 159
pericardial effusion 135
pericarditis 45
pulmonary fibrosis 162
somnolence with headache 173
transposition of the great arteries 87
cardiomyopathy
amyloid 70
diabetic 105
dilated 68, 69–70
aetiology 69
cardiac embolic stroke 12
clinical presentation 69
investigations 70
pathophysiology/pathology 69
driving 118, 119

hereditary 49
hypertrophic 66–9
aetiology 66
clinical presentation 67
complications 68
differential diagnosis 67–8
disease associations 68
epidemiology 66
investigations 67
pathophysiology/pathology 66, 67
physical signs 67
pregnancy 109
prognosis 68
treatment 68
hypertrophic obstructive 3, 4, 12, 35–6
breathlessness with exertional
    presyncope 31
exercise ECG contraindication 124
pregnancy 48
MRI 140
peripartum 109
restrictive 22, 70–1, 82
ventricular tachycardia 7, *8*
cardiotoxic chemotherapy 31
carotid sinus massage 59
catecholamines 7
cerebral abscess 85
cerebrovascular disease
hypertension 46
myocardial infarction 57
cerebrovascular events 10
chemotherapy
cardiotoxic 31
lung cancer 223
chest pain
acute central 15–18, *19*
angina 53
breathlessness
exertional presyncope 30
haemodynamic collapse 25
flu-like illness 42–6
examination 43–4
history 42–3
hypotension after myocardial infarction 23
investigations 17–18
lobar collapse 181
lung cancer 220
management 18, *19*
myocardial infarction 20
pleuritic 39, 163–5, *166–7*
recurrent syncope 35–8
examination 35–6
investigations 36–7, *38*
management 38
sickle cell disease 217
chest radiograph 244, *246*
bones 245
breathlessness 154, *155*
ischaemic heart disease *216*
left atrial enlargement 134–5
lung cancer 221, *222*
lungs 245
mesothelioma 224, *225*
pericardial effusion 135
pulmonary vasculature abnormalities 135
chest trauma 98
chest wall deformity 172, *173*
chest wall disorders 227–30
chronic respiratory failure 230
cor pulmonale 231
tuberculosis 228
see also scoliosis
Chlamydia 168
chlorambucil 210
chloroquine 210
chlorpromazine 213
chlorpropamide 213

chordae tendinae rupture 76
chronic obstructive pulmonary disease 194–7
  asthma differential diagnosis 192
  breathlessness with ankle oedema and
    cyanosis 34
  bronchiolitis obliterans 206
  chronic respiratory failure 230
  complications 196
  cyanosis 33
  differential diagnosis 195
  exertional dyspnoea 158, 159
  hypercapnic exacerbation 185–7
  intercostal tube insertion 240
  investigations 195
  lung transplantation 236
  non-invasive ventilation 234, 235
  oxygen therapy 232
  prognosis 104, 196–7
  pulmonary artery enlargement 134
  smoking 194, 196
  treatment 196
Churg–Strauss syndrome 183, 211, 212
  asthma differential diagnosis 192
cirrhosis 201
clinical data interpretation 241–5, 246, 247,
  248–9
clopidogrel 52
clubbing, finger 34, 86, 92, 161
  cryptogenic fibrosing alveolitis 204
  exertional dyspnoea 183
  haemoptysis with weight loss 175
  hypoxia 168
  myxoma 95
  ventricular septal defect 90
coal-worker's pneumoconiosis 202–4
  compensation claims 225
coarctation of aorta 47, 48, 91–2
  infective endocarditis 84
  pregnancy 109
cocaine use 31
colchicine 80
collagen disorders 134
colloid therapy 116
compensation for occupational disease 225
compression stockings 118
computed tomography (CT)
  cardiac disease 140
  conventional 247
  helical 247
  high-resolution 247
  spiral 165
  thorax 245, 247, 248–9
confusion 221
congenital heart disease 84–92
  acyanotic 84, **85**
  cardiac catheterization 136
  cyanotic 84, **85**
  MRI 140
  pregnancy 109
  recurrence risk in baby 110
congestive heart failure
  asthma differential diagnosis 192
  atrial fibrillation 59
  exertional dyspnoea 158
  hypoalbuminaemia 20
  palpitations 4
Conn's syndrome 48
continuous positive airways pressure
  (CPAP) 232–4
  complications 233
  nasal 189
  outcome 233
Cope's needle 239
cor pulmonale 20, 230–1
  bronchiectasis 197, 198, 199
  chronic obstructive pulmonary disease
    195

chronic respiratory failure 230
cyanosis 33
  parenchymal lung disease 205
  sarcoidosis complication 210
  scoliosis 228
  sickle cell disease 217, 218
  sleep apnoea 172
coronary angioplasty 143
  driving 118
  thrombolysis 56
coronary arteries
  cardiac catheterization 137
  stenting 138, 139
  trauma 97
coronary artery bypass grafting 52
  diabetes mellitus 105
  driving 118
  myocardial infarction 56
  PTCA 139
coronary artery disease 51–8
  angina 51–4
  mitral regurgitation 76
  myocardial infarction 54–8
  myocardial perfusion imaging 144
  renal disease 106–7
coronary revascularization in diabetes
  mellitus 105
coronary syndrome, acute 143
  acute pericarditis differential diagnosis 79
coronary vasospasm 18, 19
corticosteroids see steroids
cough
  asthma 191
  chronic obstructive pulmonary disease
    195
  differential diagnosis **170**
  lobar collapse 180
  nocturnal 169–72
    examination 170–1
    history 170
    investigations 171
    lung function tests 171
    management 172
    obstructive sleep apnoea 188
Coxsackie B virus 79
craniofacial abnormalities 188
creatine kinase
  biochemical marker 135, 136
  heart muscle damage 17
  traumatic heart disease 97
crocidolite 224
cromoglycates 190
Cryptococcus neoformans 219
cryptogenic fibrosing alveolitis 161, 162,
  204–5
  aetiology 206–7
  chronic extrinsic allergic alveolitis
    differential diagnosis 208
  differential diagnosis 204–5
cushingoid features in lung cancer 221
Cushing's syndrome 48
cyanosis 33–4
  breathlessness 154
  congenital heart disease 85
  Ebstein's anomaly 89
  exertional dyspnoea 183
  pregnancy 109
  right-to-left shunts 85–6
  smoke inhalation 216
  transposition of the great arteries 87
  ventricular septal defect 90
cyclophosphamide
  Churg–Strauss syndrome 212
  parenchymal lung disease 205
  sarcoidosis 210
  Wegener's granulomatosis 212
cyclosporin 210

cystic fibrosis 199–202
  breathlessness with ankle oedema and
    cyanosis 33
  complications 201
  diabetes mellitus 200
  epidemiology 200
  exertional dyspnoea 158, 159
  gene mutations 200
  investigations 200
  liver disease 201
  lung destruction 199
  lung transplantation 201, 236
  nasal potential difference 200
  pancreatic insufficiency 201
  prevention 201
  prognosis 201
  respiratory failure 201
  sweat test 200
  treatment 201
cystic fibrosis transmembrane conductance
  regulator (CFTR) 199
cytomegalovirus (CMV) 219

D-dimer 165
δ waves 4, 5
  chest pain and recurrent syncope 36
dapsone 220
DC cardioversion 14
  atrial fibrillation 61, 62, 63
deep vein thrombosis
  breathlessness
    exertional presyncope 31
    haemodynamic collapse 26
  pleuritic pain 29
  pulmonary embolism 115
defibrillator, implantable cardioverter 6, 9,
  131, 216
dermatomyositis 206
dextrocardia 159
diabetes mellitus
  angina 52
  cardiac complications 105
  cystic fibrosis 200, 201
  hypertension 46
  ischaemic heart disease risk 16
  myocardial infarction 56, 105
diabetic cardiomyopathy 105
diaphragm disorders 227–30
diaphragm paralysis 155
diethylcarbamazine 214
digitalis
  aortic regurgitation 74
  mitral regurgitation 76
digoxin
  atrial fibrillation 62
  cardiac failure 65
  Ebstein's anomaly 89
  overdose 132
  ventricular tachycardia 7
diphtheria 170
diuretics
  pulmonary hypertension 34
  syncope 10
DNase in cystic fibrosis 201
dobutamine
  hypotension after myocardial infarction 24
  stress echocardiography 141, 143
Doppler echocardiography 141–2
driving
  hypertrophic cardiomyopathy 69
  obstructive sleep apnoea 174, 190
  restrictions 118–19
drug abuse, intravenous 39
drugs
  intoxication 237
  overdose 132
dyslipidaemia 105

dysphagia 220
dyspnoea
  exertional 153, 158–60
    chronic obstructive pulmonary
      disease 185, 195
    domiciliary oxygen therapy 231
    examination 159, 183
    iatrogenic lung disease 215
    investigations 159, 183–4
    management 160, 184
    normal radiograph 182–4
    scoliosis 228
  nocturnal 153
    paroxysmal 160
  see also breathlessness

Eaton–Lambert syndrome 156
Ebstein's anomaly 33, 88–9
  infective endocarditis 84
  tricuspid regurgitation 77
echocardiography 141–3
  breathlessness 21–2
  contraindications 142
  M-mode 141
  stress 141, 143
  stroke 108
  syncope 11
  two-dimensional 141
Eisenmenger's syndrome 33, 86–7
  atrial septal defect 89, 90
  pregnancy 109
  pulmonary artery enlargement 134
  ventricular septal defect 90
electrocardiogram
  stroke 13, 14
  ventricular tachycardia 7, 8
electrocardiography (ECG) 120, 121–2,
    123–5, 126
  ambulatory 9
  atrioventricular (AV) block 122–3
  bradyarrhythmias 120, 123
  breathlessness 21
  exercise 8, 124–5
  fibrillations 4, 5
  heart block 122–3
  left axis deviation 122
  left ventricular hypertrophy 123
  myocardial infarction 17
  normal intervals 120, 121
  principle 120
  right axis deviation 121
  right ventricular hypertrophy 124
  stroke 13, 14
  syncope 10–11
  tachyarrhythmia 123
  ventricular tachycardia 7, 8
electrolyte imbalance 59
electrophysiology studies 125, 127, 128
  complications 127
embolectomy 116, 165
embolism, paradoxical 89
emphysema 196
  smoking 159
empyema 177–8
  bronchiectasis complication 198
  intercostal tube insertion 239
  pleural biopsy contraindication 239
endocarditis
  myxoma differential diagnosis 96
  non-bacterial thrombotic 92
endocarditis, infective 92–4
  aetiology 92
  antibiotic treatment 40
  aortic regurgitation 73
  aspergillus 94
  cardiac embolic stroke 12, 13
  clinical presentation 92

congenital heart disease 84
  epidemiology 92
  fever, weight loss and new murmur
    39
  hypertrophic cardiomyopathy 68
  investigations 92–3
  mitral regurgitation 76
  pacemaker complication 133
  patent ductus arteriosus 91
  pathophysiology/pathology 92
  physical signs 92
  pregnancy 49
  rheumatic fever differential diagnosis
    95
  streptococci 94
  subacute bacterial 109
  treatment 93, 94
  tricuspid regurgitation 77
endocardium
  cushion defects 77
  trauma 97
endomyocardial fibrosis 70
eosinophilic granuloma 210
epileptic fits see seizures
epinephrine 24
Epstein–Barr virus (EBV) 208
eptifibatide 54
erythema nodosum 160, 161
Ewart's sign 81
exercise ECG 124–5, 126
exercise test requirements for driving 119
expiratory positive airways pressure
    (EPAP) 233, 234
extrinsic allergic alveolitis 162, 206–8
  acute 207
  chronic 207–8
  cryptogenic fibrosing alveolitis differential
    diagnosis 205

familial Mediterranean fever 176
farmer's lung 206–7
fever
  lobar collapse 180, 181
  myxoma 95
  pleural effusion 176–8
  pleuritic pain 164
  weight loss and new murmur 38–41, 42
    investigations 40–1
    management 41
fibreoptic bronchoscopy 240–1
fibrillations, ECG 4, 5
fibronectin 208
fibrothorax 228
filariasis 213, 214
  cor pulmonale 231
flow–volume loops 244
foramen ovale, patent 89
forced expiratory capacity 243
forced vital capacity 243
foreign body
  asthma differential diagnosis 192
  bronchiectasis 199
  inhaled 154
    lobar collapse 181, 182
Friedreich's ataxia 68
furosemide (frusemide)
  accelerated phase hypertension 114
  cardiac failure 64

gas transfer 244
gastric juice aspiration 241
gastro-oesophageal reflux
  nocturnal cough 172
  obstructive sleep apnoea 188
gastrointestinal obstruction 201
general anaesthesia 110
glomerulonephritis, acute 114

glucose intolerance 47
  cystic fibrosis 201
glyceryl trinitrate
  angina 51, 53, 54
  coronary vasospasm 19
  myocardial infarction 57
glycoprotein IIb/IIIa receptor blocker 105,
    136, 138
goitre, retrosternal 185
gold therapy 213
Goodpasture's syndrome 175
gout 95
Graham Steell murmur
  aortic regurgitation differential
    diagnosis 73
  mitral stenosis 74
  pulmonary regurgitation 78
  see also pulmonary regurgitation

haemoptysis
  breathlessness
    exertional presyncope 30
    haemodynamic collapse 25
  bronchiectasis 198, 199
  cystic fibrosis 201
  fever, weight loss and new murmur 39
  investigations 175
  lobar collapse 181
  lung cancer 220
  management 175
  pleuritic pain 163
  pulmonary embolism 163
  pulmonary nodule 155, 156
  sarcoidosis complication 210
  weight loss 174–5
haemothorax
  intercostal tube insertion 239, 240
  pericardial effusion/pneumothorax
    aspiration 238
headache, morning 172–4, 188, 230
Heaf test 209
heart
  chest radiograph 244
  infective diseases 92–5
  see also cardiac entries
heart block
  atrial fibrillation 123
  ECG 122–3
  malignancy 96
heart murmur 75
  breathlessness
    ankle oedema and cyanosis 34
    exertional presyncope 32
  examination 40
  fever and weight loss 38–41, 42
  hypoxia 168
  ischaemic heart disease 20
  machinery 90
  pregnancy 48–50
    investigations 49–50
    management 50
  stroke 12–15, 108
  tricuspid valve disease 77
  see also Graham Steell murmur
heart muscle disease 66–71
heart sounds
  breathlessness with exertional
    presyncope 32
  examination 40
  stroke 108
  traumatic heart disease 97
heart transplantation 65
  cardiac catheterization 136
heart–lung transplantation 103
helium–oxygen mixture 185
hemiparesis 12, 13
hemiplegia 101

Henoch–Schönlein syndrome 211
heparin
    low-molecular-weight 136, 165
    pulmonary embolism 116, 118
hepatic failure 237
hepatomegaly 89
hepatosplenomegaly
    constrictive pericarditis 82
    cystic fibrosis 200
herpes, labial 29
herpes zoster 238
hilar lymphadenopathy 162
His bundle 123
histamine 191
HIV infection
    aetiology 218–19
    Cryptococcus neoformans 219
    cytomegalovirus 219
    fungal infections 219
    haempotysis and weight loss 174
    investigations 219–20
    Kaposi's sarcoma 219, 220
    lung disorders 218–20
    Pneumocystis carinii pneumonia 168, 169,
        218, 219, 220
    tuberculosis 219, 220
HLA-Bw 15 208
hoarseness, voice 184
Hodgkin's lymphoma *217*
Holter monitoring 11, 59, 60, 127, *129*
Hoover's sign 195
hormone replacement therapy
    angina 52
    pulmonary embolism 115
Horner's syndrome
    breathlessness 154
    lung cancer 220, 221
hydrocortisone **194**
hydroxycarbamide 214
hyperaldosteronism 112
    primary 47
hypercalcaemia
    bone pain 156
    ECG 124
    malignancy 157
    sarcoidosis 209
        complication 210
hypercalciuria 209
hypercapnia 173
hypercholesterolaemia 16
hypereosinophilic syndrome 212
hyperkalaemia 124
hyperlipidaemia
    angina 52
    hypertension 46
hypernephroma 40
hypertension 46–8, 110–14
    accelerated phase (malignant) 46, 112,
        113–14
    aetiology 110–11
    angina 52
    aortic dissection 99
    aortic enlargement 134
    aortic regurgitation 73
    atrial fibrillation 59
    clinical presentation 111
    complications 112
    differential diagnosis 112
    epidemiology 111
    essential 46, 111, 112
    examination 47
    history 46
    investigations 47–8, 111–12
    ischaemic heart disease risk 16
    left ventricular hypertrophy 111
    myocardial infarction 112
    obstructive sleep apnoea 188, 190

pathophysiology/pathology 110–11
    peripheral vascular disease 112
    physical signs 111
    pregnancy 109
    prognosis 112–13
    pulmonary embolism 118
    pulmonary oedema 111, *112*
    renal 46
    risk factors 46
    secondary 46, 111, 112
    sleep apnoea 172
    stroke 112
    treatment 112
    white coat 48, 111, 112
    see also pulmonary hypertension
hypertensive encephalopathy 113, 114
hyperthyroidism 104, 105
hypertrophic cardiomyopathy *see*
    cardiomyopathy, hypertrophic
hyperviscosity
    breathlessness with ankle oedema and
        cyanosis 33
    cyanosis 85
hypoalbuminaemia 20
hypocalcaemia 124
hypogammaglobulinaemia 158, 159
hypokalaemia
    ECG 124
    hypertension 47
    syncope 11
hypotension
    myocardial infarction 23–5
        examination 23
        investigations 23–4
        management 24–5
        prognosis 25
    orthostatic 35
        chest pain and recurrent syncope
            36, 38
hypothermia 59
hypothyroidism
    bradycardia 59
    cardiac complications 104, 105
    obstructive sleep apnoea 188
    pericarditis 43
    somnolence with headache 173
    upper airway obstruction 184, 185
hypoxia
    differential diagnosis **167**
    investigations 168–9
    management 169
    sickle cell disease 218
    unexplained 167–9

imipramine 213
immunoglobulin deficiency 197
immunotherapy 190
infection
    pacemaker complication 133
    systemic 124
    transbronchial biopsy 241
    viral 95
infective diseases of heart 92–5
inferior vena caval filters 116, 118, 165
influenza vaccination 199
informed consent for life-support 186
insulin 56, 173
intercostal artery 239
intercostal tube insertion 239–40
γ-interferon 223
interstitial lung disease 160, 161, 204–6
    amiodarone 160, **161**, 215, *216*
    hypoxia 168
    sarcoidosis differential diagnosis 210
    see also parenchymal lung disease
intra-abdominal catastrophe 26, 27
intrapericardial pressure (IPP) 80

ipratropium **194**
irradiation 205
ischaemic heart disease
    atrial fibrillation 59
    chest pain 16
        recurrent syncope 35
    chest radiograph *216*
    general anaesthesia 110
    history 20
    hypertension 46
    risk factors 16
    syncope 10
    ventricular tachycardia 6–7

Janeway's lesions 39, 92
juvenile chronic arthritis 95

Kaposi's sarcoma 219, 220
Kawasaki disease 211
Kerley B lines 162
ketoacidosis 237
Kussmaul's sign 82
kyphoscoliosis *173*
kyphosis 228

labetalol
    accelerated phase hypertension 114
    aortic dissection 100
lactic acidosis 237
laryngeal nerve palsy 220
laryngeal oedema 216
laser bronchoscopy 223
left atrial enlargement
    chest radiograph 134–5
    constrictive pericarditis 83
    mitral regurgitation 76
    patent ductus arteriosus 91
left atrial myxoma 12
left ventricular assist device 65, *66*
left ventricular dilatation 71
left ventricular dysfunction 24
    breathlessness with exertional
        presyncope 32
    renal disease 106, 107
    secondary pulmonary hypertension
        differential diagnosis 104
left ventricular failure
    dyspnoea with inspiratory crackles
        160, 163
    transposition of the great arteries 88
left ventricular function 22
left ventricular hypertrophy 4, 5, 135
    aortic stenosis 71
    chest pain and recurrent syncope 36
    ECG 123
    hypertension 47, 48, 111
    mitral regurgitation 76
    patent ductus arteriosus 91
    somnolence with headache 173
    syncope 10
left ventricular outflow obstruction 31, 32
Legionella 168
leukotriene receptor antagonists 192,
    193, **194**
leukotrienes 191
lidocaine 8
life-support, informed consent 186
Light's criteria for pleural effusions 177
liver disease 201, 237
    see also hepatomegaly; hepatosplenomegaly
living will 186
Löffler's syndrome 212
long QT syndrome 35, *37*
    chest pain and recurrent syncope 36
loop recorders, implantable 127,
    129–30
lower limb ischaemia 101

lung abscess 153
  bronchiectasis complication 198
  exertional dyspnoea 158, 159
  lung cancer differential diagnosis 222
lung cancer 220–4
  aetiology 220
  asbestos exposure 178–80, 202, 220, 224
  breathlessness 153, 220
  chemotherapy 223
  chest pain 220
  chest radiograph 221, *222*
  clinical presentation 220–1
  compensation claims for
    asbestos-associated 225
  complications 222, **223**
  differential diagnosis 222
  epidemiology 220
  haemoptysis 220
  histological cell types **220**
  investigations 221–2
  metastases 223
  pain control 223
  pathology 220
  physical signs 221
  prevention 223
  prognosis 223
  pulmonary nodule 155
  radiotherapy 223
  smoking *171*, 181, 220, 223
  surgery 223
  treatment 223
lung consolidation
  breathlessness and haemodynamic
    collapse 27
  lobar collapse 182
  lung cancer 221
  organizing pneumonia 206
  pleuritic pain 164
  sickle cell disease *218*
lung disease
  breathlessness 154
  iatrogenic 214–15, *217*
  inflammatory 170
  obstructive sleep apnoea 188
  occupational 202–4
  see also chronic obstructive pulmonary
    disease; interstitial lung disease;
    parenchymal lung disease
lung fibrosis
  amiodarone *216*
  asbestosis 202, 204
  interstitial 210
  pneumoconiosis 202, 204
  radiation-induced 214, 215, *217*
lung function
  definitions **243**
  laboratory 243
  tests 243–4
lung lobes
  collapse 180–2, *246*
  resection in bronchiectasis 198
lung metastases 156
lung parenchymal compression 81
lung transplantation 236
  bronchiectasis 198
  bronchiolitis obliterans 206
  chronic obstructive pulmonary disease 196
  complications 236
  contraindications 236
  cystic fibrosis 201
  indications 236
  living donor bilateral lobar 201
  parenchymal lung disease 205
  primary pulmonary hypertension 103
  rejection 236
  retransplantation 236
  sarcoidosis 210

lung tumour, benign 158
lung volume reduction surgery 196
lymphadenopathy
  hilar 162
  lung cancer 221
  mediastinal 157
lymphoma *217*
  sarcoidosis differential diagnosis 210

magnetic resonance imaging (MRI) 140
malabsorption in cystic fibrosis 201
malignancy 220–7
  acute pericarditis 79
  asbestos-related disease 180, *181*
  breathlessness 154
  cardiac 95, 96
  cardiac tamponade 80
  hypercalcaemia 157
  nocturnal cough 170
  parenchymal lung disease 205
  pericarditis 43, 82
  pleural effusion with fever 176,
    177, 178
  pleuritic pain 163
  pulmonary embolism 115, 118
  smoking 169–70
  thromboembolism 163
  transbronchial biopsy 241
marfanoid habitus 29
  pleuritic pain 163
Marfan's syndrome
  aortic dissection 44, 99
  aortic regurgitation 73
  pregnancy 49, 109
  pulmonary artery enlargement 134
measles
  bronchiectasis 160
  vaccination 199
mebendazole 214
mediastinal nodes
  lung cancer 222
  lymphadenopathy 157
mediastinal shift 26, 27, *175*
  mesothelioma *181*
  upper airway obstruction 185
mediastinal tumours 226–7
mediastinal widening 134
mediastinum **227**
  CT scan 248–9
mesenteric ischaemia 101
mesothelioma 153, *181*, 202, 224–6
  aetiology 224
  chest radiograph 224, *225*
  clinical presentation 224
  compensation claims 225
  complications 225
  differential diagnosis 224
  disease associations 226
  epidemiology 224
  investigations 224, *225*
  non-pleural 226
  pain control 224
  peritoneal 226
  physical signs 224
  pleural effusion with fever 176
  prevention 225
  prognosis 225
  treatment 224
metastases
  bone pain 156
  brain 221
  lung 156
  lung cancer 221, 223
  transbronchial biopsy 241
methotrexate
  cryptogenic fibrosing alveolitis differential
    diagnosis 205

pulmonary eosinophilia 212
  sarcoidosis 210
metolazone 64
midazolam 239, 240
middle ear disease 170
mitral annular calcification 76
mitral regurgitation 23, 24, 75–7
  breathlessness and haemodynamic
    collapse 26
  cardiac catheterization 136
  complications 77
  echocardiography 76, 77
  prognosis 77
  rheumatic fever 94
  surgery outcome 77
  traumatic heart disease 97
mitral stenosis 74–5
  aortic regurgitation differential diagnosis 73
  cardiac catheterization 136
  complications 75
  palpitations 4
  pregnancy 109
  prognosis 75
  rheumatic fever 94
  severity **75**
mitral valve disease
  myxoma differential diagnosis 96
  pregnancy 48
mitral valve prolapse 76
  pregnancy *50*
mitral valve replacement 75
mitral valvuloplasty 75
montelukast 193
motor neuron disease 230
mucociliary clearance 197
mumps 160
muscular dystrophy
  chronic respiratory failure 230
  scoliosis 228
musculoskeletal disorders 163
musculoskeletal pain 16, 17, 30
  acute pericarditis differential diagnosis 79
  chest pain 43, 44
  pulmonary embolism differential
    diagnosis 116
myasthenia gravis 184, 185
  mediastinal tumours 226
mycetoma 210
Mycobacterium 246
Mycobacterium avium intracellulare 219
Mycobacterium chelonea 219
Mycobacterium kansasii 219
Mycobacterium tuberculosis 174
  sarcoidosis 208
mycoplasma 176
myocardial infarction 54–8, *57*
  aetiology 54
  anterior *55*
  biochemical markers 136
  breathlessness and haemodynamic
    collapse 25
  cardiac embolic stroke 12
  chest pain 15, 16, 20, 42, 43
    recurrent syncope *37*
  clinical presentation 55
  complications 56–7
  coronary artery disease 54–8
  creatine kinase 135
  diabetes mellitus 105
  differential diagnosis 55
  disease associations 57
  driving 118
  ECG 17
  endocarditis 39
  epidemiology 55
  examination 16–17
  exercise ECG contraindication 124

myocardial infarction (*continued*)
  hypertension 112
  hypotension 23–5
  information for patients 57
  investigations 55
  myocardial perfusion imaging 144
  non-Q-wave 57
  pacemakers 132
  palpitations 4, 5
  pathophysiology/pathology 54
  physical signs 55
  prevention 57
    cardiac failure 65
  prognosis 57
  PTCA 138, 139
  pulmonary embolism differential
    diagnosis 116
  renal disease 106
  sickle cell disease 217
  syncope 10, 11
  thrombolysis 56
  treatment 56
  unstable angina 54
  ventricular tachycardia 7
myocardial perfusion imaging 143–4
myocarditis
  exercise ECG contraindication 124
  treatment 106
myocardium trauma 97
myoglobin assay 136
myxoma 95–7
  complications 96
  prevalence 95
  prognosis 97
  syndrome 97
  treatment 96
myxomatous degeneration 77

nails, splinter haemorrhages 92
naproxen 212
nasal congestion 188
nasal polyps 172, *173*
  allergic rhinitis 190
  cystic fibrosis 201
Necator 214
neck palpitations 3
neuralgic pain 220
neuromuscular disease 235
next of kin 186
nicorandil 52, 54
nicotine replacement therapies 223
nifedipine 114
nitrate, long-acting 52
nitrofurantoin 213
nitrogen dioxide
  inhalation 217
  pneumonitis 207
nitroprusside
  accelerated phase hypertension 114
  mitral regurgitation 76
non-invasive positive pressure
  ventilation 234
  see also ventilation, non-invasive
non-steroidal anti-inflammatory drugs
  (NSAIDs)
  acute pericarditis 80
  pericarditis 45
noxious fume inhalation 241
nuclear cardiology 143–4

obesity
  chronic respiratory failure 230
  cor pulmonale 231
  hypertension 46
  obstructive sleep apnoea 188
  pulmonary embolism 115
  upper airway obstruction 184

obstructive vascular disease 231
occupational disease
  allergic rhinitis 190
  asbestos exposure 178
  compensation 225
  cryptogenic fibrosing alveolitis differential
    diagnosis 205
  extrinsic allergic alveolitis
    acute 207
    chronic 208
  lung 202–4
  mesothelioma 224
oedema
  salt consumption 22
  see also pulmonary oedema
oesophageal reflux 170
oesophagitis 16, 43
opiate premedication 239, 240
oral contraceptives
  breathlessness with exertional
    presyncope 31
  primary pulmonary hypertension 103
  pulmonary embolism 115, 118
organic dust toxic syndrome 207
orthopnoea 160
  scoliosis 228
Osler's nodes 39, 92
oximetry, overnight 244
oxygen
  partial pressure 242
  saturation 137
oxygen therapy
  ambulatory 231
  complications 232
  contraindications 232
  domiciliary 231–2
  long-term 231, 232
  pulmonary embolism 116
  short burst 231, 232
  smoking 232

P waves 120, 123, 125
pacemaker 132–4
  complications 133–4
  dual-chamber 68, 132, *133*
  implantation
    bradycardia 59
    driving 118, 119
    practical details 133
  permanent 133
  syndrome 133
  temporary 132
    bradycardia 59
  ventricular lead displacement 133, *134*
palpitations
  ambulatory monitoring 4, 5
  cardiovascular examination 4
  causes **3**
  with dizziness 6–9
  ECG 4, 5
  electrophysiology studies 125
  examination 4, 7
  history 3–4
  investigations 4, 5, 6
  management 4, 6, 8–9
  paroxysmal 3–4, 5, 6
  presyncope 6
Pancoast tumour 220
pancreatic insufficiency 201
pancreatitis 17
papillary muscle dysfunction 76
  tricuspid regurgitation 77
parapneumonic effusions 177, 178
paraquat 205
parenchymal lung disease 34, 183, 204–6
  complications 205
  cor pulmonale 231

lung transplantation 205
  prognosis 205
  treatment 205
  see also interstitial lung disease
paroxysmal atrial fibrillation/flutter 6
patent ductus arteriosus 90–1
  infective endocarditis 84
patient-activated devices 127
peak flow 243
penicillamine 213
penicillin
  pulmonary eosinophilia 213
  rheumatic fever 95
pentamidine 220
pentoxyfylline 210
peptic ulcer, perforated 17
percutaneous transluminal angioplasty
  (PTCA) 138–9
  angina 52
percutaneous transluminal septal myocardial
  ablation 68, *69*
pericardial calcification 83
  constrictive pericarditis 83
pericardial constriction 22, 70, 83
pericardial disease 78–84
  acute pericarditis 78–80
  atrial fibrillation 59
  constrictive pericarditis 82–4
  CT 140
  malignancy 96
  MRI 140
pericardial effusion 45, 80–2
  acute pericarditis 79
  breathlessness and haemodynamic
    collapse 26
  cardiomegaly 135
  chest radiograph 135
  complications 82
  differential diagnosis 82
  hypothyroidism 104
  malignancy 95
  pacemaker complication 133
pericardial knock 82
pericardial rub 44, 81
  breathlessness and haemodynamic
    collapse 26
  pleuritic pain 29
pericardiectomy, surgical 82, 84, 107
pericardiocentesis 44, 79, 82, 107
pericardiostomy, balloon 82
pericarditis 16, 17
  acute 42, 43, 78–80
    complications 80
    ECG 79, *80*
    prognosis 80
  constrictive 82–4
  examination 43–4
  exercise ECG contraindication 124
  idiopathic 45
    relapsing 80
  investigations 45
  management 45
  treatment 106
  uraemic 107
  viral 45
pericardium trauma 97
periodic limb movement syndrome 172
peripheral vascular disease
  hypertension 46, 47, 112
  myocardial infarction 57
pertussis
  breathlessness with ankle oedema and
    cyanosis 33
  bronchiectasis 160
  vaccination 199
pH 242, *243*
phaeochromocytoma 46, 48